Psychology and sociology applied to medicine

SECOND EDITION

AN ILLUSTRATED COLOUR TEXT

Commissioning Editor: Michael Parkinson
Project Development Manager: Lynn Watt
Project Manager: Frances Affleck
Designer: Sarah Russell
Illustration Manager: Bruce Hogarth

Psychology and sociology applied to medicine

SECOND EDITION

AN ILLUSTRATED COLOUR TEXT

Edited by

Beth Alder PhD C.Psychol FBPsS
Professor and Director of Research
Faculty of Health and Life Sciences
Napier University
Edinburgh, UK

Mike Porter BA MPhil
Senior Lecturer
General Practice Section
Division of Community Health Sciences
College of Medicine and Veterinary Medicine
University of Edinburgh, UK

Charles Abraham BA DPhil C.Psychol FBPsS
Professor of Psychology
Department of Psychology
University of Sussex, Brighton, UK

Edwin van Teijlingen MA MEd PhD
Senior Lecturer in Public Health & Dugald Baird Centre for Research on Women's Health
University of Aberdeen, UK

FOREWORD by **Keith Millar**

ILLUSTRATED by **Robert Britton and Roger Penwill**

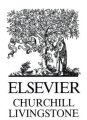

ELSEVIER
CHURCHILL
LIVINGSTONE

EDINBURGH   LONDON   NEW YORK   OXFORD   PHILADELPHIA   ST LOUIS   SYDNEY   TORONTO   2004

CHURCHILL LIVINGSTONE
An imprint of Elsevier Limited

First edition 1999 (as Porter)
Second edition 2004
    Reprinted 2005, 2006, 2007

ISBN-13: 978–0–443–07295–6
ISBN-10: 0–443–07295–7

British Library Cataloguing in Publication Data
A catalogue record for this book is available from the British Library

Library of Congress Cataloguing in Publication Data
A catalogue record for this book is available from the Library of Congress

Notice
Medical knowledge is constantly changing. Standard safety precautions
must be followed, but as new research and clinical experience broaden
our knowledge, changes in treatment and drug therapy may become
necessary or appropriate. Readers are advised to check the most current
product information provided by the manufactacturer of each drug to be
administered to verify the recommended dose, the method and duration
of administration, and contraindications. It is the responsibility of the
practitioner, relying on experience and knowledge of the patient, to
determine dosages and the best treatment for each individual patient.
Neither the Publisher nor the editors assume any liability for any injury
and/or damage to persons or property arising from this publication.

The Publisher

ELSEVIER your source for books,
journals and multimedia
in the health sciences

www.elsevierhealth.com

Working together to grow
libraries in developing countries

www.elsevier.com | www.bookaid.org | www.sabre.org

ELSEVIER BOOK AID International Sabre Foundation

Printed in China

Contributors

Charles Abraham BA DPhil
Professor of Psychology,
Department of Psychology,
University of Sussex, UK

Beth Alder PhD C.Psychol FBPsS
Professor and Director of Research,
Faculty of Health and Life Sciences,
Napier University,
Edinburgh, UK

Amanda Amos BA MSc PhD
Reader in Health Promotion, Public
Health Sciences, Division of
Community Health Sciences,
University of Edinburgh, UK

Jacqueline M. Atkinson BA PhD C.Psychol
HonMFPHM
Senior Lecturer, Department of Public
Health and Psychological Medicine,
University of Glasgow, UK

Pamela J. Baldwin BA MPhil PhD C.Psychol
Clinical Psychologist,
Working Minds Research,
Astley Ainslie Hospital, Edinburgh, UK
(deceased)

Lloyd Carson C.Psychol AFBPsS
Lecturer in Psychology,
School of Social and Health Science,
University of Abertay, UK

Sarah Cunningham-Burley BSocSc PhD
Reader and Co-Director, Centre for
Research on Families and Relationships,
Public Health Sciences,
University of Edinburgh, UK

George Deans BSc MSc PhD C.Psychol
Consultant Clinical Psychologist and
Honorary Clinical Senior Lecturer,
Department of General Practice and
Primary Care,
University of Aberdeen Medical School,
UK

Morag L. Donaldson MA PhD
Senior Lecturer in Psychology,
School of Philosophy,
Psychology and Language Sciences,
University of Edinburgh, UK

Helen Eborall BSc MSc
Research Psychologist,
General Practice and Primary Care
Research Unit,
Department of Public Health
and Primary Care,
Institute of Public Health,
University Forvie Site,
Cambridge, UK

Mary Gilhooly BS Med MPhil PhD C.Psychol
Head of School,
School of Social Work and
Primary Care,
University of Plymouth, UK

Kathy Jenkins BSc MSc
Honorary Lecturer,
Division of Community Health
Sciences, University of Edinburgh, UK

Richard Hammersley MA PhD
Professor of Social Psychology,
Health and Social Services Institute,
University of Essex, UK

Sarah E. Hampson PhD
Department of Psychology,
University of Surrey, UK
and Oregon Research Institute,
Eugene, Oregon, USA

Mike Hepworth BA AcSS
Reader in Sociology,
University of Aberdeen, UK

Jane Hopton MA Phd HonMFPHM
Research Psychologist,
McKenzie Medical Centre,
Edinburgh, UK

Gail Johnston B.SocSc PhD, Dip District
Nursing, CertEd for Health Professionals
Macmillan Lecturer,
Macmillan Cancer Relief,
Macmillan Education Unit,
Belfast, UK

Marie Johnston PhD, BSc Dip.Clin.Psych
C.Pschol FBPsS FRSE FMedSci AcSS
Professor in Psychology,
Department of Psychology
and Institute of Applied
Health Sciences,
University of Aberdeen, UK

Michael P. Kelly BA(Hons) MPhil PhD
HonMFPHM
Professor,
Director of Research and Information,
The Health Development Agency,
London, UK

Jenny Kitzinger BA MA PhD
Professor, School of Journalism,
Media and Cultural Studies,
Cardiff University, UK

Susan Llewelyn PhD F.BPsS
Reader in Clinical Health Psychology
Department of Psychology,
University College London, UK

Hannah M. McGee
PhD Reg.Psychol FpsSI C.Psychol AFBPsS
Professor, Director,
Health Services Research Centre,
Department of Psychology,
Royal College of Surgeons in Ireland,
Dublin, Ireland

Susan Michie Mphil DPhil C.Psychol FBPsS
Reader in Clinical Health Psychology,
Department of Psychology,
University College London, UK

Kenneth Mullen MA MLitt PhD
Lecturer in Medical Sociology, Section
of Psychological Medicine, Division of
Community-based Sciences, University
of Glasgow, UK

Ronan O'Carroll
BSc MPhil PhD C.Psychol AFBPsS
Professor of Psychology,
Department of Psychology,
University of Stirling, UK

Sheina Orbell PhD C.Psychol
Professor of Psychology,
University of Essex, UK

Liesl Osman PhD
Senior Research Fellow,
Department of Medicine
and Therapeutics,
University of Aberdeen,
Aberdeen, UK

Mike Porter BA MPhil
Senior Lecturer,
General Practice Section,
Division of Community Health
Sciences, College of Medicine
and Veterinary Medicine,
University of Edinburgh, UK

Nicola Stuckey BA MSc
Head of Clinical Psychology,
Astley Ainslie Hospital,
Edinburgh, UK

Edwin van Teijlingen MA MEd PhD
Senior Lecturer in Public Health and
Dugald Baird Centre for Research on
Women's Health,
University of Aberdeen, UK

Brian Williams BSc PhD
Senior Lecturer in Behavioural
Science, Social Dimensions of Health
Institute, Universities of Dundee
and St Andrews, UK

Peter Wright MA DPhil C.Psychol FBPsS
Senior Lecturer, School of Philosophy,
Psychology and Language Sciences,
University of Edinburgh, UK

Sally Wyke BSc PhD
Director,
Scottish School of Primary Care,
NHS Education for Scotland, UK

Martin Yeomans PhD AFBPsS CPsychol
Senior Lecturer in Experimental
Psychology,
University of Sussex, UK

Editorial panel
Beth Alder
Mike Porter
Charles Abraham
Edwin van Teijlingen

Foreword

Those of us who began our careers teaching Psychology and Sociology to medical students in the 1970s were faced with the unpromising task of adding to the already many hundreds of hours of didactic teaching in anatomy, biochemistry, physiology and pharmacology endured by students in the first 2 years of the then 'pre-clinical curriculum'. 'Teaching' was still an acceptable word – it would almost be two decades before the newspeak of medical education proscribed it and replaced it with 'student-centred learning'. Of course, even then, 'teaching' was a misnomer because it largely consisted of force-feeding with facts which were regurgitated at exam time and then largely and gladly forgotten. From the point of view of psychology and sociology, this was a problem because the subject matter did not readily lend itself to rote learning of 'facts'. Thought, evaluation and discussion were required, but the demands and congestion of the 'old curriculum' did not often encourage these basic academic skills. The subject matter was also often criticized as being simple 'common sense'. In bleaker moments of reflection, it often seemed that our endeavours were in the vaudeville school of medical education where, when the imparting of facts failed or required leavening, then the best that we might hope for was to entertain.

The landmark publication by the General Medical Council – *Tomorrow's Doctors* – was, of course, to put an end to vaudeville. The recommendations for sweeping curricular change in the form of student-centred learning with early patient contact and a problem-based approach have been implemented creatively across the UK medical curriculum. The active and reflective learning environment of today favours psychology and sociology, and students are fortunate that their experience of those disciplines will be so well supported by the second edition of *Psychology and Sociology Applied to Medicine*.

Only 5 years on from the publication of the first edition, the second edition continues to provide a model for the style of learning that is now established across the UK medical schools. It has all the strengths of the original – the synopses of key issues and questions, the 'Stop and Think' boxes to encourage reflection, the illustrative case studies, and the references for further in-depth reading. It also illustrates how psychological and sociological concepts, theories and methodologies inform research in virtually all areas of medicine. One can hardly imagine a more effective way to emphasize the relevance and value of these disciplines to a trainee doctor, nor a better way to encourage collaboration with psychologists and sociologists amongst those who will go on to develop research careers in medicine.

The second edition also benefits from the introduction of several new chapters. The section Society and Health introduces the important chapter on 'Quality of life', and also 'The media and health' and 'Social aspects of ageing'. In Illness and Disability we find three new chapters which reflect contemporary concerns about the increased significance of diabetes mellitus, asthma and chronic obstructive pulmonary disease and post-traumatic stress disorder. The latter chapters will be of particular value in contributing to the book's function of providing material to facilitate the General Medical Council's recommendation for the integration of the 'behavioural sciences' throughout the medical curriculum, and particularly in the later years where the student spends much time in a clinical environment. Coping with Illness and Disability introduces 'Complementary therapies', a topic of significant psychological and sociological interest which had received only brief mention in the first edition.

The first cohorts of students trained under the 'new' curriculum with its active learning environment have graduated and moved on to their pre-registration year and beyond. For many, part of their training will have been supported by the first edition of this book. Experienced consultants – a kinder way of saying older consultants – were known to be apprehensive as to how these students might differ in comparison to those who had been through the rigours of the old curriculum with its heavy emphasis on factual knowledge. While consultants' opinions may vary as to depth of knowledge of the new graduates, they seem in accord in conceding that these young doctors are more confident and competent in their interactions with patients, and show considerable awareness and understanding of the psychological and social factors relevant to their patients' care. The second edition of *Psychology and Sociology Applied to Medicine* will continue where the first left off and will support the development of these skills and understanding in those who have recently embarked upon medical training and those still at school who will do so in the years to come.

It is fitting to close this Foreword by noting that the first and second editions of *Psychology and Sociology Applied to Medicine* benefit from several chapters written by Pamela Baldwin, a clinical psychologist. It is very sad to record that Pamela died between publication of the first and second editions. In this second edition, her chapters have been updated where necessary by her co-authors, and significantly so in the case of the chapter on depression, which is now co-authored with Susan Michie. It stands as a tribute to Pamela that her work continues as a significant contribution to this textbook, and she is fondly remembered by all those who knew and worked with her.

Keith Millar
Professor, Section of
Psychological Medicine
Glasgow University Medical School
2004

Preface to First Edition

This textbook aims to provide medical students with a broad and stimulating introduction to psychological and sociological concepts, theories and research as they apply to medicine. If medicine is to be effective in maintaining people's health and well-being, it must be sensitive to the ways in which health and illness make sense within people's lives and how people understand their relationships with doctors and other health care professionals. These, and other issues, are addressed by researchers working in health psychology and medical sociology. For these reasons both psychology and sociology are seen as essential to the medical curriculum (General Medical Council, 1994).

This book has been designed and written primarily to take account of the needs of students who are embarking on the new integrated, systems-based and problem-based, medical courses which have been introduced in the UK and elsewhere.

The material is presented in accessible, two-page 'spreads'. Each spread addresses a discrete topic with its own case study, questions for further thought and key points. However, the spreads are cross-referenced so that the book also forms an integrated whole.

Of course, none of these topics can be adequately covered in two pages. Yet all can be introduced in this way. Each spread includes key references which may be followed up by the student, but individual course organisers and tutors will undoubtedly want to recommend further reading which links the material to their particular courses or modules.

The teaching and learning of psychology and sociology in relation to health, illness and medicine is often hampered by two important factors. First, psychology and sociology (unlike biomedical sciences) deal with aspects of our everyday experience. It is all too easy to believe that we already know what there is to be known about such familiar things, as for example 'Why people don't take their doctor's advice'. One of the key tasks of psychologists and sociologists is, as Fritz Heider put it, to

cut through this 'veil of obviousness'. Secondly, the very fact that people do attempt to understand and make sense of their personal and social worlds makes it difficult to conduct behavioural and social research without, in some way, influencing what they tell us and their behaviour.

Thus, for example, asking patients whether they took their medication or not may, if not carefully asked, elicit responses which patients think researchers want to hear rather than their real reasons. Asking doctors why patients don't take their medicines may start the doctor thinking about their own part in the process and change their behaviour. Such opportunities for bias and influence make it particularly important for students to think critically and to check the assumptions, methods and findings of different research studies.

The references have, therefore, been included not just to encourage students to read more deeply into a topic, but also to think critically about the reasoning and the evidence presented. Both psychology and sociology are enlivened by debate and discussion. Details of research studies are often given in boxes and students are encouraged to be critical. Evidence-based medicine is a concept that is as applicable to behavioural science as it is to clinical practice.

The book is divided into nine sections beginning with a description of normal human development and common health problems associated with the life span. The second section seeks to address the question 'How does the person develop?' and focuses on the development of some key psychological processes, for example the development of language, personality and sexuality. The third section seeks to address the question 'In what ways are our behaviour and health constrained by the social contexts within which we live?' and also includes spreads on the concepts and measurement of health, illness and disease. Section 4 presents a more specific discussion of how social and personal factors interact to

influence our risk of ill health. The topic of risk-taking behaviour is developed further in Section 5 where issues of illness prevention and health promotion are discussed in terms of both the behaviour of individuals and the behaviour of government and large organisations.

Sections 6 and 7 shift the perspective from health promotion to illness behaviour. Section 6 focuses on what people do when they feel ill or anxious about their health and on their experience of consultations and of hospitals. Doctors' communication skills are also reviewed. Section 7 selects a number of specific disorders and examines how people experience and respond to them. A range of ways of helping people to cope with illness and disability are also described.

Section 8 examines some of the problems and issues associated with different ways of organising health services, and Section 9 reviews the experience of being a medical student and a junior doctor, concluding with a discussion of basic professional and ethical issues.

It is doubtful if any introductory textbook could be comprehensive and we are aware of some important topics which have not been covered, and others which have received more of a psychological than a sociological approach, and vice-versa. We hope, however, that the breadth of coverage and the style of presentation will be attractive to students, stimulate their interest in the psychosocial aspects of health, illness and medical practice, and encourage them to pursue their interests in greater depth.

Some editorial control has been exercised by both the editorial panel and the principal editors, but final responsibility for each spread has been left to individual authors. Our thanks to the editorial panel and to our authors for responding so willingly to our comments and suggestions, and for writing to such a tight word limit.

M.P.
B.A.
C.A.

Preface to Second Edition

We were delighted with the success of the first edition of *Psychology and Sociology Applied to Medicine*. Published in 1999, it was reprinted four times and was very well received by medical and health care students. Medical care and our understanding of the psychological and sociological processes that contribute to differences in health, patients' responses to health care systems and the experiences of health care professionals has moved on since 1999. Thus the second edition has provided an opportunity for us to reflect on key topics, review recent advances and expand into new areas. We have updated the text, added some chapters and omitted others. This process has been facilitated by the expertise of our new, fourth editor, Dr Edwin van Teijlingen.

The views expressed in the preface of the first edition still hold. As new medical curricula are developed in the UK and worldwide, it is recognized that an understanding of psychological and sociological processes is crucial to optimal individual care and effective national healthcare policies. They are central to core teaching in the medical and healthcare professions. An increasingly educated patient population emphasizes the need for greater interpersonal skills amongst health professionals, and the importance of communication to understanding and initiating behaviour change.

Medical curricula in the UK and elsewhere increasingly include psychology and sociology in integrated modules dealing with care and treatment in relation to particular physiological systems or diseases. *Psychology and Sociology Applied to Medicine* seeks to make health psychology and medical sociology accessible to medical and health care students. This text also integrates psychological and sociological research findings with the delivery of care and treatment in healthcare settings. The text provides a broad introduction but focuses on key points so that medical and health care students can assimilate the material quickly. We hope that it will inspire readers to pursue the topics in greater depth. We have included recent references and often selected illustrative studies from medical and health journals rather than psychology or social science journals.

The overall format of the book remains similar to the first edition but there have been changes in both the number and content of the sections, and in the chapters within them. Section 1 takes the reader from Pregnancy to Ageing while Section 2 includes new chapters on Intelligence and Emotion. We have relocated some chapters which we feel fit better within Section 3, Society and Health, and added new chapters on Quality of Life, Media and Health and Social Aspects of Ageing. In Section 4 we consider Health Promotion and other issues relevant to Public Health. For example, new chapters on Smoking and on Eating reflect current concerns about the impact of lifestyle on public health. Section 5 includes chapters on Communication and a new chapter on Placebo. Section 6 focuses on specific health problems and issues, and includes new chapters on Depression and Post traumatic stress disorder, Respiratory disease and Diabetes. In Section 7 there is a positive perspective on how individuals, health professionals and the community help people cope with disability and health problems. A new chapter on Complementary therapies recognizes the interest people have in self-care and alternatives to traditional medicine, and a new chapter on Pain illustrates the progress in this area. Health care is always dependent on the organization of health services and this is explored in Section 8. Finally, the last section (How do you fit in to all this?) focuses on the experience of those working in healthcare settings.

We were very sad that Dr Pamela Baldwin died before this second edition was planned. She contributed greatly to the planning and writing of the first edition and her enthusiasm, insight and fluent style has been greatly missed. Her name remains attached to those chapters that have only required revision and updating.

As in the first edition, the editors have exercised some editorial control but the final responsibility has been left to the individual authors.

B.A.
M.P.
C.A.
E.v.T.

Contents

Illness and disability 104

Coping with illness and disability 130

How do health services work? 148

How do you fit into all this? 156

Pregnancy and childbirth

This textbook appropriately starts at the beginning of life, at birth. It is also appropriate to use one of the most 'natural' life events as an introduction to the behavioural sciences. The birth of humans differs from births in other mammals in our social construction of the event. Social behaviour is guided by institutions and customs, not merely by instinctual needs; and perhaps nothing illustrates this basic sociological principle better than the sheer diversity of human practices at the time of childbirth, and their responsiveness to historically changing influences. In other words, where and how and in whose presence a woman gives birth differs from one social setting to another. Human societies everywhere prescribe certain rituals and restrictions to pregnant and labouring women. For example, the place of delivery is often prescribed, be it a special village hut or a special obstetric hospital.

Pregnancy and childbirth are important life events that are often influenced by doctors. Obstetrics is an important part of medical training. Every medical student is required to attend a certain number of deliveries. Doctors may be directly involved, in providing ante-natal or post-natal care or attending the birth, or more indirectly through the provision of infertility treatment or birth-control methods, or as back-up for midwives in case something unexpected happens during a normal delivery.

The nature of pregnancy and childbirth

There are two major contrasting views on the nature of pregnancy and childbirth (see Table 1). One argues that pregnancy and childbirth are normal events in most women's life cycle. This is often referred to as the psychosocial model. It is estimated that some 85% of all babies will be born without any problems and without the presence of a special birth attendant. Many of the risks in childbirth can be predicted, and, consequently, pregnant women most at risk can be selected for a hospital delivery in a specialist obstetric hospital. The remainder of pregnant women can opt for a less specialist setting such as a delivery in a community hospital or a home delivery. A proponent of this view is Tew (1990), who discovered, to her own surprise whilst preparing epidemiological exercises for medical students in Nottingham, that routine statistics did not support the widely accepted view that increased hospitalization of birth had caused the decline in mortality of mothers and their new-born babies.

Secondly, the view most commonly held in nearly all Western societies is that pregnancy and particularly labour are risky events, where many things could go wrong. This is referred to as the biomedical model. Childbirth is, therefore, potentially pathological. Since we do not know what will happen to an individual pregnant woman, each woman is best advised to deliver her baby in the safest possible environment. The specialist obstetric hospital with its high-technology screening equipment supervised by obstetricians is regarded as the safest place to give birth. In short, this view states that pregnancy and childbirth are only safe in retrospect.

Consequently, the majority of deliveries occur in hospital. Figure 1 contrasts the percentage of home births in the Netherlands with Scotland, where Scotland reflects the trend in most industrialized countries.

Table 1 **Models of childbirth**		
Model	**Psychosocial** 'Childbirth normal/ natural until pathology occurs'	**Biomedical** 'Childbirth only normal in retrospect'
Emphasis	Normality	Risk
	Social support	Risk reduction
	Woman = active	Woman = passive
	Health	Illness
	Individual	Statistical

 STOP THINK

■ Pregnancy can be regarded as a 'normal state of health' in that it occurs without serious problems to most women in their lifetime. Pregnancy can also be seen as an 'illness' in that many women, for example, have morning sickness, experience a slowing down in physical functioning, seek medical care and/or deliver in hospital. How do you regard pregnancy and child-birth, and why?

Changing maternity care
The place of delivery

Maternity services in the 1990s in Britain moved through a period of significant change in which the need of the woman to be centrally involved in her care was given greater emphasis. This represented a change from the previous 50–60 years, when the trend was towards more hospital deliveries. For example, in Britain, an official report published in 1959 recommended that 70% of all births should take place in hospital, while a similar report in 1970 recommended 100% hospital deliveries on the grounds of safety. Political opinion changed in the late 1980s towards more choice for women, and consequently more deliveries outside obstetric units. The Winterton Report (1992) proposed a move away from total hospitalization: 'The policy of encouraging all women to give birth in hospital cannot be justified on grounds of safety.'

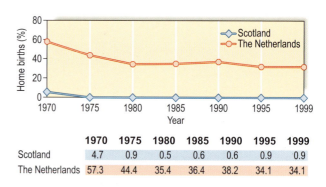

	1970	1975	1980	1985	1990	1995	1999
Scotland	4.7	0.9	0.5	0.6	0.6	0.9	0.9
The Netherlands	57.3	44.4	35.4	36.4	38.2	34.1	34.1

Fig. 1 **Percentage of births in hospital in Scotland and the Netherlands.** (Sources: Common Services Agency (Scotland); Central Bureau voor de Statistiek (The Netherlands))

The birth attendant

The two views of childbirth also differ regarding who is the desired attendant at birth. If one holds the view that pregnancy and childbirth are only safe in retrospect, then the only acceptable birth attendant is a consultant obstetrician, a specialist present just in case something goes wrong. If one holds the view that childbirth is a normal part in the life cycle of most women, then the most desirable birth attendant is the expert in normal deliveries, the midwife or the GP. Throughout history midwives have been, and continue to be, the major health-care attendants at the birthing process. Over the past 3 centuries in most industrialized countries female midwives have slowly lost control over childbirth to male doctors.

Pregnancy is often a time of great expectations and excitement relating to the birth and parenthood. Women in modern Western society have, on average, only two babies in their lifetime. At the same time, as obstetricians and/or midwives might attend deliveries many times a week or even a day, their expectations are considerably different from those of the expecting mother, and not only because the baby is not their own. Their priorities can be guided by medical requirements, hospital policies, or availability of resources. Such differences can easily lead to misunderstanding and dissatisfaction by the new parents (especially if the parties have not been able to get to know each other). Considering the role and status of health professionals (see pp. 158–159) it is more likely that the mother is disappointed than the birth attendant.

Case study

The Dutch example

The Netherlands is the only industrialized country where the proportion of all deliveries taking place outwith specialist hospitals is substantial. Every year approximately one-third of all deliveries take place in Dutch homes. Britain and the Netherlands are neighbouring countries with fairly similar levels of health-care provision and a similar quality of specialist obstetric care; perinatal mortality rates do not differ substantially between the two countries. (Perinatal mortality rate refers to the number of stillbirths (after 28 weeks' gestation) plus the number of deaths occurring in the first 7 days after the delivery, divided by all live births and stillbirths.) Other outcome indicators suggest that the Dutch programme is superior.

A number of factors have been suggested for this difference in the organization of maternity care:

- Pregnant women in the Netherlands are not regarded as patients, unless something goes wrong or the delivery is expected to be difficult for previously assessed reasons.
- Practical help is provided in the form of maternity home-care assistants, who look after the mother and new-born baby at home for up to 8 days following the birth. They wash the baby, give advice on breast or bottle feeding, look after other children in the household, walk the dog, etc.
- In case of low-risk pregnancies, the fee for a GP will be reimbursed only if there is no practising midwife in the area, and only in instances of high-risk pregnancies will the fee of an obstetrician be reimbursed.
- Midwives are trained to be independent and autonomous practitioners. They are not trained as nurses first, but attend a separate 3-year midwifery course. The importance of independent training is, first, that nurses are trained to deal with illness and disease, whilst midwives are trained to deal with normal childbirth; and, secondly, that the hierarchical relationship between nurses and doctors tends to play a part in the medical decision-making process.
- Most midwives are practising as independent practitioners in the community, similar to most dentists in Britain. As private entrepreneurs they have to be more consumer-friendly to attract customers.
- All major political parties agree that the midwife is the obvious person to provide maternity care and that deliveries should preferably take place at home.

One could, of course, argue that Britain and the Netherlands are different countries and therefore not comparable. However, the populations in these two neighbouring countries are not too different in terms of national income, the physiology of the average woman, life expectancy and many other socio-economic indicators. Although the funding of health care is different, the organization of service provision and the quality of medical care are fairly similar. For example, the majority of all deliveries in Britain and the Netherlands are attended by midwives. In fact, one can turn the question of comparability round and ask, for example: Why is the proportion of home births equally low in Britain, Germany and the USA, while their organization of health care in general, and of maternity care in particular, is so different?

What does being pregnant and giving birth mean for:
- a midwife?
- an obstetrician?
- a pregnant woman?
- her partner/husband?

Pregnancy and childbirth

- Biological events are never purely biological but always partly socially constructed.
- Where, how and in whose presence a woman gives birth differs from one culture to another.
- There are two different ways of looking at pregnancy and childbirth: (a) pregnancy is a normal event in most women's lives and (b) childbirth is a risky event and only normal in retrospect.
- Pregnant women and health professionals are likely to see the birth differently.
- Different ways of organizing health care can have profound effects on professionals and health-service users.

Reproductive issues

The practice of medicine is closely involved with reproductive issues, and pregnancy and childbirth may be the most important point of contact with the medical profession. Reproductive issues are relevant to all of us throughout our lives and for many reasons, but they have particular relevance to health. Both psychological and physical health are influenced by sexuality and fertility. A disease, syndrome or health problem that is apparently unrelated to reproduction may have been affected by a previous pregnancy, infertility problem or miscarriage. Reproductive changes over the life span particularly affect women, and from puberty onwards biological changes, social changes, and psychological changes have powerful effects.

The menstrual cycle

The biological basis of the menstrual cycle is the changing hormone production related to the ovary. It is important to be aware of the underlying biological changes even when considering people's social behaviour. Follicular stimulating hormone (FSH) and luteinizing hormone (LH) are released from the pituitary, and stimulate the growth of ovarian follicles (the follicular phase). These secrete oestradiol and as the level rises the FSH levels fall because of negative feedback. An LH surge is triggered and this provokes ovulation from the now mature ovarian follicle. The remaining follicle becomes the corpus luteum and secretes progesterone as well as oestradiol. These changes are shown in Figure 1. After ovulation, oestradiol and progesterone levels fall (the luteal phase) and the endometrial lining is shed during menstruation.

Menstrual pain is experienced by many women and may be helped by relaxation techniques as well as drugs. Menstruation may be perceived negatively, and there are religious and social taboos surrounding behaviour during menstruation. Sexual intercourse may be avoided and myths such as not washing hair during menstruation may be pervasive. Some women who are not taking the oral contraceptive pill find that they eat more in the luteal phase (Dye and Blundell 1997). Many women notice changes during different phases of the menstrual cycle. In premenstrual syndrome (PMS), symptoms such as breast tenderness, irritability or depression increase in the pre-menstrual week and improve in the post-menstrual week. There is little evidence of intellectual impairment during menstruation or in the premenstrual week (Richardson 2000).

Pregnancy

During pregnancy and childbirth:

- Women and their partners come into contact with the medical profession and health professionals, perhaps for the first time as adults.
- Admission to maternity hospital may be the first admission to hospital.
- They are experiencing a rôle transition or rite of passage.

A woman who is pregnant experiences both physical and psychological changes. These begin in pregnancy when there are physical changes in muscle tone, size and shape of the body, stress incontinence and frequency, and fatigue. She may give up work, change her role in her family, and feel that her body image has changed. There may be changes in her self-concept and feelings of self-efficacy. She may worry about being a good parent.

- Which of these changes also apply to fathers?

Childbirth

The context of childbirth is changing (see pp. 2–3) but wherever it takes place it is likely to involve the experience and management of pain (see pp. 144–145).

Many women attend ante-natal classes to prepare for the birth and many fathers are present at the birth. The delivery of a baby is an emotional event and is rated as one of the most significant events in people's lives.

Changes in mood

The transition to parenthood can be seen as a developmental crisis.

In the first post-natal year the mother:

- adjusts to the demands of a young baby
- may give up work and change her perceived status
- may have a different relationship with her partner
- may have a different relationship with her mother.

About 10% of women experience post-natal depression (Fig. 2), but there is also a similar prevalence during pregnancy (Evans et al 2001). Women who are depressed after childbirth do not necessarily see themselves as ill. Nicolson (1998) suggests that researchers have ignored women's own experiences.

Of course there are positive aspects too:

- Both partners may feel reassured about their gender role; they may feel more 'feminine' or more 'masculine'.

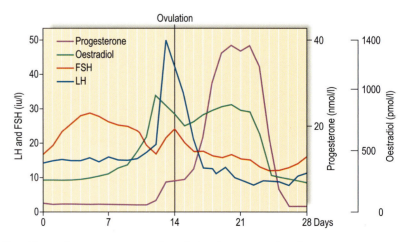

Fig. 1 **Plasma hormone concentrations during the menstrual cycle.**

- There is a high status attached to becoming a parent and they may feel more mature and confident.
- Parenting is rated as a very positive experience by most parents.

Not all pregnancies end in the birth of a healthy baby. About 20% end in miscarriage before 20 weeks. If the couple has not told their family and friends that they are expecting a baby, the loss from early miscarriage may not be recognized. About half of mothers experiencing miscarriage suffer from clinical depression. Their grief remains hidden and unspoken and it may be similar to that experienced by a woman who has been diagnosed as infertile. She may feel a loss of the image of herself as a pregnant woman and as a parent. She may believe that she may never be able to bear children, and feel guilt and anger (Hunter 1993).

The menopause
The menopause means literally the last period, but the term climacteric or perimenopause is used to describe the years either side of the menopause. Many women have several years of irregular periods and the climacteric can take place at any time between 40 and 60 years of age.

Loss of production of oestrogen, as ovulation declines, results in recognized physical changes such as vasomotor symptoms of hot flushes, night sweats and vaginal dryness; psychological symptoms such as increased depression, irritability, or low libido are often reported.

There is little association between menopausal status and psychological symptoms, and probably only vasomotor symptoms are associated with the time of the menopause.

Women may encounter more stressful events during the climacteric, and family and sociocultural factors may be more important than changes in hormones. Physical changes may cause depression in post-menopausal women, and some health problems may begin in middle age, such as diabetes mellitus, weight gain and urinary incontinence.

Different perspectives have been suggested to account for changes during the menopause.

Biomedical model
The menopause is seen as a hormone-deficiency disease. Vasomotor symptoms occur because of a decline in the levels of oestrogen produced by the ovary. These symptoms respond well to oestrogen therapy, but although all women suffer declining levels of oestrogen, not all report either vasomotor symptoms or psychological changes.

Cultural model
Society may take a negative view of the menopause. In some societies in which ageing is associated with increased status and wisdom the menopause is seen positively. Mayan Indians in rural Mexico experience loss of oestrogen production in the same way as Western women, although it occurs at a relatively early age (usually between 41 and 54 years of age). In a study of 54 women it was found that they did not report hot flushes or night sweats, nor did they suffer from osteoporosis (Martin et al 1993). The

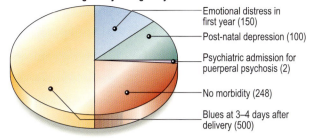

Fig. 2 **Incidence of post-natal morbidity for every 1000 women having a baby during 1 year.** (Source: Cox 1986)

interviewer was a Mayan nurse's aide and fluent in Spanish and Mayan. From their hormone levels about 80% would be expected to have hot flushes but not one of the 54 women reported them. This suggests a strong cultural component. Women may see the menopause negatively, as a loss of femininity, or positively as an end to the demands of childbearing. Health professionals may be able to promote a more positive view.

Psychosocial model
Symptoms may be associated with stressful life events. If menopausal symptoms are assessed using standardized scales it is found that life stress contributes far more than menopausal status to menopausal symptoms, and worries about work and adolescent children are major factors influencing depression. Children leaving home may be a cause of grief, but there may be just as many problems if they do not leave home and remain dependent.

Case study

Mrs Jones is 52, widowed and works part time as an office assistant. She lives with her two daughters. Anne is 25 and has a steady relationship with her boyfriend. She has a 4-week-old baby. Jane is 17 and is still at school, but has little chance of leaving with any paper qualifications. Mrs Jones is often irritable and has dropped out of her usual social activities. Anne has bouts of weepiness and lacks confidence in her abilities as a mother. Jane is disillusioned with study and stays out late in pubs. She has episodes of erratic behaviour.

How would you explain the behaviour in Mrs Jones and her two daughters, assuming either a biomedical model or a cultural explanation?

Reproductive issues

- Biological, psychological and social changes related to reproduction have powerful effects on women's lives.
- There are physical changes during the menstrual cycle and they may be related to negative psychological changes.
- Pregnancy and childbirth affect mood and relationships in both men and women.
- The menopause is an endocrinological event but it is associated with negative changes which may have psychosocial origins.

Development in early infancy

The twentieth century has seen dramatic shifts in how we view infancy. The importance of both good medical care and the right psychological environment are necessary for optimal development during childhood. Psychologists have demonstrated that even new-born infants have impressive cognitive and perceptual abilities and learning capacity. A mother goes through an intensive period of getting to know and understand her infant in the first weeks after birth, and she gains a unique insight into interpreting her baby's needs. This makes her observations of great importance should medical complications arise. It is important that doctors treating babies understand more about the baby's competence and listen to what the mother has to say. This spread will discuss changing ideas on what is meant by 'bonding', give examples of the communicative abilities of infants, and show how recognizing differences in behaviour of infants may contribute towards improving breastfeeding success.

Assessment shortly after birth

Infants who fuss and cry a great deal, or who are apathetic and unresponsive to social stimuli, can be at risk of neglect by their mothers. Tests designed to evaluate the neonate's neurological well-being can also be used to encourage mothers to become more sensitive and responsive care-givers. The Brazleton Neonatal Assessment Scale (NBAS) evaluates the neonate's neurological status and responsiveness to environmental stimuli. It is designed to be administered within a few days of birth and assesses not only the quality of some 20 inborn reflexes, but also the infant's state and reactions to stimuli such as ringing a bell or watching a moving light. If the baby is extremely unresponsive, the low NBAS score would suggest possible neurological dysfunction. If the baby is simply slow, especially when responding to social stimulation, this may be a warning sign for later emotional problems.

Because the NBAS is designed to elicit the baby's more engaging characteristics, such as cooing, gazing and smiling, it has potential as a teaching aid. Myers (1982) taught parents of healthy, full-term babies how to conduct the NBAS with their own infants and found that after 4 weeks, by comparison with an untrained control group, such parents were both more confident in their role and more satisfied with their babies. Mothers of premature and other high-risk infants similarly become more responsive in interacting with their babies. If you are sceptical about the expressive abilities of neonates (Fig. 1).

Bonding and attachment

In the 1970s a very influential view developed from the work of two paediatricians, Klaus and Kennell. They suggested that for new mothers to fall in love with their babies (referred to as maternal bonding) it was essential that only minimal separation of the infant from its mother should occur after birth. Technically maternal bonding has come to mean a rapid and irreversible change said to take place in the mother within a period immediately following birth. This 'critical period' lasts no more than a few hours or days at the most, and during this time prolonged contact between mother and baby must occur if maternal feelings are to be properly mobilized. This 'super-glue' theory of maternal love proved very influential, and failure to bond properly was frequently cited as the reason for all kinds of problems ranging from failure to thrive in infancy to cases of child abuse and adolescent delinquency. In one New York hospital this belief reached such heights of absurdity that mothers who had not held their babies after birth were given polaroid photographs to look at so they could bond adequately!

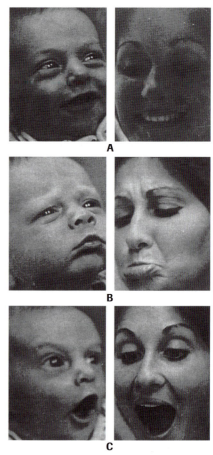

Fig. 1 **A model's happy, sad and surprised expressions, and an infant's corresponding expressions.** (Reprinted with permission from Field, Woodson, Greenberg, Cohen 1982 Discrimination and imitation of facial expression in neonates. Science 218: 179-181 Copyright 1982 American Association for the Advancement of Science)

The origins of bonding theory lay in work with animals where there is good evidence for such a critical period in the formation of maternal attachment to the new-born, but many careful studies in the past two decades have shown that there is no evidence of any

Case study

Mothers often remark that their baby looks happy, sad, or is smiling and this may be put down to harmless self-deception, but experiments (see Field et al 1982) with babies as young as 36 hours show that they are indeed able to imitate facial expressions (Fig. 1). A series of three expressions (happy, sad, surprised) were posed by an adult and observed by 74 neonates, and both baby's and model's faces were videotaped simultaneously using a split-screen technique. Observers subsequently coded the facial expressions of the infants and looked for matches to the model. The chance probability of guessing the facial expression correctly would be 33%, but surprised was correctly guessed on 76% of trials, happy on 58%, and sad on 59%. Videotapes of the model's faces eliminated shaping or reinforcing the neonate's responses as a possible explanation for the result. The authors concluded that there is an innate ability to compare the sensory information from facial expressions with the proprioceptive feedback of the movements involved in matching that expression.

long-term effects of enforced separation in the period immediately after birth. Hence a generation of doctors and nurses can be relieved of guilty feelings associated with the necessary forced separation following caesarean section or illness at birth. It is interesting that these ideas, although without scientific foundation, revolutionized practice in post-natal wards, allowing babies to sleep in cots at the side of their mothers. (For a good account of this controversy, see Schaffer 1990.)

Promotion of breastfeeding

It is widely accepted that breastfeeding conveys a number of health advantages to the baby, such as providing increased protection against gastrointestinal upset through the presence of antibodies, and longer-term influences in the form of decreased susceptibility to eczema. In a developing-world context, breastfeeding is an important contraceptive agent because the increased levels of prolactin in the mother delay the return of ovulation and therefore increase birth spacing. It is possible that other advantages of breastfeeding stem more from the act itself rather than any biochemical differences between breast milk and formula. Milk feeds are not a continuous sequence of sucking but are interrupted by removal of the bottle or breast for a variety of reasons such as choking, winding, posseting of milk, changing to another breast, etc. When filmed, feeds are analyzed to see if it is the baby or the mother who initiates the break in feeding. For bottle-fed babies the interruptions are found to be almost entirely under the control of the mother, but for breastfed infants there is a predominantly baby-determined pattern. Observations such as this, and other instances of what is known as 'turn-taking' suggest that reciprocity in the context of feeding is more evident in breastfeeding. Many psychologists have become interested in feeding because they see this kind of interaction as the source of subsequent social communication.

Despite all the obvious health advantages to the baby, regular surveys of infant-feeding practice mounted by the

■ How often have you seen a mother breast-feeding her baby ? What are the barriers that make women disincline to breastfeed publicly?
■ Find a mother with a baby under the age of 1 year and watch her 'talking' to the baby. Do you see any evidence of turn-taking?
■ What makes a baby smile? Draw two large dots on a piece of paper and hold this about 12 inches in front of the baby. Add more dots where the nose and mouth should be. Compare the response of babies at about 3 months and 8 months.

Office of Population Censuses and Surveys indicate that there are persisting regional and social class variations in the extent of breastfeeding (Fig. 2). Whereas 75% of mothers in the South of England will attempt to breastfeed at birth, in Scotland only 50% will try. By week six one-third of these mothers will have given up. Even greater discrepancies are evident from breakdown by social class, with almost 90% of social classes I and II attempting breastfeeding compared with 60% for social classes IV and V. There are also important differences in the behaviour of the babies, and how mothers interpret these seems to depend on the method of feeding. For example, bottle-fed infants begin to sleep through the night at a significantly earlier age than do breastfed babies; they are also offered solid foods at an earlier age. Breastfeeding mothers regard changes in the frequency of feeding as the most important sign of hunger in their babies, whereas bottle-feeding mothers mention changes in the avidity with which the infants suck from the bottle as most important (Drewett et al 1998).

Providing premature babies with human breast milk delivered through a nasogastric tube improves their cognitive development as measured by increases in IQ at a later age. This suggests that some component of breast milk, perhaps long-chain fatty acids, is particularly important for the optimal development of the immature brain. When intelligence (pp. 30–31) was measured at school age, in children delivered at full-term, breastfed infants were at an advantage and remained so even when the associated educational and socio-economic differences were discounted. These long-term influences on development are especially interesting examples of how early experience can exert an enduring influence in unexpected ways.

Development in early infancy

■ Babies in the first week of life can distinguish facial expressions.
■ Prolonged contact between mother and infant in the first week of life is not essential for successful mothering to occur.
■ Breastfeeding has both immediate and long-term health benefits for the baby.

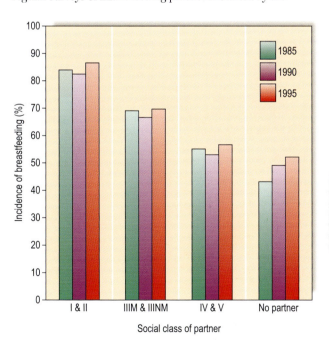

Fig. 2 **Breastfeeding by social class. (1985, 1990 and 1995, Great Britain)**. (Source: Foster N, Lader D, Cheesbrough S 1992 Infant Feeding 1997. OPCS, Social Survey Division. HMSO, London)

Childhood and child health

Childhood is a process of transition from high dependency towards autonomy. The risk of serious ill health interfering in this process has been significantly reduced in most affluent countries, but there is still a disproportionate excess of deaths and morbidity amongst the children of poorer families.

Children's health

Relatively few children in affluent countries now die between the ages of 1 and 14 years (Fig. 1), though at all ages boys are more likely to die than girls. Improvements in children's mortality have occurred steadily over the last 150 years (Fig. 2), largely as a result of improvements in living conditions, sanitation and nutrition leading to a decline in mortality from infectious disease. Immunization, fertility control, medical advances and greater access to health services have also contributed to improvements in children's health. However, deaths from injuries and poisoning remain a major cause for concern. The decline in serious infectious diseases in children in affluent countries has also meant that congenital disorders and cancers have become relatively more predominant, but they will not be discussed here (see pp. 118–119).

Minor ill health, on the other hand, is relatively common in children and can, therefore, be seen as relatively 'normal' (see pp. 36–37; 98–99). There also appears to have been an increase in self-reported chronic illness among children since data were collected in Britain from the early 1970s, with respiratory illness being the main problem.

Psychological health and well-being

There is evidence that adverse family factors, such as a marriage with low mutual support, are related to behavioural problems in children aged 3 years, and to the onset of behavioural problems when older. However, patterns of problem behaviour, such as sleep disturbance, challenging behaviour and temper tantrums, do not always

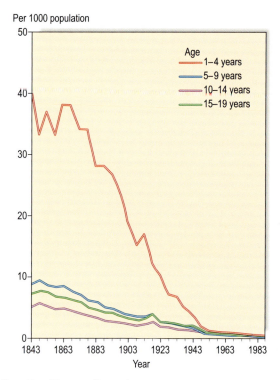

Fig. 2 **Trend in mortality under 20 years 1841–45 to 1986–90, England and Wales.** (Source: Woodroffe et al 1993)

disappear if stress factors are reduced. Counselling and psychotherapy approaches to behaviour problems would suggest that learned patterns of behaviour are often deeply internalized in the subconscious and may be difficult to change (see pp. 20–21; pp. 130–131). Furthermore, neglect and abuse of children is a sizeable problem, and is a known predictor of depression and emotional/behavioural problems later in life for both men and women.

Single mothers are particularly at risk of financial hardship and depression (Brown and Moran 1997), and both poverty and maternal depression are associated with greater risk to children's health and well-being, but care should be taken in interpreting these associations to avoid blaming the single parent.

Accidents

Although the childhood death rate from accidents in the UK has been falling, accidents are the major cause of death in children and, like most other causes of death in children, are strongly associated with social class.

Under the age of 5 years, most accidents occur in the home, with fires being the most common cause of death, and scalds and falls being common causes of injury. From 5 years onwards, most childhood accidental deaths occur on the roads, though the number of road-traffic accidents has fallen slightly despite an increase in the volume of traffic. Children from social class V are more than four times as likely to die as pedestrians than children in social class I. Although mortality from injury and poisoning has also declined in all social classes, the differential in mortality for children aged 0–15 years in social classes IV and V has increased compared with children in classes I and II (see pp. 42–43).

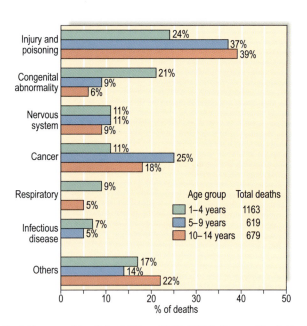

Fig. 1 **Causes of death in childhood (UK, 1990).** (Source: Woodroffe et al 1993)

Studies of children's ability to comprehend danger suggest that children younger than 7 years of age can be taught that something specific is dangerous but that they are unable to generalize from this understanding. For example, being told not to touch a specific fire will not be related to other fires. Furthermore, younger children do not have the ability to interpret traffic speed.

Although accidents are the major cause of childhood death, they are, fortunately, relatively rare. However, accidents which result in injury are relatively common and also class related. Injuries to children in social class IV and V are also likely to be more severe. Factors which help to explain this association are:

- overcrowding: leading to higher risk of falls or burns/scalds
- relative deprivation: leading to older and less-safe cooking equipment, fires, wiring, furniture and safety equipment
- unprotected roads, particularly fast arterial roads
- inadequate play facilities
- difficulty supervising children in high-rise blocks.

Risk of specific cause of accidental death and injury varies by sex and age. At all ages, boys are more likely than girls to die from an accident or to have an accidental injury, with road-traffic accidents accounting for an increasing proportion of accidents involving boys as they get older. Three types of explanation have been suggested:

- Boys are subjected to more 'rough and tumble' play and risk-taking than girls.
- Parents are more likely to supervise girls than boys.
- Boys are more 'accident prone' because they are encouraged to be more active.

Accidents to children occur more frequently in households where the mother is depressed. Brown and Davison (1978) suggest that as the mother becomes depressed she pays less attention to, and takes less interest in, her children. In order to attract her attention, the children behave more aggressively or problematically, but she withdraws further, which elicits even more extreme behaviour, leading to the increased risk of an accident arising from their behaviour and her lack of supervision.

It has been suggested that attempts to educate parents about the risks of accidents and to encourage them to take more responsibility for supervision leads to victim blaming, and to feelings of guilt and defensive anger. What do you think about this and can you think of a more appropriate childhood accident prevention policy.

Respiratory illness

On average, a child aged 5 years will have from six to eight respiratory illnesses per year. These illnesses account for about 80% of consultations with general practitioners by this age group, which is about five times the frequency of consultation for other common conditions. About 30% of all consultations for children aged 11 years are for respiratory disease.

As with accidents, there is a strong relationship between social class and respiratory illness. Dampness in houses is a significant predictor of the incidence and severity of respiratory illness in children, even when allowing for cigarette smoking (pp. 54–55). In contrast, whilst the incidence and prevalence of asthma has been increasing in the UK in recent years making it the most common chronic disease in children, there appears to be no clear relationship between asthma and social class.

Poverty, illness and child development

Children in households with low incomes are more likely to experience ill health, and to spend more time absent from school. This in turn can affect their chances of performing well at school and consequently lead to reduced employment opportunities and to poorer health in later life.

In recent years, policy attention has focused on promoting parental support. Research into the provision of emotional, social and financial support has found that, in the short term, such interventions improve parental self-esteem and lower rates of childhood behavioural problems and injury (Patterson et al 2002). We await the results of longer-term follow up.

Case study

In a study of a Glasgow housing estate, Helen Roberts et al (1993) found that mothers saw accidents as just one element of their generally risky insecure lives. They pointed to defects in the design and upkeep of their environment that contributed to the high accident rate: balconies with gaps that small children could fall through, poor kitchen design, inappropriate electrical wiring and switching, inadequate thermostatic control of immersion heaters, dangerous window design and inadequate locks, inadequate play facilities, inadequately protected roads and repair work, broken glass left by glaziers, inadequate rubbish stores and refuse collection.

The researchers concluded that only a small minority of parents were irresponsible and that professionals and contractors were often responsible for not admitting the design faults and putting them right.

Childhood and child health

- The health of children in affluent countries has improved considerably over the last 100 years.
- These improvements have largely arisen from improvements in sanitation and standards of living.
- Accidents, and particularly pedestrian accidents, are the major cause of death in children.
- Respiratory illness is the major cause of morbidity in children.
- Both accidents and respiratory illness are strongly related to social class and poverty.

Adolescence

Adolescence describes a period of transition between childhood and full adult roles. This used to be rapid after puberty and sometimes involved a formal initiation rite, but many people in their mid-twenties have still not taken on all adult responsibilities, as they may still not have left home, are unlikely to have children and may have several shorter long-term relationships and jobs rather than a sole marriage or career. The ages at which different adult activities are permitted vary. Thus, adolescents are expected to behave in some ways like adults and in other ways like children. Parents and children often disagree about which roles are appropriate at a given age. Since the 1950s there has also been increasing identification of 'youth' as a distinct and positively valued life phase, which has changed rapidly (Table 1).

The physical changes of puberty are important but the psychological changes are caused by the difficulties of adolescent roles. Adolescents have near-adult intellectual abilities (although not necessarily adult knowledge or experience) and soon acquire adult physical abilities. More important developmental issues are emotional, sexual and moral ones. Parents and children can often disagree about which behaviours are appropriate and at what age. The influential theorist Eric Erikson (1968) described adolescence as a time of forming adult identity.

Two sources of strain are:

- having to choose and adjust to adult roles. Many adolescents experiment with a variety of roles and behaviours before settling down with what suits them. This experimentation often includes activities which seem extreme to adults; for example, young fashions often offend older sensibilities.
- disputes over rights and responsibilities. Adolescents often complain that adults expect them to have adult responsibilities without adult freedoms: to be responsible enough to baby-sit, but not responsible enough to choose when to have sex. Adults often feel the opposite, that adolescents expect adult freedoms without adult responsibilities: to be free to choose what time to come in, but not to be willing to help with housework.

Despite these strains, most adolescents have a fairly untroubled time and get on relatively well with their parents and Table 2 shows how parenting styles can affect children.

Table 1 **Life for young people today has changed compared to 25 years ago**	
More	**Less**
Celebrate diversity	Marriage
Brands	Permanent jobs
Travel	'Local community'
Money	Social class
Video games	Left–right politics
Text messaging	
Serial monogamy	
Body decoration and body concerns	
Reality TV	
Recreational drug use	
Clubbing	

Most adolescents' interests and aspirations are similar to adults'. For example, West et al (1990) found that the most popular leisure activities for 18-year-olds were watching TV, listening to music and reading, hardly rebellious activities! Furthermore 78% of them had always been in work or education.

However, about 20% of adolescents will experience more problems (see Coleman and Hendry 1999). Many troubled adolescents abuse drugs or alcohol, engage in some criminal activities, may do poorly or drop out of school, and are also likely to be depressed or unhappy. They are also likely to engage in behaviour inappropriate for their age, although not considered a problem for older people. Both sexual intercourse and drinking alcohol are considered age-inappropriate for people under 14 (note this is not just a legal definition, but a social norm). For most, this is a temporary phase lasting a few years, but some troubled adolescents become adults with problems. Early intervention can help some adolescents, but there is also a risk of labelling someone as mentally ill, drug-addicted or delinquent, actually making problems worse (pp. 60–61).

The two most common social psychological explanations of risk-taking in adolescents are that they have a sense of invulnerability and that they do not think in abstract ways about the future consequences of their own actions. More sociological explanations have suggested that risk-taking behaviour is a part of some youth sub-cultures that provide

Table 2 **Effects of combined parenting styles on adolescent development**		
Two dimensions of parenting style	**Hostile** Cold, neglects or ignores child's needs, uses punishment to control behaviour	**Loving** Warm, accepts child's needs, attends to child, uses praise to control behaviour
Authoritarian Makes strict, rigid unrealistic demands on child's behaviour	*Parent is consistently strict and punishing.* Some parents may be physically or sexually abusive. Adolescent develops internalized anger: neuroses, depression or anxiety, suicide attempts.	*This extreme combination of styles is unlikely because rigid demands require ignoring child's needs.* In less extreme form, the child may become an 'over-achiever' in an unsuccessful effort to please the parent.
Authoritative Has clear expectations for behaviour but these are flexible, realistic and negotiable	*This combination of styles is unlikely because hostility precludes clear flexible expectations.*	*Parent provides good guidance.* **The ideal combination** likely to lead to well-adjusted adult.
Permissive Makes few demands on behaviour and provides few guidelines for child	*Parent largely ignores child's behaviour and punishes inconsistently.* Some parents may be physically or sexually abusive. Adolescent develops externalized anger: acting out behaviour, delinquency, drug abuse.	*Parent treats child too much as an equal: child is 'spoiled'.* Major role conflicts, less extreme acting out behaviour. Child forced to 'be the parent'.

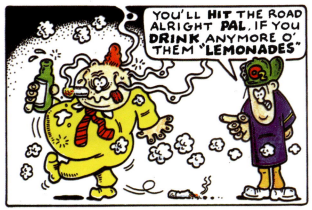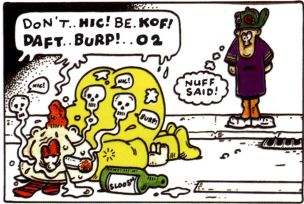

Fig. 1 **Health education information designed for young people is now widely available.** This cartoon dealing with the effects of 'alcopops' is reproduced with permission from the Health Education Board for Scotland, from O$_2$, Issue 3, 1994.

STOP THINK

Are you an adolescent? Your first response may be no, yet as a student you probably experience role conflict when you are told to take responsibility for your own learning while having the curriculum imposed on you. You probably have also experienced the strain and uncertainty of having to cope with practical and emotional matters on your own.

Are there activities which are still not appropriate for people of your age? Consider or discuss with classmates what age is too young for the following activities:

- sexual intercourse
- living with a sexual partner
- marriage
- having a child
- having a credit card
- taking a bank loan
- drinking alcohol
- smoking cannabis
- moving out of one's parents' house
- buying your own home
- studying medicine
- studying computer science

identity and meaning within a larger or dominant adult culture that is seen as irrelevant, unrewarding (or even punitive) and meaningless to their experience and life chances.

Youth is perceived as a time of resilience when a young body can cope with overindulgence: young people will take exercise more because of concerns about attractiveness than health. Even a simple review of the health statistics tends to support this. With the exception of accidents for boys, young people are generally much healthier than older people, and recent evidence has shown that there is no class gradient in health at age 15 years (West et al 1990).

Health care needs of adolescents

Adolescents are a special target for prevention and health-promotion programmes (Fig. 1). Drug abuse, alcohol abuse (including accidents while intoxicated) and suicide are among the leading causes of death in adolescents. Adolescents may

also have special health concerns related to their rapid physical development, including concerns about their sexual development, acne, allergies, fatigue, headaches, and concerns about body size, diet and exercise. Many adolescents are somewhat uncomfortable about their bodies and they may find aspects of health care exceptionally embarrassing.

The provision of health care to adolescents can be problematic as they do not fit easily into child or adult services.

Case study

Jane is 14 and comes on her own to your practice asking for the morning after pill, because she has had unprotected sex. At first she says that this was with a boy she had just met. When you do not judge this and ask her whether she has had sex before, she tells you that really it was her steady boyfriend, who is 18; she has been having sex with him about twice a week for about 3 months. They have been using the withdrawal method, but it 'went wrong'. She says he will not use condoms and she is reluctant to because she says birth control is against her religion. She seems very happy with their relationship. She is very afraid of her parents' reaction if they find out she has a steady boyfriend, never mind that he is older and having unlawful, and unprotected, sex with an under 16-year-old. This case poses you the following ethical problems:

- You have a legal obligation to disclose harm to a minor. Is unprotected sexual intercourse with an 18-year-old such harm?
- You are not supposed to provide medical treatment to someone under 16 without parental consent.
- Is it ethical to persuade someone who is against it to use contraception?
- You are supposed to respect patient confidentiality.

What do you discuss with Jane, and what do you do?

Adolescence

- Adolescence is a period of transition between child and adult roles.
- Strain can occur when there is conflict over appropriate roles and behaviours.
- Most adolescents are fairly untroubled.
- About 20% go through a period of delinquency or problem behaviour.
- Morbidity and mortality rates are low, and they make little use of health-care facilities.
- Special health problems are substance abuse, risky sexual behaviour, depression and suicide.

Adulthood and mid age

This section considers the psychosocial changes that occur in adulthood and their relation to health and illness.

Most children long to be grown up, and grown-ups are seen as having rights and privileges that are strongly desired by children (see pp. 10–11). However, they do not always recognize the accompanying responsibilities of adulthood. Young adults grapple with problems of budgeting, relationships, demands of work and study. Health is probably better in early adulthood than at any other time of life. As people get older they may begin to worry about the negative consequences of ageing. This realization may not be inevitable and may occur at different ages for different people, or, indeed, for men and women. At some point the anticipation of the next birthday may be tinged with apprehension about the ageing process.

The ages between 17 and 40 years are often described as early adulthood and, until relatively recently, would be regarded as the prime of life. Individuals and society emphasize growth and development on each birthday. In the UK, the 18th birthday is seen as being culturally important. Other important milestones may be the legal age of consent to sexual intercourse, drinking alcohol in pubs, or voting. It is also a healthy time of life and young adults are the age group that are least likely to consult doctors apart from health related to reproduction (see pp. 4–5).

Marriage

During adulthood most people will form a relationship with the opposite sex. Many cohabit, though most (76% of women and 71% of men) expect to marry. The number of single parents is increasing (Fig. 1) and the age at marriage is getting later (Social Trends 2002). Homosexual partnerships may serve the same function as heterosexual marriage and are becoming increasingly accepted in our society.

There is considerable evidence that men benefit from marriage in terms of physical and mental health, but for women being married can have disadvantages. Being single, widowed or divorced is associated with lower rates of depression in women than it is in men. Blaxter (1987) found that men living with a spouse had lower illness scores than

men living alone, but for women there was no difference. The protective effect of marriage for men could be linked to social support.

Although marriage appears to be good for men's health, men suffer more severely from loss of their wives by bereavement or breakdown of marriage, and they are more likely to suffer from a range of health problems.

Patients who consult with physical symptoms may be having marital problems, and sometimes these can disrupt their medical treatment. These may involve depression associated with childbirth or sexual problems, or major health and social problems if the wife has been physically abused. A marital separation may be followed by depression and would certainly impede recovery from illness or surgery. Knowledge of the psychology of relationships can help us understand the context of change in health and illness.

Many people live in single households (Fig. 2). In the UK in 2001, 24% of all households consisted of one single person. In 2000, 34% of adults were single, 53% were married and 12% were divorced or widowed, and the proportion of women who are divorced or widowed increases with age (Social Trends 2002).

Single women tend to be viewed negatively by society. Women may lack confidence in their ability to survive by themselves. The maintenance of our identity comes from others, and our feelings of self-worth may be closely linked to the emotional support received in a relationship. However, being single and independent may be advantageous to some women compared with being a traditional wife, and it may be easier for them to avoid emotional and sexual complications.

If a single or widowed woman is ill there may be practical problems. Women often earn less than men and they may not have employment that has generous sick pay arrangements. The absence of a partner at home may make convalescence difficult.

Transitions

One perspective on ageing has been given by Erikson. His theory suggests that mid age is a time of conflict between generativity (guiding the next generation) and stagnation (concern with own needs). Mid age will be associated with

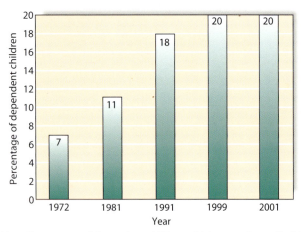

Fig. 1 **Percentage of dependent children with lone mothers.** (Social Trends 32, 2002 edition. Stationery Office, London. (http://www.statistics.gov.uk/statbase)

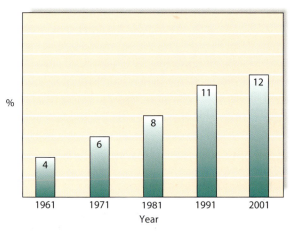

Fig. 2 **Percentage of those living alone (2002).** (Social Trends 32, 2002 edition. Stationery Office, London)

different patterns of health and illness, and assessment of a middle-aged patient may have to include their relationship with their own increasingly ageing parents as well as their dependent teenage children.

Men are sometimes said to go through a 'mid-life crisis'. Half of the men in a study of forty men aged between 37 and 41 years identified a period of uncertainty, anxiety and change (Levinson 1978). They saw mid-life as a last chance to achieve goals but others saw mid-life as a dead end, and life as pointless. Men at this stage also become aware of changing physical strength and vigour. Yet the years between maturity and the beginning of old age may be regarded as the prime of life, and a time when many men are at the peak of their careers and are still in good physical health. For these people illness is unexpected and may be perceived as being 'unfair'. It may also be seen as being a failure of medical care or as a result of an unhealthy lifestyle.

- Do you see mid age as the prime of life? What age do you think your health will start to deteriorate?

Preventive health in adulthood

The time perspective of the young adult may be limited to the demands of their jobs, marriage and bringing up families, but in mid age people may make positive plans for retirement. As people enter mid age they may increasingly focus on preventive health measures and may begin to prepare for retirement. At this time there may be an intense interest in health, shown by joining clubs or fitness programmes and attending for screening. Stressful events may occur with relative frequency in mid adulthood and there has been much interest in the link between coping with stress and heart disease in mid age (see pp. 104–105). If elderly parents die or suffer chronic illness when their offspring are mid aged, this may focus attention on illness (and health).

Youth and beauty are culturally associated and the association is perpetuated by media images. A youthful physical appearance is a source of power for women, although men's power depends on wealth and occupation. This has been described as the double standard of ageing. The Association of Graceful Ageing, Health and Moral Attractiveness developed in the 1920s illustrates the anxieties that are reflected in the belief that a healthy mid age will somehow postpone the ageing process. Physical attractiveness bears little relationship to health in reality. Those who are physically attractive may be assumed to be healthy even though they are not.

There are noticeable changes in physical appearance with increasing age, such as greying hair and loss of skin elasticity.

In an ageist society these become negative attributes and generate a vast cosmetic industry. However, greying hair and cragginess of features in men may denote increasing maturity and competence.

Child rearing may dominate the ages between 20 and 45 and much of the contact between adults and the medical profession may be about the health of the children. The mother may consult her general practitioner frequently, and this will allow a relationship to develop, which may be valuable when she becomes older and more likely to be ill herself.

- At what age do you think adults consider concealing their age?
- Why should there be a double standard for ageing for men and women? Is it changing?

Health changes and age

The menopause has been held to be responsible for the increase in women's psychological problems in mid age but the evidence for a causal relationship is weak (see pp. 4–5).

The best predictor of psychological well-being in older people is physical well-being. The best predictor of physical well-being is material deprivation (Gannon 2000).

Sensory abilities progressively decline in adulthood. People's sight deteriorates and a sure sign of reaching mid age is when newspapers are read at arm's length. Sometimes patients at outpatient clinics or admitted to hospital may not carry reading glasses with them, and may not be able to read simple instructions or consent forms.

Hearing also declines slowly but there is little loss of psychomotor skills during mid age.

On the plus side, knowledge, confidence and maturity increase with age and as yet are still valued by society. As medical technology increases we are likely to live longer, so the mid-age adult should have many healthy and productive years before an extended third age in retirement.

> ### Adulthood and mid age
> - The age of entry to adulthood is usually considered as being about 18 years, but there are differences in social, cultural and psychological milestones.
> - Marriage is more beneficial for health in men than in women. Marital problems may affect health.
> - In mid age, adults become increasingly interested in preventive health.
> - Adults spend much time in parenting in mid age and their main contact with the medical profession may be through their children, or their elderly parents.
> - Physical events such as the menopause and changes in sensory abilities signal the ageing process, but are not directly related to loss of function in mid age.

Case study

40-year-old Mr Harris and his wife (who works part time as a care assistant) have three children at school, four parents living and an elderly grandmother of 90. Mr Harris lost his job as a printer when his firm was modernized. How would you expect him to view middle age? His wife is concerned about the health of her father, who is a heavy smoker. She is grieving for the loss of her younger sister who died of breast cancer. How would you expect her to view mid age?

Ageing, society and health

Health in old age

It is widely believed by many health-care professionals that most old people are physically frail and suffer from multiple disorders. While it is true that the prevalence of disease increases with age, most old people live independent and mobile lives, free from major incapacitating disease (Sidell 1995). Problems with hearing and vision increase with age, and taste and smell sensitivity decrease. However, only about 4% of the over-65s reside in long-stay care, and most of those are over 75 years old. Perhaps one of the reasons health-care professionals think that all old people are infirm and ill is that this is the group they encounter most frequently.

Examples of ageism are not difficult to find. In 1962, a British physician wrote in *The Lancet* that it is 'normal' for people over the age of 75 to be:

frail and unsteady, dozing by day and wakeful by night, confused about people and places, forgetful and untidy, repetitive and boring, selfish and petty perhaps and consumed by a fear of death.

STOP THINK Which statements do you think are true?
- Most old people are frail and infirm and a high proportion reside in institutions.
- Old people have no interest in or capacity for sexual relations.
- Intelligence declines with age.
- Old people are incapable of learning new things.
- Depression is a major problem in the elderly.
- Most old people are poor.

If you think that all of these statements are true then you appear to accept the 'myths' of ageing. Myths are stereotypes that predispose us to think about and act towards people in particular ways.

The ageing mind

It is commonly believed that all old people are senile, incapable of learning new things, depressed, and that intelligence declines with age. It is, of course, true that all old people are 'senile' – the word means 'old'. But, to what extent do our intellectual capacities decline with age?

At one time there appeared to be a substantial body of evidence showing that intelligence declines with age (pp. 30–31). The evidence was drawn from cross-sectional studies of performance on intelligence tests. These studies fairly consistently showed that older cohorts, compared with younger cohorts, performed less well on the intelligence tests. However, as the findings from longitudinal studies emerged, the picture changed quite dramatically (Schaie 1996). When the same individuals are tested over time, there is very little change in test performance, i.e. intelligence does *not* decline with age (Fig. 1).

Does the ability to learn decline with age? There is little information about learning in old people. However, there is now much research on human learning and problem solving which compares different age groups.

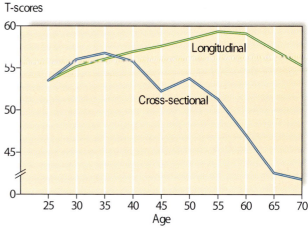

Fig. 1 **Graph showing findings from cross-sectional and longitudinal studies of intelligence and age.**

Learning requires two things: a person has to get the information 'in' and then, when tested, they must get the learned material 'out'. If the performance of old people is worse than that of younger subjects one must devise an experiment to find out which aspect of learning accounts for the differences in test performance. Most studies of what is called 'pacing' have shown that old people need longer to get the learned material 'out'. In pacing studies the experimenter varies the amount of time that subjects have to produce the answer. If no time limit is set, performance on learning tasks of older and younger subjects is similar. However, reducing the amount of time to recall the answer leads to decrements of performance for older people (Bromley 1990). Thus, it appears that it takes longer for older people to search their memory stores to retrieve information. Doctors should, therefore, allow more time for older patients to 'find' the answers to questions. Repeatedly filling the silence with another question will lead to a breakdown in communication (see pp. 94–95).

Another interesting area where older and younger subjects differ is in the ability to filter-out irrelevant information. This is sometimes referred to as the 'cocktail party' effect. When young people go to a party they have little difficulty filtering out the irrelevant conversations taking place around them. Older people find this difficult. Studies involve asking subjects to listen to headphones in which one message is played to the left ear and a different one to the right. The subject is asked to follow only one message (so-called 'dichotic listening experiments'). As people age, test performance indicates that more and more information from the 'wrong' ear appears in the test (Stuart-Hamilton 1994).

These findings are relevant to the practice of medicine:

- When taking a case history or explaining something to an older patient one should ensure that there are as few distracting and 'irrelevant' noises about as possible; patients find it stressful to have to struggle to listen to and concentrate on one particular conversation.
- It is not uncommon for middle-aged patients to visit their GPs asking to have their hearing tested or for wax to be removed from their ears. Testing often reveals no wax and little decrement in the acuity of the patient's hearing. The patient goes away frustrated and still convinced that he or she is going

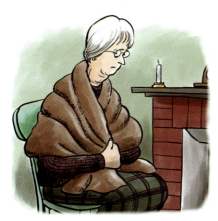

Fig. 2 **Image of ageing presented in a health promotion leaflet.**

deaf. Explanation of this 'central processing' phenomenon usually provides reassurance.

Will all old people eventually develop dementia and suffer from depression? Only a minority will develop dementia. Epidemiological studies indicate that roughly 1% of the 65–75-year-olds and 10% of those over 75 will develop dementia (Ineichen 1987). Depression is also not as common amongst the elderly as some have made out. A literature review has noted that old people are not more prone to depression than younger ones. Yet one continues to see books stating that depression in the elderly is a major health hazard.

Sexuality

Another common belief is that old people are not interested in, and have no capacity for, sexual relations (see pp. 28–29). Although there have been few studies on sexuality in the elderly, those that exist have found that older people are interested in sex. However, opportunities for sexual relations are often limited, especially for women. Widowed and divorced men often marry younger women and this greatly reduces the numbers of sexual partners available for older women. Although there is much talk of 'toy boys', the reality for older women is that sexual relations with younger men are still frowned upon in society (Bytheway 1995).

Health-care professionals often feel uncomfortable talking about sexual matters with older people. This may have to do with powerful incest taboos which make it hard for us to think about our parents as sexual beings. We may generalize these feelings about our parents to all older people.

Uneasiness about sexuality in elderly people may also be the reason why health-care professionals fail to provide opportunities for sexual relations for old people who live in residential care.

Poverty and old age

What is your image of old people? Is it like Figure 2 which appeared in a health promotion leaflet? This is certainly a prevalent media view of old people.

Poverty is a relative concept, and research does show that, as a group, elderly people are financially worse off than younger people. This is particularly true of Britain in comparison with some European countries. In Britain, nearly three out of five older people live in or on the margins of poverty compared with less than one-quarter of those under pension age (Walker 1993). Furthermore, many elderly do not claim the benefits to which they are entitled because they resent the intrusion of means testing into their private lives.

While one would not wish to belittle the problems faced by those elderly people who have minimal financial resources (and hypothermia can indeed be a severe risk for them), the danger is that old people themselves will be 'blamed' for their poverty. Rather than ask questions about the way society is structured, for example, with people forced to retire at 65, we may lapse into the view that old people are poor because they did not save for their old age (see pp. 52–53).

Working with old people

How many health-care professionals choose to specialize in areas related to old people? A review of studies on attitudes to the elderly amongst doctors and medical students revealed that most preferred to work with younger people (Palmore 1977). Few medical students say they want to specialize in geriatric medicine. This is interesting given that, except for those specializing in paediatrics and obstetrics, most specialties involve care of the elderly. Most people with cancer or cardiovascular disease are old.

Beliefs and behaviour

False beliefs about ageing may have very negative effects on old people. They may also lead to unrealistic fears for the future in adults. Society may come to view the elderly as a burden, rather than a resource. More importantly, the behaviour of doctors may be influenced by negative stereotypes of the elderly.

> ### Ageing, society and health
> ■ Most elderly people can, and often do, live independent and mobile lives.
> ■ Myths or stereotypes held by health-care professionals can limit the self-esteem and independence of older people.
> ■ There is no evidence that intelligence declines with age, but recall may take longer.
> ■ Opportunities for sexual relations are often limited, particularly for older women.
> ■ Older people are more likely to be poor than younger adults, but are often too 'proud/independent' to claim the benefits to which they are entitled.

Case study

Two persons in similar physical condition may be differentially designated dead or not. For example, a young child was brought into the emergency room with no registering heartbeat, respiration, or pulse – the standard 'signs of death' – and was, through a rather dramatic stimulation procedure involving the co-ordinated work of a large team of doctors and nurses, revived for a period of 11 hours. On the same evening an elderly person who presented the same physical signs, with – as one physician later stated in conversation – no discernible differences from the child in skin colour, warmth, etc., arrived in the emergency room and was almost immediately pronounced dead, with no attempts at stimulation instituted. A nurse remarked later, 'They (the doctors) would never have done that to the old lady (attempt heart stimulation) even though I've seen it work on them too'. During the period when emergency resuscitation equipment was being readied for the child, an intern instituted mouth-to-mouth resuscitation. This same intern was shortly relieved by oxygen machinery, and when the woman arrived, he was the one who pronounced her dead. He said that he could never bring himself to put his mouth to 'an old lady like that' (Sudnow 1967).

Bereavement

In the course of their career, doctors will often have to care for people who are coming to terms with the loss of someone through death. The terms bereavement, grief and mourning are often used interchangeably to describe a person's reaction to loss. The processes occurring after the death, during which individuals learn to adjust to the loss, are known as bereavement; grief can be described as the emotional response to that loss, while mourning refers to the expression of grief (Stroebe and Stroebe 1987). The bereavement period can provide the opportunity for doctors to assess the needs of the surviving spouse or family, and to intervene where appropriate with relevant back-up and services (Cartwright 1982).

Determinants of grief

Many factors can affect the way in which someone reacts to being bereaved. These may precede the bereavement, for example, a childhood experience, a previous life crisis like divorce or mental illness, or the nature of the relationship between the bereaved person and the deceased. The reaction may also be influenced by the bereaved person's present circumstances, for example, their age, sex, religion, type of personality or even cultural background. Reactions may also be determined by the circumstances of the bereaved after the death, for example, the amount of support they have, and other stresses in their life, such as young children. Such determinants have been referred to as the antecedent (previous experience), concurrent (present circumstances) and subsequent determinants of grief (Parkes 1975).

Cultural and religious beliefs affect how people display grief and feel they should behave during bereavement. Strict rules govern the preparation of the body after death and the rituals associated with burial and mourning among different ethnic groups (Firth 2001) (pp. 128–129).

The mourning process

In the same way that the dying process has been described as a series of stages (Kubler-Ross 1970), the process of mourning has similarly been defined as a series of phases or stages that must be passed through by the bereaved before grief can be resolved (pp. 128–129). The initial phase of numbness gradually gives way to feelings of pining, yearning and searching, as the bereaved person seeks to recover what has been lost. When the intensity of this second phase diminishes, it is replaced by feelings of depression, disorganization and despair when it becomes apparent that the loss is irretrievable. Finally, the bereaved person moves to a phase of recovery and reorganization when he/she begins to adjust to a new way of life without the deceased (Parkes 1975, Bowlby 1998). Worden (1991) prefers to describe the process as a series of tasks that must be worked through. He describes these as accepting the reality of the loss, working through the pain, adjusting to an environment in which the deceased is missing and moving on with life. More recently, the Dual Process Model suggests that bereaved people move between confronting grief (loss-orientated behaviour) and avoiding grief (restoration-orientated behaviour) (Stroebe and Schut 1999). Although these theories can be a useful way of beginning to understand the complexity of the grief process, individual reactions will vary and may not conform to a specific pattern.

Normal grief

Normal grief reactions can include a range of different feelings, moods, symptoms and behaviours. Worden (1991) has classified examples of these under four headings. These are illustrated in Figure 1.

Risk factors

Faulkner (1995) suggests that the reaction to loss may not be normal if:

- a difficult relationship with the deceased has existed before the death, for example, the bereaved person may have been over-dependent on the dead person or disliked them
- the death has been violent (e.g. murder) or sudden or unexplained (e.g. suicide)
- the nature of the bereaved's involvement in the death has been unsatisfactory, for example, the bereaved person may not have had time to say goodbye, may not have visited the person before the death or may not have been present at the death
- the bereaved person has previously experienced difficult losses, for example, divorce or mutilating surgery (Faulkner 1995).

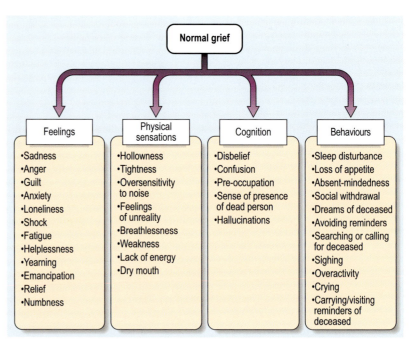

Fig. 1 **A typology of normal grief.** (Worden 1991)

Pathological grief reaction

Pathological, abnormal or complicated grief reactions occur when the bereaved person is unable for some reason to express or work through their grief, which prevents their recovery from the loss and adaptation to life without the deceased. These reactions can be excessive and prolonged, or absent and short lived. Such reactions can be classified as absent, delayed, chronic, masked or exaggerated grief.

Delayed or absent grief

The bereaved person is unable to mourn the loss. This may be conscious, when the bereaved person's situation makes it difficult for them to grieve freely, for example, in the case of a mother who carries on normally for the sake of her children. It can also be unconscious, when the bereaved person does not believe that the death has occurred, for example, when there has been no definite confirmation as in the case of soldiers missing during a war. This may be called absent grief (Faulkner 1995). Delayed grief reactions are often triggered by other losses occurring a long time after the death, e.g. a later divorce or other unrelated loss (Worden 1991).

Case study

Ethel was a 61-year-old woman whose husband Jack had died 6 months earlier after a sudden heart attack. At around the same time her youngest daughter, Ruth, had left home to start a university course in a city about 30 miles away from where they lived. Her two elder children were both married and living abroad. Previously a lively woman, with many and varied interests, Ethel had shared most of these with her husband as they both enjoyed early retirement. Lately, however, Ethel had become withdrawn and morose, and seemed to have lost all interest in anything. She had stopped going to the clubs of which she was a member and preferred instead to spend her days looking at old family photos or going through her husband's belongings, which she refused to part with. She constantly phoned her daughter in tears and said she did not want to carry on living without her husband. As a result Ruth felt guilty at having left her mother to cope alone, and at a loss to know what help to give her. Eventually, Ruth asked the family general practitioner for help. She suggested that Ruth phone a local voluntary bereavement counselling service. After a few visits from a trained counsellor, Ethel began to come to terms with her husband's death. Although she knew that her life would no longer be the same without her lifetime partner, she realized that she had to make a new beginning for her own and her family's sake. Ruth was relieved that her mother was now able to resume some of the hobbies she used to enjoy, and her own life at university became happier.

Write down the factors you think might have influenced the way Ethel reacted to Jack's death.

■ Think about how you would cope with Ethel if you were Ruth.

■ Think about the counsellor's task in helping Ethel through the grief (see pp. 130–131).

Chronic grief

The bereaved continues to experience the immediate pain of the loss months or even years later. They therefore are unable to move on in the grieving process and adapt to life without the deceased. Usually chronic grief reactions occur in people who have had ambivalent relationships with the deceased (Parkes 1975).

Masked grief

The grief reaction is masked by the development of physical or somatic symptoms that appear to the bereaved to be unassociated with the loss. Often these are physical symptoms that replicate those experienced by the deceased and these commonly appear on the anniversaries of the loss (Worden 1991).

Exaggerated grief

The grief reaction is excessive and intense. In these cases the bereaved's experience may develop into a serious psychiatric illness, e.g. clinical depression or an acute anxiety state (Worden 1991).

Other losses

Persons may react to other losses or illnesses in the same way as they would to a bereavement. For example, reaction to a cancer diagnosis (see pp. 96–97), amputation, miscarriage, still birth, physical dependency, divorce, unemployment or even relocation to a new town or city. With these losses the grief experienced and exhibited by the person may be as intense and as debilitating as grief expressed at a death. For these reasons health professionals may miss or fail to appreciate the extent of a person's distress. This may mean that the person experiencing the loss is not offered the help that they need to come to terms with it.

Bereavement care

The amount of support available for the bereaved varies greatly according to the setting where patients and their relatives are cared for. Doctors working in general hospitals may not have the time or resources to follow up carers during bereavement. Often this is done by general practitioners or community nurses, who are able to visit the bereaved at home. Not every bereaved person will want or need professional support at this time. The majority rely on family and friends or find their own ways of coping.

In cases where the grief reaction is problematic, the doctor should recognize his/her limitations and summon the help of someone who is specially trained in bereavement counselling. In some extreme cases, it may also be necessary to refer the person on to a clinical psychologist or psychiatrist (see pp. 130–131; 134–135).

Bereavement

■ Bereavement refers to the situation of someone who has experienced the loss of a loved one and grief is the emotional response to the loss.

■ Normal grief can be described as a series of stages a person must work through until they adapt to life without the deceased.

■ The way people react to a loss will depend on their past experiences and present circumstances.

Personality

Most people would agree that everyone has a unique personality. This is another way of saying that there are individual differences in behaviour. Personality is difficult to define but many psychologists would agree that it is made up of stable internal factors that are relatively constant over time and that account for individual differences in behaviour. Some characteristics, like shyness, are more obvious at certain ages, and young teenagers may be especially shy about talking about their developing bodies. It is suggested that something within us determines our behaviour but, as we shall see, external circumstances are also powerful. If someone behaves 'out of character', we should look for causes that might be related to health, such as drug abuse, the onset of dementia, or a break-down in a relationship.

There are many different personality theories and these influence how behaviour is viewed. For example, patients who complain about minor symptoms may be regarded as having a low pain threshold. But patients may also complain because they have learned that complaints are rewarded by attention from professionals and family. Complaints might also reflect unconscious conflict. None of these approaches is right or wrong but must be seen as a more or less useful way of looking at individual differences.

One view is that people have a fixed personality that is deep inside but covered up like layers of an onion. If only we could strip away the layers we would uncover the 'real' person lying within. The layers give colour or characteristics to a person. This is sometimes known as trait theory.

Trait theory

Individuals are thought of as having many different traits. These traits can be described by different sets of adjectives relating to behaviour. Hans Eysenck and colleagues used factor analysis (a statistical technique that investigates correlations between different variables, and looks for clusters of association which suggest an underlying structure) to identify two main super factors (Fig. 1):

- **Introversion–extroversion**. People who score highly in extroversion are sociable, lively, assertive, in contrast to introverts, who are more retiring and controlled.
- **Neuroticism–stability**. Those who score highly on neuroticism show anxiety proneness, guilt feelings, have low self-esteem and experience low mood.

They then added a third dimension, psychoticism, which can be considered as being at right angles to the other two in Figure 1.

- **Psychoticism–impulse control**. Those scoring high on psychoticism are aggressive, cold, and lack empathy.

These trait theories describe differences but we also want to know why people are different and if these descriptions allow us to predict behaviour. Personality traits may be linked to coping behaviours (Ferguson 2001)

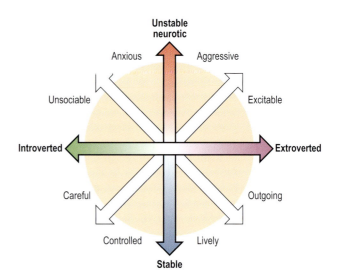

Fig. 1 **Dimensions of personality based on Eysenck's theory.**

STOP THINK

- Contrast your behaviour as a student and as a son or daughter. Are they different? Are your views of yourself different from those of your parents?

This exercise stresses the importance of the situation in determining personality. The correlation between personality and actual behaviour is actually low. This ties in with the social learning theory approach (see pp. 20–21).

A patient who seems very timid and anxious when consulting a doctor may be dynamic and forceful at home or at work. This may be because the sick rôle encourages subservient behaviour and deference to doctors.

We do not always agree with everyone about the characteristics of a person. Consider your reaction if you were told that you were unpunctual. Would this be a fair comment? You might feel that you were always on time for appointments with patients and always turned up in time for ward rounds. However, you might realize that your time-keeping at lectures was not so good and that your partner had complained that you were unreliable. Mischel (1968) suggested that far from having consistent traits that are stable over time and situations, we behave in particular ways according to the situation.

Is it the person or the situation?

The answer is neither one alone but most likely personality results from an interaction between the two. It is hard to imagine an extroverted personality appearing as a shrinking violet, but among people who know you well there will be some common agreement about the kind of person you are.

Life events including illness can have a marked effect on the way people behave. The threat of a second myocardial infarction may change a person's approach to life. Disfigurement of the body, especially of the face, can lead to a loss of self-esteem and lack of social confidence.

STOP THINK

■ To what extent do you think that people's physical appearance influences their personality?

Types of personality theories

Some theories are known as 'ideographic theories' because they seek to identify an individual's unique characteristics. These are more often used in clinical contexts. They contrast with 'nomothetic theories' such as the trait theories. These consider that people differ in a number of different traits or characteristics common to everyone. These are often used in large-scale research studies.

Psychodynamic theory

The approach taken by Freud and psychoanalytic theory is ideographic.

His theory is based on the assumption that behaviour is influenced by the unconscious mind. Using an iceberg analogy he described the part above water as representing the conscious experience, and the bulk below as representing the unconscious experience. The unconscious is accessible through the technique of free association and is revealed in dreams and memories of early childhood.

Freud's theory of personality describes three major systems. The *ego* is conscious and is in touch with the real world. The *id* is childlike and demands that its needs be fulfilled. The *super ego* is the individual's conscience and tends to be authoritarian. The three work together but may also be in conflict. The ego has to reconcile impulses from the id and the super ego. There are no actual physiological systems or parts of the brain that correspond to these systems, but Freudians use them to explain individual behaviour.

There are many scientific arguments against the acceptance of Freudian theory of personality. There is little scientific data, no statistical analysis, and the theory is based on patients who were rich middle-class women living in Victorian Vienna. However, it has intuitive meaning, some doctors find it clinically useful and it is important to be aware of psychodynamic theories. They have also been influential in modern literature!

Personality traits

Five basic traits appear to be constant across age groups and cultures. These are: neuroticism, extroversion/introversion, openness to experience, agreeableness/antagonism and conscientiousness.

Neuroticism has been linked with greater symptom reporting, more complaints about health and health worries, and more frequent consultations.

Extroversion has been associated with fewer physical and psychological symptoms, and better perceived health status. Jerram and Coleman (1999) found all five traits were related to health reports and health behaviour in a study of 50 people aged 75–84 years.

Case study

Mr McDuff was very competitive at work and worked hard to become the top salesman in his area. He drove aggressively and always appeared in a hurry. He was impatient of others and many people thought that his manner to his colleagues was unnecessarily rude. At home he was quiet and never raised his voice, although he had young teenagers in the house. He visited his mother, who lived nearby, twice a week and she regarded him as quiet, home loving and dominated by his wife. Why does this description sound rather unconvincing? Which aspect of his behaviour would be associated with vulnerability to heart disease?

Vulnerability to specific diseases

Personality differences may predict people's behaviour to illness but there has also been much interest in the relationship between individual differences and vulnerability to specific illnesses. Lively controversies have arisen over the relationship between psychosocial and organic factors in cancer and cardiovascular disease. It has been suggested that some people have particular personality characteristics that make them more prone to cancer, known as 'Type C personality'. Gossarth-Maticek et al (1984) assessed a sample of 1353 elderly Yugoslavian patients and monitored them over 10 years. Significant characteristics of those dying of cancer included 'rational and anti-emotional behaviour' and a high level of 'traumatic life events involving chronic helplessness'. Gossarth-Maticek does not define these terms and they are difficult to interpret. This study and other studies have been severely criticised by Pelosi and Appleby (1992). The definition of personality types is imprecise, and the methodology and analyses are unclear. In the Yugoslavian study a 100% follow-up was claimed after 10 years. Some of these criticisms have been addressed by Eysenck (1992), but the link between cancer, personality and therapy remains unclear.

Behaviour patterns may be linked to heart disease and a pattern of behaviour known as Type A has been associated with risk of heart attacks (see pp. 104–105). Feelings of hostility appear to be most closely associated with increased risk of heart attacks but the claims are contentious. Although Type A and Type B have been described as personality types, they are better thought of as behaviour patterns that can be modified by interventions. Changing Type A behaviour is often incorporated into rehabilitation programmes following mild heart attacks.

What is personality?

■ There are many different personality theories but they should not be seen as being either right or wrong but as different in their approach.
■ Trait theory suggests that behaviour is determined by personality traits which may cluster into factors such as extroversion.
■ The situation may influence behaviour more than individual characteristics.
■ Freudian psychoanalytic theory suggests that our behaviour is influenced by unconscious motives and these develop during our childhood.
■ Individual differences in Type A behaviour may be related to vulnerability to heart disease.

Understanding learning

Learning is not just about acquiring facts or knowledge. Social skills, beliefs and values are also learned. We learn how to respond emotionally, how to recognize symptoms and, as children, we learn appropriate (and inappropriate) ways of behaving (Fig. 1). If we understand how behaviour is learned we may be able to change it. We may wish to change to a more healthy life style, to learn how to monitor our own glucose levels, or to overcome a phobia. Understanding learning has been of central concern to psychologists, and the source of much debate (Eysenck 1996).

Learning can be defined as a relatively permanent change in behaviour. Behaviourist theories of learning assume that there are laws of learning that are fundamental to all animals, and that humans are no different in this respect. Behaviourism suggests that learning results from stimulus–response associations. A stimulus can be any change, such as the sight of food or a moving ball. A response is a reflex action such as salivation, or a muscular response such as catching the ball. Of course much learning is cognitive – such as the acquisition of knowledge and concepts that is taking place as you read this book.

Theoretical background
Operant conditioning

One kind of learning, known as operant conditioning, was described by an American psychologist, B. F. Skinner. In operant conditioning, the likelihood of a response occurring again is increased if the behaviour is followed by a reinforcement. Thus, the behaviour is controlled by its consequences. The principles of operant conditioning have been established through experimentation on animals such as rats and pigeons, as well as humans (Table 1).

If a goal results from an accurate kick, then the motor responses leading up to the kick will be reinforced. In this case the reinforcement would be in the form of satisfaction and approval by the team and fans. Success in walking following an amputation would be rewarded internally by feelings of mastery and enhanced self-efficacy, and externally by the approval of others. Praise (especially from medical staff) can be a very powerful reinforcer.

Classical conditioning

Operant conditioning is contrasted with classical conditioning described by a physiologist, I. Pavlov. In classical conditioning an initially neutral stimulus becomes associated with an involuntary response by its association with a previously conditioned stimulus. Pavlov worked with dogs, who naturally salivate at the sight of food. After pairing a bell with the food, the dogs learned to salivate at the sound of the bell alone.

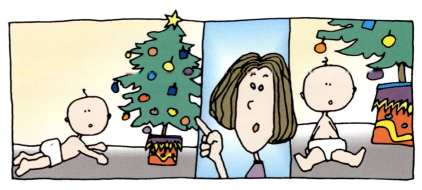

Fig. 1 **If an infant approaches the Christmas tree decorations it will be restrained: this will decrease the frequency of approach**. In practice punishment is a very poor way of changing behaviour and often it arouses emotional responses. What does the baby do when it is not allowed to touch the tree (or approach medical equipment)?

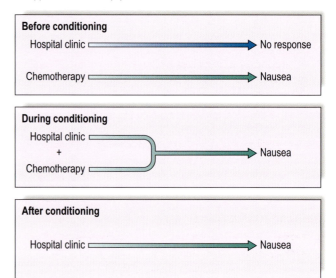

Fig. 2 **Classical conditioning applied to nausea and chemotherapy.**

These principles were later tested with human emotional responses.

Watson and Raynor (1920) used classical conditioning to produce a phobia in a 9-month-old child known as Little Albert. Before the experiment he had no fear of white rats but was frightened by loud noises. In the experiment the loud noise was paired with the presence of a white rat. After six pairings Albert showed a fear response in the presence of the white rat alone. Fear had now become a response conditioned to the previously neutral stimulus of the white rat. Moreover the fear generalized

Table 1 **Principles of operant conditioning**			
Principle	**Definition**	**Effect on behaviour**	**Example**
Positive reinforcement	Provides positive, pleasant consequences	Increases probability that the response will occur again	Verbal praise in rehabilitation
Negative reinforcement	Removes unpleasant conditions	Increases probability that response will occur again	Adjusting gait to avoid pain in walking
Punishment	Removes a positive reinforcer or applies an aversive stimulus	Decreases the probability that response will occur again	Vomiting after eating poisonous fungi
Extinction	Removes positive reinforcer	Decreases the probability that response will occur again	Ignoring tantrums in waiting room
Shaping	Reinforces successive approximations to the one required	Gradually increases approximation to desired behaviour	Teaching someone with a learning disability how to feed themselves

to other furry animals. White rats and loud noises are not an everyday occurrence but white coats may be associated with painful injections. The fear of pain may become associated with the white coat (and its wearer) and generalize to white coats worn by any staff.

Some patients may develop conditioned responses to the sight or smell of hospitals. If hospital treatment has been associated with nausea, as, for example, in the case of chemotherapy for cancer, the mere sight or smell of hospital can induce nausea or even vomiting (Fig. 2).

In practice, operant conditioning and classical conditioning probably both occur in many learning situations. Food elicits salivation but also acts as a reinforcer.

- Does the behavioural approach reduce people to passive objects being manipulated by health professionals?
- What reinforcements do you think would be appropriate for medical staff to use in a hospital setting?
- If someone is on a medically advised weight-reducing diet, success will be reinforced by praise from doctors, family and friends. Why is this not an effective reinforcer and why is it so hard to resist eating crisps and chocolate?
- If playing a fruit machine (or the National Lottery) gave too few prizes, people would soon stop playing. Why?

Observational learning

This model suggests that behaviour patterns can be learned by watching other people's behaviour. Many clinical skills are learned in this way. Both voluntary and involuntary responses can be learned by modelling.

Children who were going to be admitted to hospital were shown a film of an unstressed child going into hospital, undergoing surgery and going home. Compared with others who were shown an unrelated film they showed less anxiety both before and after the operation (Saile et al 1988). The closer in age and sex the model was to themselves, the more imitation took place. However, the films may have reduced the anxiety of the parents as much as the children so that the child had a very powerful model of an unanxious parent to imitate as well! In the same way, anxiety or embarrassment shown by a doctor will be quickly picked up and learned by a patient. Doctors and medical staff are powerful models.

Practical application

Behaviour therapy has been widely used to modify undesirable behaviour patterns.

Systematic desensitization

Systematic desensitization or graded exposure would treat a phobia such as Albert's learned fear of furry animals by gradually exposing the person to the feared object while replacing the anxiety with a relaxed condition. This can be achieved by reassurance or relaxation training. In a diabetic outpatient clinic someone with a needle phobia might be treated by such methods so that they can tolerate injections. Initially this might be done by imagination alone, by visualizing the object, and once this is achieved without fear, the syringe could be introduced in the form of a picture. Later it might be shown in vivo, firstly at a distance and then gradually brought nearer (see pp. 110–111).

Cognitive behavioural therapy (CBT) tries to alter behaviour by undoing the learning of maladaptive behaviour and by learning new behaviour patterns (pp. 134–135). It is based on theories of classical and operant conditioning.

Principles of learning have also been used in theories that enhance coping with stress, such as rational emotive behaviour theory (REBT) and biofeedback.

Learning factual material

Medical students find that they have to learn and recall difficult material (see pp. 26–27). Various strategies have been proposed to help this. *Mnemonics* can be associations of two words or letters, or a word and a visual image. *Rehearsal* can establish words in long-term memory, and this is most effective if they are *organized*. Many students make lists, or mind maps of a topic.

Case study

Night waking in children can be a problem for both child and parents. An otherwise healthy and happy child of age 2 years woke up regularly at night, and early in the morning. His parents were becoming exhausted because of broken sleep; they were becoming irritable with each other and their work was suffering.

The parents were asked to monitor their behaviour when the child woke up. They described how they gave the child a drink, read him a story and sometimes took him into their own bed to settle him. It was pointed out that these were acting as reinforcers, as well as the drink filling his bladder causing soaking nappies in the morning.

The parents then left him to cry for longer before responding and gave him minimal attention in the night. Reinforcers were given for sleeping through the night such as giving cuddles and toys in his own bed, not the parents'. Within a few weeks the broken nights were fewer and the child's behaviour was further reinforced by having happy, rested parents.

Understanding learning

- Learning is a relatively stable change in behaviour and may occur by operant conditioning, classical conditioning or observationally.
- Operant conditioning has been used to change health behaviour and is based on principles of reinforcement, punishment, extinction and shaping.
- Principles of learning have been used in behaviour therapy to modify undesired behaviour patterns.

Perception

Why do we perceive what we do? How does the brain process information so that what we see or hear is what we create, not what is actually 'out there'? This spread shows how perception is not a passive process, but is active, creating and constructing our world. Whereas *sensation* (the stimulus which impacts upon the sense organs) provides the raw data about the environment, it is *perception* which provides meaning.

The main emphasis in this spread will be on visual perception, but these points also apply to other types of perception such as auditory, olfactory or tactile perception.

The main features of perception

- **Perception is knowledge-based and partly learned.** Early works of art show that artists (and young children) have to learn about perspective; likewise, your perception of pathological signs on a slide under a microscope improves with medical education.
- **Perception is inferential.** When we see part of an object, like the top half of a person sitting at a table, we perceive them as a 'whole' person, not half a person.
- **It is categorical.** We tend to categorize what we see, so that a variety of clinical signs are perceived as a disease in a patient, even though they may not in fact be related.
- **Perception is relational.** What we perceive as small or large depends on context. A 2 cm flesh wound on an adult is seen as less serious than the same size of wound on a child.
- **Perception is adaptive.** We tend to perceive significant things better than insignificant things. For example, we notice a car which is moving more than we notice a stationary vehicle: this is more important for our survival.

What are illusions, and why are we subject to them?

Illusions demonstrate how creative a process perception is, because the stimuli are ambiguous, or presented in a context which distorts our perception. Figure 1 (a, b) illustrates this.

We are subject to illusions, not because we are unintelligent or not paying attention, but because the brain interprets reality in the light of our prior experience.

How do we recognize what is perceived?

Recognition is organizing what is perceived into something meaningful by using past experience. A number of theories exist to explain:

- **Bottom-up processing.** The perceptual system is assumed to analyse a stimulus into a set of features and then the brain matches it to other sets already existing in the brain. If a match occurs, then recognition occurs. In examining a rash, a general practitioner takes note of the shape, type, size, colour and distribution of spots on the skin, then matches them to previous cases of measles that he has seen, or the colour illustration and description of measles that he has seen in a textbook.
- **Top-down processing.** The context creates expectancy and sets up what is known as 'perceptual set'. We 'see' what we expect, or want to see, and recognition occurs. For example, the general practitioner learns from the patient that he has been in contact with someone suffering from German measles. This creates an expectancy, and a perceptual set when examining the patient's rash. It can sometimes lead to misdiagnosis when the expectancy is strong.

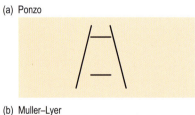
(a) Ponzo

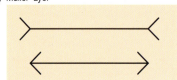
(b) Muller–Lyer

Fig. 1 In these two figures, the sets of horizontal lines are the same length, but we see them as differing lengths according to the rest of the drawing.

STOP THINK

- What factors may help to explain why one 45 year-old man perceives his symptoms of dyspepsia as severe and serious, whereas another similarly aged man perceives them as trivial? (See also pp. 88–89)

- **Both mechanisms together.** In trying to read a page of poor handwriting we may use both processes: puzzling out what each letter looks like, as well as guessing meaning from the context. Figure 2 shows how you do this.

How do we influence perception?

We control our perception by paying attention to different aspects of our environment. Attention is the directing and focusing of perception. It may be:

- **Selective.** We attend more to stimuli that are changing, repeated, intense and personally meaningful. Certain words catch our attention, for example our names, words connected with significant interests, or important concerns such as words like 'sex'.
- **Divided or focused.** Our ability to divide attention is limited, although it can be improved with practice. It is easier to divide attention if two different types of stimuli are used. For example, you can probably look at pictures and listen to music simultaneously, but it is hard to read and listen to someone talking at the same time.
- **Negatively affected by stress and fatigue.** When we are tired, or when there are more demands being placed upon us than there are resources to meet those demands, our attention may decrease. This can have disastrous results. Tired doctors are more likely to make errors because they are no longer able to pay full attention to all the details of a particular set of diagnostic signs.

The relevance of the psychology of perception to medicine

The brain is an active component of the perceptual process. Brain damage

What does this squiggle mean?

Analysis of features alone will not tell you.

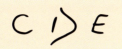

Context is also needed.

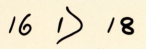

Fig. 2 **Interpretation in context.**

will result in perceptual distortion, hence an early indicator of organic damage may be perceptual disturbance.

There is often no such thing as the 'correct' way to perceive something: perceptions vary because the perceptual process is a creative one. Most of the time we do not notice this, but sometimes the differences are critical. A pathologist may carry out a post-mortem examination, with an assumption about the cause of death. It may lead them to seek, identify and report an incomplete set of evidence. A second pathologist may discover another, highly significant sign which can change the course of the police enquiry completely.

We are prone to see what the context indicates we should see. Given ambiguous cues we 'recognize' things according to our expectations.

Attention can be divided, with practice. When you start to acquire a skill (e.g. taking blood from a patient) it is almost impossible to do anything else at the same time, such as talking reassuringly to the patient. In time, however, the skill of attending to both aspects of the patient encounter simultaneously can be learned.

Social perception
Past experience
We may be influenced by our previous experience when making a diagnosis (see Case study). Our perception may also be influenced by our past experience. For example, we tend to be more positive towards physically attractive people. In studies of social perception people were asked to

choose the company with whom they would prefer to watch television. Most expressed a preference for people who were not physically disabled. In many cases this may be due simply to a lack of experience with disabled people. Congenital deformities may, at first, seem distressing but as you become familiar with such patients you will find that the deformity becomes less distressing and less pertinent. In a sense you no longer 'see' the deformity. Instead you are able to see past these to the people within.

Cognitive constructs
Our impression of people depends on our cognitive constructs. These include sociability, likeability and intelligence. The constructs that we use depend on the context and the people. You will use different constructs when forming impressions of people that you meet at a party from those that you use when seeing patients in an outpatient clinic. Sometimes we make errors in assuming that the behaviour of hospital patients is because of their personality rather than the situation of being ill in hospital (see pp. 100–101). On the other hand you may also attribute a patient's behaviour to having a particular disease rather than the fact that he/she really does behave in that manner.

Schemas
We have many expectations of other people's behaviour. These are called *schemas*. For example, students expect certain standards of behaviour from their lecturers and doctors expect certain behaviour patterns from their patients. Schemas influence what we see even if the behaviour has not occurred. The diagnostic process may

involve schemas. When you make inferences you may fill in the gaps about the relationship between symptoms. You use schemas in order to do this. The trouble is, you can make inferences which are in fact not true. You may assume that a patient from a certain part of the country will have certain characteristics which may not be the case, or you might assume that because someone is of a particular sex that individual will behave in certain ways.

We also have schemas about ourselves, called *self schemas*. We retain information about ourselves and this may influence our selective perception.

Patients have schemas too. Anxious patients may believe that they are unable to cope. Depressed patients may have negative self schemas in which they view themselves as inadequate, hopeless and worthless. These schemas influence what they see, think, feel and do. Patients who are depressed will be much less able to solve day to day problems than other people because they do not believe themselves capable of doing so.

Case study

We see what we expect to see
A junior doctor, just starting in obstetrics and gynaecology, admitted a pregnant woman late one afternoon. She was complaining of stomach pains. The doctor had herself been in hospital on and off during her pregnancy with a series of minor complaints. She carried out a physical examination, as well as asking for an account of her symptoms, and then recommended bed rest. A second junior doctor was covering the ward at night and was asked to check the patient. His aunt had recently been admitted for an ectopic pregnancy. He immediately suggested an ultrasound scan, although the scanning unit was closed for the night. As a result, a life-threatening ectopic pregnancy was detected, and a successful operation was immediately carried out.

Perception

- Perception is an active, creative process.
- Perception depends on the brain's ability to interpret the senses.
- Attention is part of the perceptual process, and it too can be affected by a variety of psychological factors such as previous experience, motivation, and fatigue.

Emotion

Emotions are transient feelings that we experience as happening to us, rather than being initiated by us. They can be positive or negative, and more or less intense. They differ in cognitive complexity and tone. Regret requires more sophisticated representations of reality than does fear, and embarrassment is distinct from guilt. Emotions involve physiological changes and affect our thinking and actions. They can be communicated to others through facial expression, body language, eye contact and non-verbal sounds, as well as through language. Others can be affected by our emotional states, even when we try to hide them, because we are not always able to control non-linguistic channels of emotional communication.

In the late 19th century, William James in the USA and Carl Lange in Denmark both independently argued that perception of events (e.g. learning that one has an inoperable tumour) can lead automatically to physiological changes and that awareness of these changes leads to the experience of emotion. This is known as the James–Lange theory of emotion. The theory highlights the role of physiological arousal in emotional experience, but is too simple to provide a good understanding of emotions. For example, how can this theory explain the feelings of emotion reported by people who have spinal injuries that block physiological feedback to the brain? Schachter (1964) argued that, while physiological change is necessary for emotion, the nature of emotional experience depends upon interpretation of arousal. This is known as the 'two-factor theory of emotion'. It implies that the same physiological arousal could lead to different emotions, for example, anger or happiness, depending on how the person interprets the situation in which they experience arousal. Schachter also pointed out that the social context, and, in particular, others' behaviour, can strongly influence how we interpret physiological arousal and, thereby, what emotions we feel. Thus, emotions are, in part, socially created between people.

We do not have a complete explanation of the generation and regulation of emotion. The physiological bases of emotion are complex. Emotional responses often involve fast responses to something that is either unexpected or highly positively or negatively valued. This raw and fast character may be due to neural pathways that are routed through the amygdala rather than the cortex. This capacity for rapid response could have provided an evolutionary advantage. The amygdala is connected to the cortex, which is involved in the cognitive or interpretative aspect of emotions. Hormones and neurotransmitters play an important part. The release of adrenaline, noradrenaline and dopamine create arousal, central to many emotions. Dopamine and oxytocin may also be important in the regulation of positive versus negative emotional states (Greenfield 2000).

The perception of basic emotions in others' faces may also be biologically determined, rather than learnt. This was first suggested by Charles Darwin in 1872 but has only been systematically studied since 1965, when Paul Ekman began his research into the recognition of emotion from facial expression, across cultures. Ekman proposed that six primary emotions were expressed using the same facial expressions across cultures: fear, anger, disgust, sadness, enjoyment or happiness, and surprise. There is strong evidence indicating cultural agreement for the first five. Ekman (1993) notes that when 70% or more of the people from one cultural group judge a picture of a facial expression to be one of these five emotions then evidence indicates that a similar percentage in another cultural group will recognize the picture as expressing the same emotion. Figure 1 shows some of the basic facial features used to express happiness, anger and sadness across cultures. However, understanding other people's emotions involves much more than recognition of primary emotions.

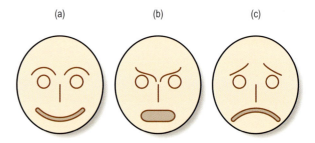

Fig. 1 **Universally recognised facial expressions of emotion. (a) Happy; (b) angry; (c) sad.**

Different cultures have different 'display rules' for the expression of emotion. Emotional expression that would seem appropriate at a wedding or funeral in one culture could be offensive in another. Display rules may also determine different use of emotional expression depending on power relations or gender. For example, women are expected to smile more than men in many Western countries, even when they are not experiencing positive emotions (Deutsch et al 1987), but this gender difference is not observed across all cultures.

Psychologists have argued that positive and negative emotions may operate separately so that one can feel happy or amused even in the midst of sadness. The left and right cerebral hemispheres appear to be specialized in relation to emotional expression, with the left hemisphere dominant in processing positive emotions such as happiness while the right hemisphere is more involved in emotions such as fear and sadness (Davidson et al 1990). This has implications for coping. It suggests that positive emotions may be nurtured in upsetting and distressing circumstances, and may help people deal with frightening and threatening situations.

Chronic negative emotions may endanger health in two ways. First, people may be less concerned about the health risks of smoking, drinking and drug taking if they feel unhappy and worthless (see pp. 84–85; 78–79; 76–77). Second, negative emotions may affect the cardiovascular and immune systems directly (see pp. 104–105). For example, people who show chronically high levels of hostility towards others are more likely to suffer from coronary heart disease. People's personality influences their emotional experience. People high in agreeableness and low in neuroticism are more likely to form good relationships with others and experience fewer negative emotions, including anxiety and hostility.

When breaking bad news, the emotions of health-care professionals and the recipient affect what is heard and understood, and how the recipient responds (pp. 96–97). Emotions are also important in other consultations. A patient visiting their doctor may be worried because they think they have a serious illness. They may be embarrassed about their body or their lack of knowledge. They may feel humiliated if the doctor highlights their lack of understanding and may be intimidated by the doctor's powerful social position. They may also experience the doctor as friendly and leave the consultation feeling pleased by the resolution of a problem. Such feelings affect whether patients consult (pp. 88–89), what they say in consultations (see pp. 94–95) and whether or not they adhere to doctors' advice after consultations (see pp. 92–93).

How people think about or represent symptoms and diagnoses affects their emotional responses. This, in turn, affects how they cope and how well they recover or adapt (see pp. 132–133). A useful model for understanding how people react to threatening information is Leventhal's 'self regulation' or 'parallel processing' model (Leventhal 1971, Leventhal et al 1997). As Figure 2 shows, people may have different representations of the threat or danger and may also vary in their experience of emotion (e.g. fear). People may deal with their emotions (e.g. fear) independently of their thoughts about the threat (i.e. danger). If a patient perceives their illness or the information they have been given as very threatening, or their abilities to cope with it as very poor, they may focus on managing their emotion at the expense of managing the danger.

Emotion-focused coping strategies include avoiding thinking about the threat, denying its existence or distracting oneself by intense involvement in other activities that reduce fear in the short term. However, such coping responses may lead to behaviour detrimental to health, such as delays in seeking health care and non-adherence to recommended

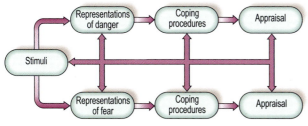

Fig. 2 **Leventhal's parallel processing model.** (Source: adapted with permission from Leventhal et al 1997)

treatment. This has important implications for the use of fear appeals in health-promotion campaigns (see pp. 74–75) (Ruiter et al 2001). To help people manage the danger as well as the emotion, it is important to introduce threatening information in a way that prevents people from being overwhelmed by emotion and to help them recognize and develop their coping strategies. Problem-focused coping strategies include problem solving, action planning, expressing emotion and seeking social support.

Patients' emotional response to threatening news is unpredictable. They may express their distress as anger, which may include anger against the 'messenger'. If this occurs, the clinician–patient relationship is vulnerable and must be preserved by patience and understanding. Clinicians should be prepared for such reactions and be

confident in their skills to manage them. If patients are upset, they are unlikely to understand or remember what is said to them or to follow advice given. It is, therefore, important to acknowledge and deal with the distress. Clinicians should ensure that they are not frightened of patients' distress and that they have the skills to listen, understand and respond appropriately. The clinician should be able to explore reasons for distress and to check that the patient would like to continue the discussion. If patients do not express distress, it should not be assumed that they are not feeling strong emotions. Sensitive questioning is required to elicit patients' thoughts and feelings (see pp. 130–131).

- Imagine you are told you need to be admitted to hospital for major surgery. List some of the emotions you might experience. Think about how you might respond to these emotional experiences. What kind of support would be helpful to you? How might your emotions be conveyed to staff on the ward? How might they respond to your emotion?

Case study

George is recovering from a myocardial infarction in hospital. He is feeling frightened and upset. A nurse notices this and talks to him. He begins to explain some of his worries and the nurse says 'Don't worry about those things now – you just relax and get well'. He talks to a doctor on the ward and the doctor says 'There's no need for you to be worried. You're on the mend and everything will be fine'. Although both clinicians want to cheer George up, they make him feel rejected and isolated because he has no-one to talk to about his feelings. This may affect his decision to enter into a rehabilitation programme and his recovery. A more helpful response from the clinicians would be to have acknowledged George's upset and allowed him to talk through the problems he is worried about and what he might do about them. This would have provided social support and encouraged problem solving.

Emotion

- Emotions involve physiological arousal and cognitive interpretation. They often involve fast responses to something that is either unexpected or highly positively or negatively valued.
- Facial expressions of some basic emotions are recognized across many cultures but cultures also have their own 'display rules'.
- People can experience positive emotion even when they are upset or stressed. This can be important to effective coping.
- Chronic negative emotion can damage physical and mental health.
- If people lack the capabilities to deal with issues prompting strong emotions they may seek to control their emotions rather than reality. This can lead to denial and other emotion-focused coping strategies.
- Emotional experience affects how we respond to other people. Thus emotional management of consultations is crucial to patients' responses to doctors and, thereby, to the effectiveness of consultations.

Remembering and forgetting

We are all familiar with lapses of memory – not being able to put a name to a face, forgetting to keep an appointment or poor recall during an exam. Psychologists have learned a great deal about the process of memory this century both through laboratory-based experiments and by studying patients with brain damage, which results in unique forms of memory loss. Although a very simplified view, the diagram outlined in Figure 1 is a useful summary of a widely held model of memory. Items are initially held in a short-term memory (STM) store and whether they become permanently represented in a long-term memory (LTM) store will depend on a host of factors, such as how important and interesting they are, and whether we engage in active rehearsal strategies to encode items into permanent memory.

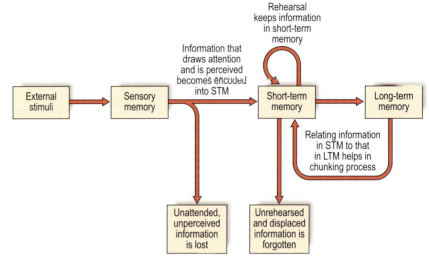

Fig. 1 **Memory: short-term and long-term storage.**

Stages of memory

If we listen to a list of unrelated words read out to us, and then are required to recall the words immediately, items presented either first or last are better remembered than those in the middle. This better recall for the more recent items is because we are retrieving them directly from the short-term memory store. If we were to delay recall of the word list by 30 seconds, then this recency effect disappears (Fig. 2).

Even items which do successfully enter into long-term memory may not be recalled when we need them, but are recalled much later. This illustrates the problem of *retrieval*.

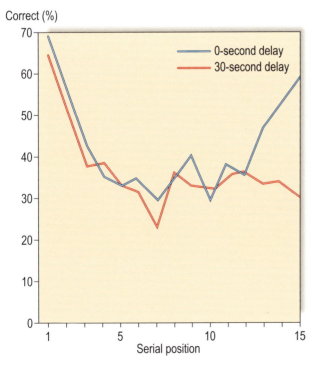

Fig. 2 **The recency effect and short-term storage.**

If a book is stored in a library and we lose the catalogue slip, then the book is very difficult to find. This problem of memory loss is clearly very different from being unable to locate the book because it was never stored correctly in the first place. A good practical illustration of this distinction is the difference between testing your knowledge about anatomy by *recall* (describe the structure of the brain) and *recognition* (which of the following is part of the limbic system – medulla, amygdala, motor cortex?). Multiple choice exam questions have already carried out the retrieval part of remembering, leaving only the recognition component to be necessary.

When we consider the problems of forgetting and the poor memory of head-injured and elderly patients, and we are trying to devise methods to aid recall, we need to have clear ideas about the stage at which the process is disturbed. Is it the initial learning that is defective or do those with poor memories simply forget more quickly?

How much can we remember?

Realizing that we have seen a film previously, but only about 10 minutes before its end, or revisiting a childhood home and having a flood of forgotten memories are powerful experiences that may tempt us into thinking that we do indeed store all events, and, given the right conditions, could retrieve such memories. Although there are well-documented cases of people with exceptional memories (one fascinating account is provided by the Russian neuropsychologist Luria), there is no scientific evidence to support this 'videotape' view of memory. To acquire permanent representation in memory we need to organize the new material and establish connections with the existing LTM store. Hence the use of mnemonic techniques that rely on devices such as learning a list of items in relation to an easily remembered rhyme, or first-letter mnemonics such as Richard Of York Gave Battles In Vain for the colours of the visible spectrum. Memory 'tricks' like this should not be scoffed at and have proved useful in helping elderly patients remember people's names.

- Can you recall the moment you first encountered a younger sibling? Your first day at school? Why are such memories more enduring?
- What were you doing on March 15th last year?

Helping patients to remember better

When patients have been asked to recall what they have been told during a consultation, they have been found to forget almost half (see pp. 92–93). Memory for medical advice as opposed to diagnostic information can be particularly poor, especially in the case of highly anxious or elderly patients. Statements made early in the consultation are more likely to enter LTM (the primacy effect) and those at the end are remembered better initially but then tend to be forgotten (the recency effect). General or abstract statements are more difficult to remember than more specific concrete suggestions. Researchers have concluded that patient recall is aided by following some simple rules:

- Give the most important information early in any set of instructions.
- Stress importance of relevant items (e.g. by repetition).
- Use explicit categorization under simple headings (e.g. 'I will tell you what is wrong . . . what treatment you will need . . . what you can do to help yourself').
- Make advice specific, detailed and concrete rather than general and abstract.

Memory after traumatic brain injury

Memory problems often follow accidental trauma from a closed head injury. In their most dramatic form, the patient

---

Case study

HM is an engineering worker who in 1953, in his late twenties, was operated upon in an experimental procedure intended to relieve his incapacitating and worsening epileptic seizures. The operation involved a radical bilateral medial temporal lobe resection, destroying the anterior two-thirds of the hippocampus, as well as the uncus and amygdala. It was successful in alleviating the epileptic symptoms, but left HM with a profound memory impairment. Although he can remember events he experienced and facts he acquired up to 2 years before his operation, he can remember essentially nothing that has occurred since. He recalls nothing of day-to-day events in his own life or the world at large. He does not know what he had for lunch an hour ago, how he came to be where he is now, where he has left objects used recently, or that he has used them. He reads the same magazines over and over again. He has learned neither the names of doctors and psychologists who have worked with him for decades nor the route to the house he moved to a few years after his surgery. Yet despite such difficulties he is not intellectually impaired. His language comprehension and production and conversational skills are normal; he can reason competently and do mental arithmetic. His IQ measured in 1962 was an above-average 117 – higher than the 104 measured pre-surgery in 1953. This neurological dissociation supports the idea that the temporary retention of information in working memory and the permanent storage of new information depend on different brain mechanisms (for a more lengthy account of HM's problems see Hilts 1995).

---

may be unable to recall not only the events leading up to the accident, but for many years prior to that. This memory loss extending backwards in time is known as retrograde amnesia, as distinct from the inability to form new memories, which is known as anterograde amnesia. Such a patient may well report themselves as 10 years younger than they are, and be unable to recall all the events of those 10 years, such as marriage, birth of children, employment, etc. At the same time, they will repeatedly need to be told why they are in hospital, and the names of the nurses and doctors caring for them. Eventually these years of memory loss will be recovered, indicating that the problem was difficulty of retrieval, but they may be left with enduring deficits of memory which may be secondary to attentional or concentration difficulties. The exact nature of the deficit will require extensive testing by a neuropsychologist. (A collection of essays dealing with the effects of brain damage can be found in Sacks 1986.)

- How would you set about establishing the extent of retrograde amnesia in a patient for whom you have no autobiographical information?

Organic amnesia

Permanent memory loss is a very serious problem necessitating continuous care of such patients. These instances of organic amnesia may be due to long-term alcohol abuse and development of Korsakoff's syndrome, to the brain damage from viral encephalitis, or to other surgical interventions. In all such cases where the memory loss is primary and not secondary to other cognitive deficits, patients are likely to have suffered damage to components of the limbic system, with the hippocampus being a key structure. One such case has been very widely reported in the scientific literature (see Case study).

Remembering and forgetting

- The distinction is clear between registration, retrieval, recall, and recognition processes in memory.
- Different kinds of memory mechanisms underlie STM and LTM, as shown by the serial position effect and the nature of the amnesic syndrome in brain-damaged patients.
- Improving memory recall by means of mnemonic aids is especially useful for unconnected items and events.

How does sexuality develop?

Sexual identity and behaviour are fundamental in the development of the person and the relevant influences are diverse and complex. The nature of sexuality is such that it has an important effect on health and well-being, and is, in turn, strongly influenced by these factors.

Gender identity

Biological influences

Gender identity (whether you feel male or female) usually coincides with sexual identity indicated by chromosomes, hormones, and sexual organs, but this is not always the case. Biological indices can occasionally be abnormal so that gender may be ambiguous or contradictory.

The sex chromosomes determined at conception, and the subsequent hormonal activity in the fetus, set the pattern for development of the internal and external sex organs, and the sexual differentiation of the brain. There are exceptions. For example, abnormal chromosomes may give rise to a definite gender identity, but altered sexual organs and atypical social and sexual behaviour, or a fetus with normal chromosomes may be exposed to unusual levels of hormones in utero. Some mothers given progestogens to prevent abortion had daughters who developed genital abnormalities, and atypical sexual and social behaviour.

Cultural factors

During puberty, gender identity becomes linked to sexual activity. There is often a period of sexual experimentation before individuals feel confident of their orientation. In the development of homosexual orientation, there is some evidence for a genetic factor: monozygotic twins show higher concordance than dizygotic twins, but cultural factors and individual learning experiences will also determine attraction to a partner.

Social and cultural influences

Psychological influences on gender start at birth with the family, where interactions are determined by the perceived sex of the baby (Fig. 1). This process quickly extends to peers, school and the media. It is thought that a core gender identity is fixed by about the age of 4 years.

Cultural pressures may delay the acceptance of sexual identity, since in many societies variations from the norm are not accepted. It many take a long period of adjustment and considerable courage to 'come out', accepting one's own

sexuality and letting others know. Fear of one's sexuality being discovered may lead to secretive or reclusive life styles, and can be the source of enormous distress.

The development of sexual activity

Although some sexual behaviour (genital play and stimulation) is seen in infants, the level of activity rises before puberty and this takes the form of sexual play with other children or solitary genital stimulation (masturbation). Peers are the major source of knowledge about sexual behaviour.

The age at which sexual intercourse first takes place varies not only from culture to culture, but across time and according to class. The average age of first intercourse has fallen in the last 40 years in the UK from 21 to 17 (Table 1). In the 1960s, surveys in Europe showed that sexual activity including intercourse took place at an earlier age in working-class males and females than amongst the middle classes. By the 1970s, the differences were disappearing.

An increasing proportion of young people have sexual intercourse aged less than 16 years (Wight et al 2000) and studies have found that sexual intercourse before the age of 16 is often regretted.

The most common pattern of long-term sexual partnership is heterosexual monogamy. Although in many societies polygamy is part of religious and cultural structures, in practice many men do not take more than one wife at a time,

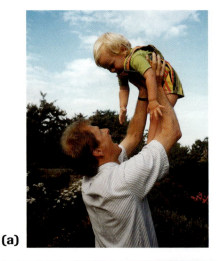

(a)

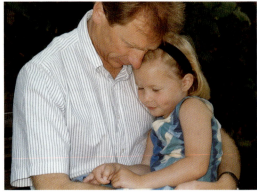

(b)

Fig. 1 **Parents play with their offspring in different ways according to the child's gender**. More 'rough and tumble' games with boys (**a**); more talking and cuddling with girls (**b**). This difference can be seen from birth.

> **STOP THINK**
> ■ Transvestism (most commonly males dressing in female clothing) has always taken place in many societies, either as entertainment for others or in secret. Many cross-dressers have no wish to change their sexual identity, but get pleasure from cross-dressing. Sexual excitement is sometimes involved, but cross-dressing is also done in private to comfort the individual and to relieve stress. What does this say about society's sex-role stereotypes and expectations of men?

Table 1 **Age at first sexual intercourse by age at interview**

Age at interview	Women		Men	
	Median age at first intercourse	% (No.) reporting first intercourse before age 16	Median age at first intercourse	% (No.) reporting first intercourse before age 16
16–19	17	18.7 (182/971)	17	27.6 (228/827)
20–24	17	14.7 (184/251)	17	23.8 (271/1137)
25–29	18	10.0 (152/1519)	17	23.8 (268/1126)
30–34	18	8.6 (116/1349)	17	23.2 (235/1012)
35–39	18	5.8 (73/1261)	18	18.4 (181/982)
40–44	19	4.3 (55/1277)	18	14.5 (150/1042)
45–49	20	3.4 (37/1071)	18	13.9 (115/827)
50–54	20	1.4 (13/933)	18	8.9 (61/684)
55–59	21	0.8 (6/716)	20	5.8 (35/603)

Analysis was based on weighted data

(Source: Wellings et al. BMJ 311: 417–420, 1995)

through lack of either availability or resources. Worldwide, the pattern of human attachment is often serial monogamy (one partner after another) rather than lifelong monogamy. The high rates of divorce in the industrialized world are one example of this.

Sexual activity continues through adulthood into old age (see pp. 14–15). While the sexual behaviour of young adults and those in middle age are discussed (see pp. 28–29), and form the subject of films and plays, the needs of older people are seldom portrayed. Sexual interest continues in this age group, although functioning changes: for example, in postmenopausal women, reduced oestrogen may cause thinning and dryness in the vagina, making intercourse more painful. In men, ageing is associated with increased time to achieve an erection, longer refractory periods and increased need for tactile rather than psychic stimuli. For men these changes are most marked after the age of 70 or so. It may be difficult for older people to discuss sexual problems with a doctor because their interest in sex is sometimes seen as inappropriate.

Sexual problems

Sexual difficulties can arise through problems in functioning (e.g. erectile difficulties in the male, or failure to achieve orgasm in the female);

incompatibility (differences in appetite or style of sexual activity); problems of fertility (inability to conceive, or fear of conception); psychosocial problems arising through sexual behaviour (e.g. problems of sexual identity or problems with the law); and sexually transmitted infections (see HIV, pp. 106–107). A number of medical conditions give rise to sexual problems. Most common among these are multiple sclerosis, cardiovascular disease, diabetes, epilepsy and renal disease. A person who is dependent on alcohol is also likely to experience sexual problems, and there are prescribed drugs that carry loss of interest, or problems in functioning, as unwanted secondary effects. For example, drugs given to reduce blood pressure may cause erectile and ejaculatory difficulties in men. Psychological factors, especially anxiety and depression, frequently affect sexual interest and performance (see pp. 110–113).

Sexual problems arising from conditions treatment may be overlooked by doctors through their own embarrassment or that of their patients. Yet many sexual problems can be effectively treated by a combination of approaches: medical intervention (e.g. changing a drug (e.g. viagra), the use of hormones), surgical interventions (e.g. vascular surgery), or counselling (see pp. 130–133).

Case study

A 29-year-old woman came to see her general practitioner (GP) because of infertility. Karen stopped the contraceptive pill 2 years ago but had not conceived. She was well, and reported no relationship difficulties. Her 34-year-old husband, Chris, was a marketing manager on a short-term contract.

Before referral to the infertility clinic, the GP wanted more information and asked to see each partner separately. Both said that the frequency of sexual intercourse was low. Karen assumed that this was due to her husband's tiredness through overwork and did not want to put extra pressure on him. Chris acknowledged that he was very anxious about work, had resumed heavier drinking again with a recurrence of gastritis, and was experiencing erectile difficulties. Afraid of impotence, he did not initiate sex, but wished that Karen would do so sometimes. He was too embarrassed to say this to her.

Instead of referral for infertility, they went to a sexual problems clinic for five sessions. There was a ban on intercourse at first to take the pressure off both partners. With the therapist as intermediary, they began to communicate honestly about their own worries and expectations of sex. Chris was given advice on anxiety management and targets for reduced drinking. In their homework non-threatening goals were set for increasing sexual activity, which included Karen taking the initiative sometimes. By the fourth session, Chris was drinking less, and the frequency of intercourse had increased to two or three times per week. Karen conceived 7 months later.

How does sexuality develop?

- Sexual development is influenced by biological, social and cultural factors.
- Difficulties can arise in sexual function, compatibility, fertility, psycho-social function, or as a result of sexually transmitted disease.
- Medical and psychological disorders can interfere with sexual function.
- Sexual problems can be effectively treated by medical or surgical interventions, or by counselling, (e.g. behavioural psychotherapy).

Intelligence

What is 'intelligence'?

Intelligence has been described as the ability to: learn from everyday experience; think rationally; solve problems; act purposively and engage in abstract reasoning. However, a precise definition of intelligence that relates directly to the measurement of mental ability and to everyday skills has been difficult to achieve. Some psychologists focused on 'general intelligence' to refer to a hypothetical common ability while others have distinguished between different types of intelligence. Assumptions about intelligence may affect how we treat others and, for a very small minority of people, their intelligence limits their capacity for self-care.

'Intelligence' is a value-laden term. No one wants to be categorized as unintelligent and stereotyping patients or students as 'intelligent' or 'unintelligent' has consequences for how they are treated. When someone is perceived to be unintelligent people may think it is not worth explaining things to them, resulting in communication breakdown, loss of confidence and uninformed decision making. This can be especially problematic when we want to encourage self-management and adherence amongst patients (see pp 92–93).

What do intelligence tests measure?

Intelligence tests are a type of aptitude test, that is, they are designed to assess how well a person will be able to learn or acquire skills in the future. All aptitude tests depend, to some extent, on prior experience and learning. Intelligence tests have been designed to identify individual differences in general reasoning abilities while other aptitude tests, such as tests of musical ability, focus on particular abilities.

Psychologists have distinguished between 'crystallized' and 'fluid' intelligence. Crystallized intelligence is based on skills and knowledge learnt within particular cultures. Fluid intelligence is the capacity to reason and solve problems. Fluid intelligence enables us to learn from experience, and experience enables us to use fluid intelligence more effectively. Tests that measure abstraction and generalization primarily assess fluid intelligence. For example, the Raven Progressive Matricies Test involves a series of pattern matching problems. Carpenter et al (1990) examined the reasoning required by this test. They concluded that the test measures the ability to infer abstract relationships and patterns from data and assesses the capacity to decompose problems into sub-tasks and hold multiple sub-tasks in mind simultaneously.

Tests that assess vocabulary, general knowledge and scholastic attainment provide information about crystallized intelligence. For example, the Wechsler Adult Intelligence Scale (WAIS) has 11 sub-scales. Six of these combine to generate a 'verbal intelligence' score: (i) information; (ii) comprehension; (iii) arithmetic; (iv) similarities; (v) digit span and (vi) vocabulary. The other five allow calculation of a 'performance' score: (a) digit symbol; (b) picture completion; (c) block design; (d) picture arrangement and (e) object assembly sub-scales generate. Items in this test draw on culture-specific learning, assessing crystallized as well as fluid intelligence. For example, 'What is the capital of Spain?' (comprehension) and 'How are a comb and a brush alike?' (similarities). A children's version

of the test (the Wechsler Intelligence Scale for Children, WISC) is used to assess performance and progress at school.

Intelligence tests are often scored so that the average (or mean) score is 100 and the standard deviation is 15. This means that 68% of the population have scores, or intelligence quotients (IQs), between 85 and 115 and 95% score between 70 and 130. A score of 148 is required to become a member of MENSA, a society that only admits those with exceptionally high IQs, and people scoring less than 70 (2 standard deviations below the mean) may have learning disabilities and need special help in school and with everyday living.

Scores on intelligence tests tend to be stable. Successive test scores correlate highly and children's scores, e.g. at age 6, predict adult scores, e.g. at 18, (r = 0.8), although an individual's score may change over time. Children's scores also predict performance at school and the number of years they stay at school (r = 0.5–0.55). However, other determinants are also important. IQ scores can predict various measures of job performance such as supervisor ratings and samples of job performance but other characteristics such as interpersonal skills, particular knowledge and aspects of personality are probably of equal or greater importance to job performance. Task-specific assessment is usually required to make accurate predictions about how someone will perform on job-related tasks or aspects of everyday living.

Some psychologists have suggested that IQ tests provide inadequate assessments of differences between people's intelligence. Guildford (1967) mapped out 120 separate mental abilities and Gardner (2001) has suggested that as well as verbal, logical/mathematical and spatial intelligence (which are measured in tests like the WAIS), we should also consider musical, body-kinetic, interpersonal and intrapersonal intelligence.

Is intelligence genetically determined?

Performance on intelligence tests is affected by many factors. Those with closer genetic relationships tend to have more similar scores. The correlation between the IQ scores of monozygotic (MZ) twins brought up in the same family is 0.9 while the correlation for MZ reared apart is 0.7–0.8. By contrast, the correlation between genetically unrelated children reared together in adoptive families ranges from 0.0–0.2. This does not mean that performance on intelligence

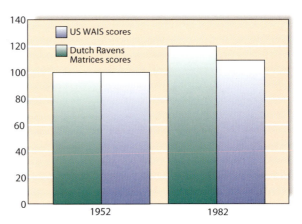

Fig. 1 **The Flynn effect**

tests cannot be changed. One of the mechanisms by which genetic make-up affects performance is through the selection of environments that enhance particular skills. By manipulating the environment and learning experiences we can change performance, including intelligence test performance (Neisser et al 1996).

Group differences on intelligence scores

Most intelligence tests have been standardized for sex, that is, items producing different scores for men and women have been eliminated. Consequently, it is unsurprising, that, in general, men and women tend to have equal intelligence scores. Differences have been found between other groups such as black and white Americans, with the white mean being about 10 points higher. A range of explanations have been proposed for this difference. Most controversially, it has been suggested that there may be differences in the black and white gene pools that confer a different range of intellectual abilities. This explanation is problematic if other factors affecting performance are unequal between the two groups. By analogy, imagine two plants with the same genetic make-up planted in soil that is either rich or poor in nutrients. The plants will grow to different heights even thought height is genetically determined. If the environment relevant to intelligence test performance differs, on average, for black and white Americans then group performance might differ, even if the two populations share the same intelligence-relevant genes. A larger proportion of black Americans live in poverty which is associated with poor nutrition, less adequate parenting and a lack of intellectual resources and stimulation during development. In addition, only one generation ago, black Americans did not have equal civil rights (in relation to voting, schooling etc.) and continue to suffer discrimination (Neisser et al 1996). Can we assume that the environment (analogous to the soil) is the same for both black and white Americans?

Another explanation for group differences is that intelligence tests are based on a particular cultural background so that people brought up in a different culture are disadvantaged (see Box).

Health and intelligence

In 1997 Whalley and Deary (2001) traced more than 2000 children born in Aberdeen in 1921. Mental ability scores based on childhood tests converted into IQ scores were found to be positively related to survival to age 76 years in both women and men. Overcrowding in the person's school catchment area, estimated from the 1931 UK census, was weakly related to death. Such data suggests that intelligence scores are related to mortality. However, intelligence scores and socioeconomic status (SES) are also correlated. For example, the correlation between one's parents' SES and one's own IQ is about 0.33. Mortality and morbidity rates are inversely related to SES.

A number of environmental factors can affect intelligence and health. For example, malnutrition, exposure to lead and ante-natal exposure to alcohol are all associated with lower IQ scores. Associations between lower IQ and ante-natal exposure to aspirin and antibiotics have also been reported (Zigler and Valentine 1979).

Are we getting more intelligent?

Yes! This is known as the Flynn (1987) effect. Average scores on intelligence tests have increased over time.

> **Box 1** **Black intelligence test of cultural homogeneity**
>
> Williams (1973) suggested that questions such as the following might provide a more culture-fair test of vocabulary for black American children than those included in the WISC.
> 1. 'Nose opened' means (a) flirting (b) teed off (c) deeply in love (d) very angry.
> 2. 'Blood' means (a) a vampire (b) a dependent individual (c) an injured person (d) a brother of colour.
>
> The answers are 1. (c) and 2. (d).

Interestingly, the largest gains are on tests focusing on fluid intelligence. For example, Raven's Matrices IQ scores in The Netherlands increased by 21 points between 1952 and 1982. This implies that if we transported a person with an average IQ today back in time by 70 years they would be regarded as exceptionally intelligent (e.g. scoring up to 149). By comparison, US WAIS scores, which reflect crystallized as well as fluid intelligence, have risen by about 3 points per decade (see Fig. 1). Similar effects have been observed in other countries. This may be due to better schooling and in a more visually sophisticated and information-rich culture; they might also be related to improved nutrition. Alternatively, as Flynn (1987) suggests, these gains may mean that intelligence tests only measure a particular type of problem-solving ability that may not have important implications for cultural development and achievement.

Does intelligence decline with age?

No. It appears that as we get older we also get wiser. On many tests of intelligence, especially those of crystallized intelligence, IQ increases with age, peaking around the mid 50s. Older people, including those in their 80s, can draw upon knowledge built up over their lives. Younger people may outperform older people on tests focusing on fluid intelligence, especially when these are timed tests. The best predictor of an older person's IQ score is likely to be their IQ score when they were younger.

Can we boost intelligence?

During Project Head Start, a series of pre-school schemes run in the USA in the 1960s, children were provided with extra teaching and play opportunities designed to enhance the intellectual content of their environment. Participating children in such schemes had higher intelligence test scores than similar children not involved. However, once the schemes ended, these differences tend to fade and disappear by age 11–12. However, children taking part were less likely to be assigned to special education, less likely to be held back in school and less likely to leave school than matched children who did not have extra pre-school input (Neisser et al 1996).

> ## Intelligence
> - Intelligence can be defined as the ability to learn from everyday experience and to think rationally.
> - Psychologists distinguish between fluid and crystallized intelligence.
> - 68% of the population have IQs between 85 and 115.
> - People with closer genetic relationships tend to have similar IQs.
> - Average group differences in IQ are not helpful in predicting an individual's intelligence.
> - IQ is associated with mortality, but both are associated with SES.
> - Average scores on intelligence tests have increased over time (the Flynn effect).
> - Older people do better than younger people on tests of intelligence that draw on their experience.

Development of thinking

Do children simply know less than adults or do children and adults think in qualitatively different ways? For example, are children just as capable as adults of understanding why they are ill or why they should take their medication, if they are presented with the relevant information? Or do children under a certain age lack the necessary concepts to make sense of such explanations? Questions like these are addressed by psychological research into cognitive development, which investigates age-related changes in intellectual abilities.

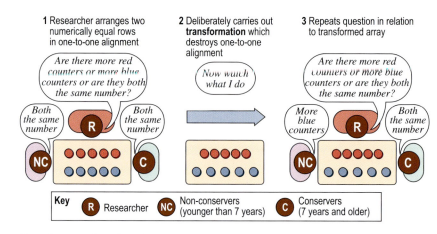

Fig. 1 **Conservation of number task.**

Differing views of cognitive development

Jean Piaget (1896–1980) revolutionized the study of cognitive development by arguing that young children do not just know less than older children and adults, but that they view the world in radically different ways. For example, Piaget argued that until the age of about 7 years, children are not able to reason logically and lack fundamental concepts in such areas as number and causality.

Most researchers agree with Piaget's general claims that:

- Cognitive development is influenced by an interaction between biological and environmental factors.
- Children play an active role in acquiring knowledge.
- Children's thinking is sometimes qualitatively different from adults'.

On the other hand, many researchers (e.g. Donaldson 1978) have challenged certain aspects of Piaget's views and have argued that he has tended to underestimate:

- young children's conceptual understanding
- the influence of contextual factors
- the extent to which children's performance depends on their familiarity with the specific content of reasoning tasks.

To illustrate these differing views, we will consider two aspects of cognitive development: understanding of number and of causality.

Understanding of number

To investigate children's ability to reason about numerical relationships, Piaget used tasks like the one in Figure 1. He found that children younger than about 7 years typically changed their answer when the question was repeated after the transformation, and he described these children as 'non-conservers'. In contrast, children of about 7 years and upwards typically succeeded on the task and were therefore classed as 'conservers'. Piaget interpreted young children's failure to conserve as being symptomatic of their inability to reason logically: they lack an understanding of general principles, such as that the number of objects in a set is independent of their spatial arrangement.

However, other researchers have found that young children's performance on conservation tasks can be improved by modifying the way the task is presented. For example, when the transformation was carried out by a 'naughty teddy' character who likes to 'mess up games', many more 4- to 6-year-old children responded correctly than when the transformation was carried out deliberately by the researcher (Donaldson 1978). In interpreting this finding, Donaldson argues that the deliberate nature of the transformation in Piaget's version of the task misleads children into inferring that it is relevant to the question which follows it, and thus into misinterpreting the question as referring to length. This type of reasoning is characteristic of what Donaldson terms *embedded* thinking, in which the child actively attempts to make sense of the total situation by attending to non-verbal cues as well as to what is said and by making inferences about other people's intentions. Young children, according to Donaldson, are capable of reasoning logically, but they are most likely to demonstrate this in contexts where they can exploit their understanding of human purposes and where non-verbal cues support the spoken message.

Understanding of causality

With respect to children's understanding of causality (see Donaldson and Elliot 1990), Piaget argued that until the age of about 7 years children show:

- an inability to distinguish between causes and effects
- a tendency to 'psychologize' by inappropriately explaining physical phenomena in terms of human motives.

For example, when they were asked to complete sentences, they tended to reverse the order of the cause and effect, as in: *That man fell off his bicycle because . . . he broke his leg.* Also, when Piaget interviewed children about the causes of various phenomena, they gave explanations which were not simply incorrect but were of the wrong type, in that they tended to explain physical phenomena in psychological terms, for example: *Why do the clouds move across the sky? . . . Because they want to.*

However, the phenomena which Piaget asked children to explain were ones for which information about causal mechanisms was not directly accessible to them, so it may be that they psychologized as a last resort. Several studies have shown that when children are presented with demonstrations of physical phenomena involving familiar principles (e.g. that an object will fall if a supporting object is removed), even 3-year-olds tend to give explanations in terms of physical causes. Similarly, when they are explaining events with which they are directly involved, children as young as 3 years show an ability to distinguish appropriately between causes and effects. Thus, it appears that young children do have a basic understanding of causality, but that their ability to apply their understanding depends on the context and on their knowledge of specific causal phenomena.

Understanding of illness

How do these findings and arguments relate to children's understanding of illness? Some researchers have argued that children's developing understanding of illness is consistent with Piaget's account of the development of causal reasoning (see Table 1). It is important to be aware of the types of explanations of illness that are typically given by children at particular stages of development, since this can be helpful in alleviating misunderstandings and anxieties. For example, young children who believe that all illnesses are caught through contagion or contamination may be anxious about coming into contact with children with non-infectious illnesses, such as epilepsy or leukaemia.

On the other hand, the typical stages in understanding the causes of illness may not represent the limits of children's ability to understand explanations of illness.

Table 1 Developmental changes in understanding of causes of illness	
Approximate age	**Explanations of illness**
4–7 years	Contagion: illness caused by proximity to ill people or to particular objects Illness viewed as punishment for own misbehaviour
7–11 years	Contamination: illness caused by physical contact with ill person Illness caused by germs
Over 11 years	Internalization: processes (e.g. swallowing, inhaling) through which external causes influence internal bodily processes Psychological factors can influence physiological processes Multiple, interacting causes

Based on studies: Bibace and Walsh 1980; Kister and Patterson 1980

Since most young children do not receive much tuition about the causes of illness, it may well be that the typical stages merely reflect what they have had the opportunity to learn. For example, most childhood illnesses are infectious so it is perhaps hardly surprising that young children tend to overgeneralize the concepts of contagion and contamination.

The case study suggests that children's understanding of medical phenomena may sometimes be influenced by their personal experience. However, other research has indicated that the extent of children's medical experience (duration of illness, frequency of hospitalization) does not affect their understanding of the causes of illness (Kury and Rodrigue 1995). Therefore, in order to communicate effectively with children about health and illness, health-care professionals need to be careful neither to overestimate the knowledge of children with prior medical experience, nor to underestimate the extent to which children's understanding could potentially be enhanced by presenting explanations geared to their individual cognitive levels. (For further discussion of clinical applications see Rushforth 1999.)

STOP THINK

■ What would you do/say to help a 4-year-old child who was worried about catching appendicitis from the child in the next bed?

Development of thinking

■ Young children do not simply know less than older children and adults: they sometimes think in qualitatively different ways.

■ Piaget's view that these differences reflect an inability in children younger than 7 years to reason logically and to understand fundamental concepts (such as those of number and causality) has been challenged.

■ Young children's cognitive abilities depend not only on their underlying concepts but also on the context in which tasks are presented.

■ Children are most likely to understand explanations which:
  – take account of their existing level of understanding
  – are linked to their own experiences and immediate concerns
  – are presented with appropriate non-verbal contextual support.

Case study

Children's understanding of their blood

When a 3-year-old girl with leukaemia joined a playgroup, the staff were concerned about how to explain her illness to the other children, and a group of researchers decided to investigate this topic (Eiser et al 1993). They interviewed healthy 3- and 4-year-old children about their knowledge and experiences of blood, and then gave the children an explanation of the functions of different types of blood cells, illustrating their explanation with drawings. Although on the whole the children had difficulty understanding the explanation, the children who showed most understanding were those who had mentioned a personal experience involving blood.

The researchers also interviewed the 3-year-old girl with leukaemia. In the course of her treatment, she had received more extensive and more frequently repeated explanations about blood than the healthy children had, and these explanations obviously had clear personal relevance to her. Her knowledge of the structure and function of blood was found to be much more advanced than that of the healthy children: 'she knew that blood . . . is full of red cells which make new blood, white cells which fight infection, and platelets which stop bleeding. 'Sometimes the platelets don't come and then you keep bleeding.' About the leukaemia, she said that she was 'full of bad cells – they just come'. (Eiser et al 1993, p. 535).

Although this explanation includes some misunderstandings and some of the phrases may be simple repetitions of adults' speech without full understanding, and although we do not know how typical the explanation is of other 3-year-olds who are receiving treatment, it is nevertheless extremely impressive for such a young child and it suggests that young children's ability to understand explanations of illness may be much greater than has often been supposed.

Understanding groups

The effectiveness of medical staff depends on team work. No doctor works completely alone. So, if doctors are going to be effective they need to know how best to work with and in groups. Groups can also have negative effects, which can be controlled, if understood, and groups influence our social and personal identity. Becoming medical students, and eventually joining the medical profession, results in more changes in people than just occupational category: they become different people, with different identification, interests and loyalties.

What are groups?

Groups are essential and pervasive. Each of us belongs to many groups of different kinds. It has been estimated that we each have membership of about 100 groups, ranging from our family, our nationality, or our professional group, to the gang of personal friends. A group can be defined as consisting of three or more people who interact with each other, have shared goals and relationships, have mutually agreed ways of doing things, and a shared identity.

Features of groups
Conformity

In groups we all tend to be conformists. Most people will usually conform to group opinion, despite having private reservations. Conformity is sometimes seen as negative: for example, it can be as a result of real or imagined pressures. A conformist might also be defined as a person who has managed to avoid being defined as a deviant. Yet conformity can be important and valuable. To an extent we all conform when we learn professional skills. We do as others do when we learn to become a competent professional, but there may be negative influences, as for example when we fail to challenge an incorrect but popular opinion.

There are three underlying dynamics of conformity:

- normative pressures (be like others to get rewards or avoid punishment)
- informational pressures (group provides useful information)
- inter-group pressures (support group versus other groups).

These pressures are especially acute when we are being monitored or when it's not clear what's going on, like when we join a new group.

Obedience

Most people obey authority. In one well-known psychological experiment, carried out by Milgram (1963), subjects were asked by a respectable-looking experimenter to administer electric shocks to volunteers. The prediction was that 1/1000 would obey. However, in fact two-thirds did as requested. (The shocks were not in fact real!)

Factors which influence the likelihood of obedience are not only similar to those affecting conformity, but also include the perceived benefit of obeying the person in authority.

Many human systems depend upon obedience of authority, e.g. the armed services. To some extent hospital medicine relies on obedience to authority to ensure that there is a clear and appropriate understanding of responsibility for patients. If consultants are ultimately responsible for patient care, they must be able to trust that junior medical staff will carry out instructions. Automatic obedience, however, is not wise. Occasionally, senior staff make errors in their instructions, and young doctors need to think critically as they work, and be courageous enough to question a wrong decision.

Deviance

Groups do not easily tolerate people who do not conform. Dissenters are:

- normally unpopular, because they threaten the cohesiveness of the group and challenge its opinions
- likely to be rejected by the group because they are threatening and produce feelings of discomfort for others
- usually seen as particularly valuable by the group if won over
- need one another to survive the hurt of rejection by a group, possibly by setting up a new group of their own
- offer alternative and new solutions
- challenge the group to explore, elaborate and justify its position.

Structure

- Groups consisting of people who are very similar to each other are called homogenous groups. These groups often get on well together, and quickly establish working practice. However, they may be poor at innovating or dealing with difficult problems. Groups with many different types are known as heterogeneous. These often take time to settle down, and may experience conflict, but may be able to generate better solutions in the long run.
- Groups which function well have both social and 'task' aspects; that is, there is a social, interpersonal aspect to the group as well as its formal, stated objective or 'task'; a group which only completes tasks may seem efficient, but it engenders little loyalty and does not survive long (see Figure 1).

Inter-group conflict

Sometimes groups conflict with one another. Inter-group conflict is very common and occurs between rival football clubs, different schools, NHS professional groups, and nations. While competition may be healthy, if it escalates, conflict can lead to serious disputes, even war, and eventually genocide. This can happen when one group thinks itself so superior to another that total annihilation of the other group is legitimate. This stems from all the above features of groups.

- Consider groups in places where you have been, for example, in a tutorial or work group. Most groups or teams tend to show the above features, especially if the team has worked together for a long time. You may also have noticed that group members tend to do different things to keep the team functioning (Fig. 1). Also, different people tend to behave fairly consistently in one group, but may also behave differently in another group.

Which one are you? Have you noticed that your role changes depending on what group you are in? Why?

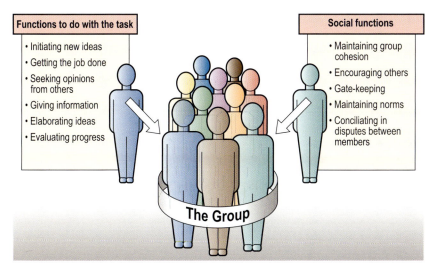

Fig. 1 **Typical roles in a group.**

'In-groups' and 'out-groups' are formed where the 'in-group' feels good about itself and simultaneously superior to, but persecuted by, the 'out-group'. Perhaps the 'out-group' consists of deviants who were rejected by the 'in-group' because they would not or could not conform. Alternatively they may have disobeyed the leader of the 'in-group', or be different in some way, for example, by racial origin or sex.

One notable feature of inter-group conflict is stereotyping, whereby members of the 'out-group' are lumped together and seen as bad, weak or aggressive, or as possessing admired but feared characteristics such as intelligence, cunning or sexuality. Individual differences between people are minimized: hence all white people are seen as mean, all women as petty, all football supporters as hooligans, and so on.

Group therapy

Therapy is often carried out in groups. Obviously if many people can be helped by one trained professional, instead of individual half-hour sessions, this has economic benefits. Membership of groups has also been shown to have psychological benefits. Support from other people may come from self-help groups (see pp. 138–139) but there may also be more formal groups set up in hospital or general practice.

Group therapies may take one of four basic approaches or a combination that may be pragmatically chosen on the basis of the composition of the group. The *analytical approach* might analyze motives for the group members' behaviour; an *interpersonal approach* might provide an opportunity for social learning where people can learn from each other how to cope with a particular condition; an *experiential approach* might generate emotional experiences, which it is hoped will resolve emotional difficulties; and a *didactic approach* might impart new information and teach new skills.

The evidence for the benefits of group therapy compared with individual therapy is positive. For example, membership of a group increases the chances of stopping smoking, and membership of cardiac rehabilitation provides social support, which increases the likelihood of adhering to a programme.

Case study

Inter-group conflict

The medical staff of a large inner-city general practice decided to establish an asthma clinic in order to respond to the increasing numbers of patients coming to the surgery for help. Part of the strategy of the clinic included the assessment of patients within their own home environments, which would be carried out by the community staff in the practice. The medical staff then announced the plan to the health visitors and district nurses, without consulting them about the feasibility of the assessment procedures. Some nurses tried to carry out the assessments as requested, while others declared the whole strategy to be unworkable given other time constraints. One of the nurses who was eager to implement the strategy was criticized heavily by the others, and soon afterwards gave in her notice. Some of the medical staff felt some sympathy for the nurses and suggested that the plan had been implemented too hastily, but they were accused by the others of being behind the times. Each group of staff considered the other group to be thoughtless, unprofessional, selfish and lazy. The atmosphere in the practice became unpleasant and hostile, so that even the patients began to notice it. Only the appointment of a practice manager, who agreed to review the whole issue, allowed the situation to calm down and return to normal again.

Understanding groups

- People take on a role when they join a group often without being aware of it.
- Groups encourage conformity and give us a sense of belonging.
- Groups may punish non-conformers by making them feel odd, unwanted and rejected.
- Groups can be a force for good, encouraging patriotism, team-work, loyalty and identity.
- Inter-group conflicts also underlie most forms of industrial dispute, religious and political rivalry, war and even genocide.

Concepts of health, illness and disease

Health and illness are concepts that relate to social and moral values as much as they relate to disease. Medicine is particularly concerned with identifying and treating diseases. This model of disease is called biomedicine, drawing as it does on medical sciences with an emphasis on biological abnormality. Biological abnormalities are not found for all diseases (e.g. some mental illness), and biomedicine is only one way of looking at the ill health that people experience. It is also important to understand how people feel when they are ill, and what their own interpretations of their symptoms are (Radley 1994). In this way, health care can be provided more sensitively, doctors can get a fuller picture of what ails their patients, and patients can be part of the process of identifying what is wrong with them and what can be done about it.

Health has also become an important concept in recent years, especially through an increasing emphasis on promoting well-being as well as preventing illness (Crawford 1987). However, health is not easy to define. Health, illness and disease mean different things to different people. We will consider the extent to which these concepts are as much social (that is to do with society) and personal as they are to do with biology.

Disease

Defining disease may at first seem to be quite straightforward. However, changes in medical knowledge may alter our understanding (e.g. many diseases are now thought to have a genetic component) and new symptoms and diseases may appear or be discovered (e.g. HIV/AIDS, chronic fatigue syndrome). Typically, in Western medicine, disease refers to pathological changes diagnosed by signs and symptoms: it is considered to be objective and defined by doctors. Yet, as the above examples show, definitions are not fixed but change over time in the light of new knowledge and experience. Homosexuality used to be defined as a disease but is now much more socially accepted as a lifestyle choice; alcoholism used to be seen as

immoral, but it is now often typified as a disease. Heart disease, while existing before the twentieth century, was seldom considered a specific cause of death until this century. We are increasingly able to define disease at earlier and earlier stages, or even identify risk factors for disease. This can lead to many more people being defined as diseased, even in the absence of any symptoms. So, it is possible to feel quite well but for disease to be present.

Armstrong (1994) has argued that normality plays a crucial role in how medicine defines disease. If the definition of normal relates to what is statistically normal, or an average measure, it is not always clear-cut where the normal becomes the abnormal or pathological. What is normal for one person may not be normal for another, or whole populations may display some kind of pathology which, while representing disease or risk of disease, is normal in some sense. Normality can also be seen as being socially rather than biologically defined. Here, normality is viewed more in terms of what is considered acceptable or desirable. Mental illness, for example, is very much rooted in culture, and what is considered abnormal behaviour varies across cultures. An extreme example would be the labelling of political dissidents as mentally ill, as occurred in the former Soviet Union. There are also concerns about possible overdiagnosis of mental illness amongst some ethnic minority groups, such as Afro-Caribbean men in the UK. Some disabled people challenge the medical definitions of their conditions and argue that it is society that disables them (see pp. 116–119). Disease, then, is not such a straightforward concept.

Biomedicine is only one way of understanding disease. Humoral theories, elaborated by Hippocrates, present disease as an imbalance between four humours. Echoes of such understandings are still present today, for example, in the promotion and use of cough expectorants and laxatives. Other systems of medicine, such as Indian Ayurvedic medicine or Chinese medicine, also stress the importance of balance. These are complex,

professionalized systems used in other cultures to explain disease (as well as health and illness) and organize health care. Patients and doctors may work within several systems of belief at any one time.

Illness

Illness is a subjective experience and as such will be defined and responded to differently by different people. How people interpret bodily experiences may have no direct relationship with the presence of a medically defined disease. People's own experience, as well as their wider knowledge, is drawn from their own culture (for example, their 'lay referral network' as well as wider values within their society) and from other sources of knowledge – the media, their doctors or other healers. People's own beliefs are important to understand as these may influence whether they seek health care, the type of health care they seek, and also their reasons for seeking professional advice (see pp. 86–87).

Importantly, illness can be thought of as a moral category, especially in a society that emphasizes personal responsibility for health (Crawford 1987). People like to think of themselves as healthy. Research, such as Cornwell's detailed study conducted in the East End of London (Cornwell 1984), has found that many people consider that having the right attitude is important in preventing illness and maintaining good health; this attitude means that you should not 'dwell on illness'. She found that people produced what she termed 'public accounts' when she first started interviewing residents in the area. Because of the moral imperative to be seen as healthy, people wanted to prove the legitimacy of illness by describing it as normal, real or a health problem that was not illness (Fig. 1).

As her study continued, she found that people became much more prepared to talk about a whole range of experiences that they felt had affected their health. Getting behind these 'public accounts', Cornwell found that people discussed their experience of illness as part of their everyday lives, affected by their social

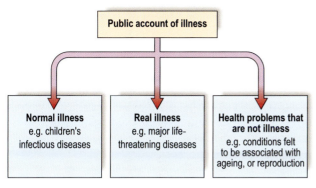

Fig. 1 **Public accounts of illness** (Cornwell 1984).

roles (work, domestic commitments) and their experience of health services. She called these 'private accounts'. Since doctors often only have a short time with their patients, it is important that they allow for the tendency of people to provide 'public accounts', and that they realize that patients' underlying concerns and worries may be much less clearly and openly expressed (see pp. 88–89).

Health

A negative view of health would define it as the absence of disease. However, the World Health Organization (1946) offers a more positive definition: a 'state of complete physical, social and mental well-being and not merely the absence of disease or infirmity'. The Health and Lifestyle Survey, conducted in England and Wales (Blaxter 1990), found this holistic view of health was often echoed in what people *themselves* said about being healthy. However, concepts of health differ across the life course. The survey found that younger men thought of health as physical fitness, while younger women emphasized energy and coping. In middle age the emphasis moved towards notions of mental and physical well-being, while older people stressed the ability to do things, as well as contentment and happiness (Fig. 2).

Large-scale surveys and other smaller, in-depth studies have found that people define themselves as healthy despite experiencing symptoms. A study of working-class women in the North East of Scotland (Blaxter and Paterson 1982) found that the grandmother generation (average age 51 years) had low expectations of what good health was – it was being able to carry on and being able to work, despite experiencing

disease and illness. In other words, they had quite functional definitions of health, and their norms of health were low.

Practical application

Within society and between cultures, there are varied concepts of health, illness and disease. All concepts are inherently social, and it is important to recognize this in practice. Doctors and patients may have different views about health, and patients may not reveal their subjective experiences in the belief that these are not important. However, if medicine is to deal seriously with the patient in the context of his or her family and social relationships, then listening to and understanding his or her perspective becomes a prerequisite for good practice.

STOP THINK
- What does being healthy mean to you? What do you think it may mean to someone who is 75 years old?
- What impact might defining something as a disease have on a patient?
- Why is it important to understand the patient's own beliefs?

Case study

Making sense of illness

People always try to make sense of misfortune and illness is no exception. Research conducted by Williams (1984) identified how the diagnosis and experience of chronic illness affected people's sense of identity. They then made sense of their own illness by considering its causes within the context of their own life experiences. This helped them answer the question 'why me?' In one case study presented by Williams, Gill considers her arthritis to have been caused by stress – something built up over the years as well as related to specific difficult life events:

. . . 'I'm quite certain that it was stress that precipitated this . . . not simply the stress of events that happened but the stress perhaps of suppressing myself while I was a mother and wife; not "women's libby" but there comes a time in your life when you think, you know, "where have I got to? There's nothing left of me".'

Concepts of health, illness and disease

- Health, illness and disease are social concepts.
- Health and illness are defined differently by different social groups.
- Someone can perceive themselves to be healthy yet at the same time experience illness and disease.
- People initially provide 'public' accounts of their experience and concepts of illness in contrast to more 'private' accounts as their trust in the interviewer/doctor grows.
- Medical science plays a crucial role in defining disease, but these definitions change over time.

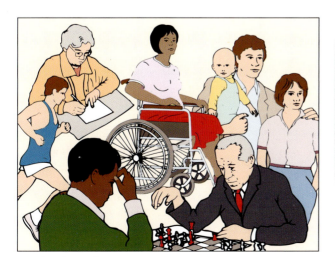

Fig. 2 **Health means different things to different people as it is not just the absence of disease**.

Measuring health and illness

The measurement of health and illness has become increasingly important as doctors, health-service agencies and governments have tried to assess the effectiveness of treatments and the performance of health services. However, measuring health and illness can be problematic.

Mortality

All births and deaths in developed (and in many developing countries) are legally required to be registered so that, together with census data, accurate counts can be made of birth and death rates, and of population change. Mortality rates, particularly infant and maternal mortality rates, are often used as proxy measures of a country's health and development (see pp. 40–41).

Life expectancy also provides a summary figure of health in an area or country and approximates to a measure of average length of life. Figure 1 summarizes overall life expectancy for selected countries. 'Years of life lost prematurely' is a recently developed concept that provides an indication of the potential of health promotion and effective treatment to reduce the number of people who die younger than the national average life-expectancy figure.

Crude death rates are calculated by dividing the total number of deaths by the number of people in the population. However, because older people and men are more likely to die over a given time-period than younger people and women, allowance is normally made for the age and sex of the population when making comparisons between areas. Age/sex-specific death rates show the proportion of deaths in a particular age group specifically for men and women.

Cause-specific death rates are also useful. Cause of death is entered on death certificates and then coded using the International Statistical Classification of Diseases and Health Related Problems (ICD). However, care in their interpretation is required because of different reporting procedures and fashions between countries and regions, and changes in medical knowledge and fashion over time can lead to 'apparent' differences. Coding errors can also occur.

Standardized mortality ratios (SMRs) are commonly used to compare death rates for specific sub-groups in a population. An SMR is the ratio of the number of observed deaths to the number of expected deaths (which would have occurred if the study population had experienced the same mortality as a reference population – allowing for age and sex differences). An SMR of 100 indicates that observed deaths equals the expected number of deaths (average mortality). An SMR >100 indicates that observed deaths exceed expected deaths, and an SMR <100 indicates that observed deaths are lower than expected deaths. For example, Figure 2 shows that in England in 1991–93 men aged 20–64 years in social class III non-manual had average 'all cause' death rates, whereas social class I and II men were about 30% below average, social class III manual and IV men were about 17% above average and

social class V men were 89% above the average for men in this age group (Drever et al 1996). SMRs are useful summary indicators of mortality in a sub-population or specific social group, and social scientists have used SMRs particularly to investigate social inequalities in health (see pp. 42–43).

At the hospital unit level, 'avoidable deaths analysis' has been developed to provide comparative data on individual doctor and unit performance, thereby providing a way of identifying poor standards of practice.

Morbidity

Whilst death is (generally) a certain and countable event, mortality rates do not tell us much about illness or health in a population. Illness, morbidity and health are, however, considerably more difficult to define, and hence to measure, than death.

Consultation rates with doctors are sometimes used as a proxy measure of illness in a population. Measured as the number of consultations over a defined time-period in a given population, consultation rates suffer from a number of limitations. In many countries it may be difficult to define and measure the denominator population from which the consulters came. Use of a doctor is strongly influenced by availability of doctors in a particular area and psychological, social and cultural factors strongly influence people's decision to consult a doctor (see pp. 86–87), and these may change over time.

Community morbidity rates are also calculated in the UK using survey data collected in general practice, including diagnosis/reason for consultation. Such data can reveal changing trends in the incidence and prevalence of different diseases/problems (see Box 1) but similar caveats to those outlined for consultation rates need to be borne in mind. Moreover, GPs vary considerably in their tendency to diagnose particular diseases.

Referral rates to hospital and hospital admission rates (by diagnostic groups) provide some information on patterns and trends in morbidity, but these too vary by referrer practice, supply of hospital services and admission and discharge practice.

Disease registers, which hold details of the identity of every person

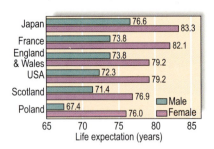

Fig. 1 **Life expectancy at birth (1993).**
(Source: WHO 1996 World Health Statistics Annual 1995. WHO, Geneva, Table B-3.)

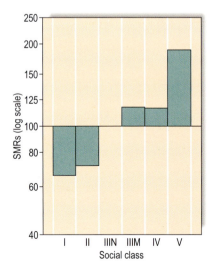

Fig. 2 **SMRs from all causes by social class (based on occupation) for men aged 20–64 years, England and Wales 1991–1993.**
(Source: Drever et al 1996)

diagnosed with a particular disease (e.g. cancer), its type and its treatment, provide excellent individual, longitudinal data for research, but they are expensive to set up and to maintain.

In the UK, the General Household Survey (GHS) is a national sample survey of households which, once a year, asks questions about chronic and acute illness. Whilst the GHS provides a regular picture of ill health, the sample size makes it difficult to examine differences in morbidity at regional or district level.

A large number of self-report instruments have been developed to measure the impact of specific diseases and illness on health (Bowling 1995a), most of which incorporate a variety of scales designed to assess the physical, psychological and social effects of the disease (see Case study).

A number of instruments have also been designed to measure health and well-being more generally (Bowling 1997). For example, the SF-36 has become a commonly used evaluative instrument – for example, to assess the effectiveness of secondary prevention clinics for coronary heart disease (Campbell et al 1998). The SF-36 has been shown to be reliable and valid (Box 2) and covers eight health 'domains':

- limitations in physical activities because of health problems
- limitations in social activities because of physical or emotional problems
- limitations in usual role activities because of physical health problems
- bodily pain
- general mental health (psychological distress and well-being)
- limitations in usual role activities because of emotional problems
- vitality (energy and fatigue)
- general health perceptions (see pp. 48–49).

Overall, it is important to be clear about the purpose for which measurement instruments have been designed and how this relates to their use. If using instruments in a new context or population it is important to make sure that they are valid and reliable. Care should also be taken not to

assume that these instruments measure health or ill health comprehensively – they are summary indicators. Finally, care should be taken when comparing the results of studies using different instruments.

Case study

Fitzpatrick (1994) has illustrated the problem of measuring changes in the health of people with rheumatoid arthritis. Four different instruments were used to measure the degree of change in dimensions of health.

Table 1 **Degree of change indicated by four different health-status instruments***

Dimension	Effect Size**	Dimension	Effect Size**
Mobility		*Mood/Emotions*	
AIMS	0.43	AIMS	0.83
HAQ	0.38	NHP	0.59
NHP	0.27	FLP	0.61
FLP	0.69		
Pain		*Social*	
AIMS	0.73	AIMS	0.06
HAQ	0.53	NHP	0.24
NHP	0.38	FLP	0.60

AIMS = Arthritis Impact Measurement Scales; HAQ = Health Assessment Questionnaire;

NHP = Nottingham Health Profile; FLP = Functional Limitations Profile

*From a sample of patients with rheumatoid arthritis considered to have improved over a 3-month period.

**Effect size = difference between mean score at time 1 and mean score at time 2, divided by standard deviation at time 1. Effect size of 0.20 or less considered small, 0.50 moderate, and 0.80 or higher, large.

(Adapted from Fitzpatrick R, 1994)

The NHP reveals little change in mobility, pain, or social well-being, whereas the FLP shows high change in mobility, mood, and social well-being. The AIMS reveal little change in social well-being, but considerable change in pain and mood. Which instrument is to be preferred?

STOP THINK Could one instrument measure the health of people being treated for:

- angina?
- depression?
- eczema?

Box 1 **Incidence and prevalence**

Incidence: the number of new cases of people diagnosed with a particular disease/problem over a particular time period, usually a year.

Prevalence: the number of people with a particular disease/problem in the population at a particular point in time.

One way of thinking about these terms is of a river flowing into a reservoir. The reservoir is the prevalence, the flow of the river into the reservoir the incidence.

Box 2 **Reliability and validity**

An instrument is **reliable** if it reproduces the same results if tested twice on the same population (test–retest reliability). The instrument should also be internally consistent and inter-rater reliable.

Validity relates to the extent to which an instrument actually measures what it sets out to measure. The main aspects of validity are:

- Face validity: the instrument appears to be appropriate and clear, and to give sensible results
- Content validity: the items in the instrument appear to be comprehensive and appropriate
- Criterion validity: the results derived from the instrument correlate well with results from a previously validated 'gold-standard' instrument
- Construct validity
  – convergent: the instrument (or items within it) correlates with similar related variables
  – discriminant: the instrument (or items within it) does not correlate with dissimilar variables

Measuring health and illness

- Infant and maternal mortality rates and life expectancy are useful indicators of a country's overall health and development.
- Mortality rates need to be adjusted for the age and sex of the population.
- Disease-specific mortality rates can reveal trends in specific disease, but tell us little about illness or morbidity in a population.
- Measurement of morbidity ranges from measures of health-service use to instruments measuring self-reported perceptions of illness and self-report measures of health, well-being and functional ability.
- Considerable care should be taken when using instruments for measuring health and when interpreting their results.

Changing patterns of health and illness

Births and deaths in Britain are recorded by the Registrar General. The data provided on birth and death certificates are compiled by the Office of Population Censuses and Surveys, which publishes annual reports showing the incidence of disease and deaths due to specific causes and a variety of statistics relating to use of hospital and outpatient services. These reports are public documents and can be consulted in libraries and on the web.

Changes in life expectancy

Over the last century there has been a marked decline in premature death throughout the developed world. In 1888, a new-born baby girl in England and Wales had an average life expectancy of just over 40 years. By 1930, this had risen to just over 60 years, and by 1999 it had reached 80 years (Fig. 1). However, if a child survived into middle age, life expectancy even in 1888 was quite high. A 45-year-old woman in 1888 could, on average, expect to live to nearly 70 years of age, and in 1999 she had an average life expectancy of over 80 years.

The major cause of increase in life expectancy is a dramatic fall in the death rate for infants during their first year of life. In 1888 in England and Wales, out of every 1000 infants under the age of 1 year 145 died. By 1930 this figure had been more than halved to 68 infant deaths and the rapid decline continued until the present-day rate of five to six infant deaths per 1000. At the beginning of the 21st century almost all new-born babies in the UK can expect to live through childhood. In many developing countries in the world, life expectancy at birth remains below 50 years of age because of high rates of infant mortality. According to McKeown (1979)

 STOP THINK ■ If you were going to practise medicine in a developing country today, what sorts of ill health would you expect to encounter and what sorts of intervention would you become involved in?

the most important factor leading to changes in infant and child mortality has been a dramatic improvement in child nutrition and maternal nutrition over the past century.

Diseases that have declined

Another way to look at the changing nature of health and illness is to compare rates of death due to particular causes over the years. In order to examine the relative importance of different diseases over time, we need to take account of the fact that the population structure might also have changed over time. For example, cancers are more common in the older age groups and if the proportion of older people in the population has increased whilst the actual rate of cancer has stayed the same, we are likely to make the mistake of assuming that the rate of cancer is increasing. This could be very misleading. In order to calculate real changes in the rates of different diseases over time we can calculate what are called standardized mortality ratios (SMRs) (see p. 42). These enable us to examine changes over time and consider the possible causes of these changes (Table 1). Over the past century, death rates due to nearly all causes have declined. Striking changes in death rates have occurred for tuberculosis and influenza. SMRs for tuberculosis have changed from 867 in the period 1891–1895 to four in 1986–1990; however, they are now on the increase. Similarly, SMRs for influenza have changed from 514 in 1891–1896 to seven in 1986–1990. A very important improvement in health has been due to our ability to control the spread of infectious disease and fight it more effectively when we are infected.

An important debate surrounds the explanation of changing rates of infectious disease. A great deal of medical research effort has been devoted to the identification of viruses and bacilli, and to the development of vaccines and cures during the last 100 years. For example, the tubercle bacillus was first identified in 1880. However, the introduction of the BCG vaccination to prevent infection did not take place until the 1950s. It can be seen from Table 1 that deaths due to tuberculosis had dropped dramatically long before the introduction of the BCG suggesting that some other factor, such as improved nutrition, public health

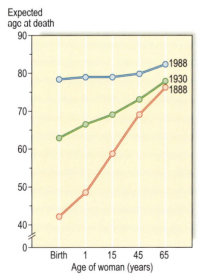

Fig. 1 **Average life expectancy for a woman at different ages in 1888, 1930 and 1999 (England and Wales)**, (Source: Registrar General's Mortality Statistics 1999)

Table 1 **Standardized mortality ratios for selected causes of death, 1890 to 1990 in England and Wales**					
Cause of death	**1891–1895**	**1921–1925**	**1946–1950**	**1961–1965**	**1986–1990**
Tuberculosis	867	393	157	20	4
Influenza	514	359	57	36	7
Digestive diseases	750	263	114	75	79
Diseases of the respiratory system	526	250	93	94	60
Diseases of the genito-urinary system	309	226	113	60	35
Diseases of the skin, sub-cutaneous tissue, musculo-skeletal system and connective tissue	671	381	127	97	182
Malignant neoplasms	–	–	96	103	115
Diseases of the heart	–	–	93	89	63
Cerebrovascular disease	–	100	92	95	60
Suicide	137	125	106	112	74
(Source: Registrar General's Mortality Statistics, HMSO)					

measures and housing conditions, or changes in the nature of the bacillus, must have contributed to the decline (McKeown 1979) (see also Fig. 1, p. 62.)

Deaths due to some causes have not changed a great deal over the years. The SMR for diseases of the heart, cerebrovascular disease and suicide have shown a steady but undramatic downward trend over the last 50 years. Although the rate for suicide has gradually declined over the years, it reached an all-time high during the years of the economic depression, 1931–1935, with an SMR of 150. The only cause of death to show an upward trend over all the years it has been recorded is malignant neoplasm or cancer. Over the last 20 years, death rates amongst women from cancer of the trachea, bronchus and breast have increased steadily, whilst amongst men death rates for cancer of the prostate have increased steadily.

STOP THINK
■ Bearing in mind the impact of immunization on death rates from tuberculosis, speculate on how important vaccination against HIV might eventually prove to be.

Current common diseases

Whilst SMRs are very useful for examining trends in the rates of disease over time, if we want to know which are the most common causes of death in a population we need only examine the rates per head of population (see Table 2). In 1999, deaths certified as due to disease of the circulatory system accounted for 40% of all male deaths and 39% of all female deaths. Treatments for these conditions are an important area of research, and survival rates are improving. However, an understanding of the causes of heart disease and cancer remains important and they have been linked to a variety of socio-economic. cultural and behavioural factors. Figure 2 shows recent changes in the incidence of lung

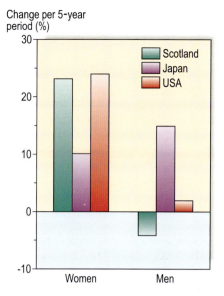

Fig. 2 **Change in lung cancer incidence 1972–1987** (Source: Registrar General's Mortality Statistics 1994)

cancer in Scotland, Japan and the USA. These changes may be closely linked to changes in the tendency of men and women to smoke cigarettes, which may in turn be related to cultural changes in the past 30 years.

An important consequence of increases in life expectancy and in the prevalence of diseases for which cures are unknown is that medical practice is increasingly concerned with the management of chronic ill health and the prevention of disability amongst a population whose average age is on the increase.

STOP THINK
■ What implications do the changing patterns of mortality have for the demographic structure of the population and health care over the next 50 years?

Changing patterns of health and illness

■ The single factor which most accounts for our improved life expectancy at birth in the UK is that at the start of the 21st century almost all new-born babies can expect to live through childhood. This has occurred largely as a result of improvements in nutrition.

■ Over the last century infectious disease has declined dramatically. This may be a result of: (a) changes in people's susceptibility to infection; (b) changes in the nature of the biological agents; (c) the introduction of medical treatments.

■ In 1999, diseases of the circulatory system accounted for 39% of all deaths. Malignant neoplasms accounted for 25% of all deaths.

Regular UK statistical bulletins concerning mortality and morbidity are on the HMSO website: www.hmso.gov.uk/HPSSS/INDEX.HTM

Table 2 **Death rates per million population in England and Wales in 1974, 1991 and 1999 by cause of death**						
Cause of death	Women			Men		
	1974	1991	1999	1974	1991	1999
Diseases of the circulatory system	6118	4533	3985	6149	4570	4216
Neoplasms	2771	2833	2689	2244	2559	2439
Diseases of the respiratory system	1816	1043	1666	1458	1054	2008
Accidents. violence and poisoning	496	427	395	379	223	221
Diseases of the digestive system	292	285	373	309	361	442
Diseases of the nervous system	126	203	186	132	213	197
Diseases of the endocrine system	113	170	132	178	200	151
Mental disorders	28	145	–	47	282	–
Diseases of the genitourinary system	179	97	120	153	115	153
Diseases of the musculoskeletal system	30	44	36	83	135	99
Diseases of the blood	27	38	32	47	45	37
(Source: Registrar General's Mortality Statistics, HMSO, 1999)						
Note: 1999 figures are for England only.						

Social class and health

In clinical practice, we are particularly concerned with the health of individual patients. When clerking a patient we ask about occupation with an expectation that what we are told – bus driver, publican, lawyer, computer programmer, cleaner – will tell us something about the risks associated with work. We may also make an instant appraisal of their lifestyle and material circumstances. Whilst there are significant differences between individual bus drivers and individual lawyers, there is also strong evidence that people's health is closely associated with their occupation (see pp. 56–57), their occupational group and their social class.

What is social class?

Social class is a general measure obtained by combining occupational groups roughly equivalent in skill and 'general standing in the community' to form occupational classes in the UK; these can be seen as an indirect indicator of education, income, standards of living, environment and working conditions. The Registrar General's occupational measure of class (Table 1) is most commonly used in health research even though it does have some flaws – for example, it does not include people who are unemployed nor deal adequately with women's occupations. Other important categorizations, which use information on employment status and occupational data, are socio-economic group (SEG) and socio-economic status (SES). In 2001 a new classification, the NS SEG, was introduced to overcome some of the drawbacks of the Registrar General's classification, but this has yet to be linked to mortality and morbidity data.

Social class and health

Over the last 100 years there have been great improvements in the health of the UK population (see pp. 40–41). However, inequalities between different sections of the population still exist; one form of increasing disparity that has received particular attention is social class inequality in health (Bartley et al 1998, Davey Smith et al 2000, Scambler 2002). Death rates for the UK can be calculated for occupational classes by combining data collected on birth and death certificates with occupational data collected at the Decennial Census. Although reproductive and adult mortality rates for each social class have been decreasing over the last 100 years, there has, however, been an increase in the disparity in mortality rates between social class I through to social class V.

Figure 1 illustrates the current gradation in all-cause standardized mortality ratios (SMRs) (see pp. 38–39) from social class I through to social class V. Class differentials exist in each of the 14 major cause-of-death categories used in the International Classification of Diseases. When married women are classified according to their husband's occupation, similar if smaller differentials also appear. Only one cause of death for men, malignant melanoma, and four for women, including breast cancer, show a reverse trend.

In general, the evidence suggests that disparities in illness, and especially chronic illness, are at least as wide as disparities in death. These facts are not challenged; controversy lies in their interpretation and in the implications of different interpretations for policies of preventive or corrective action. In the 1990s the influential Research Working Group on Inequalities in Health produced *The Black Report* (Townsend et al 1992). Four major theoretical explanations were presented, which were to become the matrix for future debate in this field.

Explanations for these relationships – the four hypotheses

Cultural/behavioural explanations

These explanations stress individual or lifestyle differences, rooted in personal characteristics and levels of education, which influence behaviour and are, therefore, open to alteration through health-education inputs leading to changes in personal behaviour. Cultural and behavioural explanations suggest that lack of knowledge, and lack of long-term goals, give fewer possibilities of making maximum use of health and other services, and of taking preventive health measures (see pp. 62–63). Their main focus has been on the health-related behaviours of cigarette smoking, diet (including alcohol consumption) and lack of exercise:

- There are higher rates of smoking among manual groups, which will contribute to ill health.
- There is lower consumption of vitamin C, carotene and fibre, along with a higher dietary sodium/potassium ratio among the manual occupational classes. There are lower rates of vegetable intake, but elevated rates of the consumption of saturated fats.
- People in manual occupations take less exercise than those in non-manual groups.

Table 1 **The Registrar General's social class classification**			
Social class	**Description**	**Examples**	**% of population**
I	Professions Business	Lawyers Large employers	5
II	Lesser professions Trade	Teachers Shopkeepers	20
III (nm)	Skilled non-manual	Clerical workers	15
III (m)	Skilled manual	Electricians Lorry drivers	33
IV	Semi-skilled manual	Farm workers Machine operators	19
V	Unskilled manual	Building labourers	8

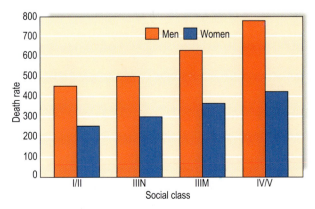

Fig. 1 **Age standardized death rates per 100 000 people by social class, men and women aged 35–64, England and Wales, 1980–92.** Adapted from Harding et al 1997.

Materialist or structuralist explanations

These explanations emphasize the role of economic and associated socio-structural factors, for example, the labour and housing markets, in the distribution of health and well-being. Proponents of this explanation believe that social structure is characterized by permanent social and economic inequality, which exposes individuals to different probabilities of ill health and injury:

- Poor-quality and damp housing has been shown to be associated with worse health and particularly with higher rates of respiratory disease in children (pp. 8–9).
- Low socio-economic status, low pay, and insecurity produce inadequacies in diet and dietary values.
- All-cause mortality has been shown in one study to be directly related to income, with the age-adjusted relative rate of the poorest group of subjects being twice that of the richest group. The rate increased in a stepwise fashion between these extremes (Davey Smith et al 1990, Bartley et al 1998).

Social selection

These explanations argue that the occupational class structure is seen to act as a filter or sorter of human beings, and one of the major bases of selection is health: physical strength, vigour, or agility. In this hypothesis, health determines social class.

- Illsley (1986) found that women who were taller and in better health than the other members of their class of origin were more likely to marry into a higher social class and have lower rates of prematurity, stillbirths and first-week infant deaths.
- Goldberg and Morrison (1963) reached a similar conclusion in the case of schizophrenia. They found that while the fathers of schizophrenics had the same social class distribution as that of the general population, patients with schizophrenia were disproportionately concentrated into social class V.

Artefact explanation

This suggests that both health and class are artificial variables produced by attempts to measure social phenomena and that, therefore, the relationship between them may itself be an artefact – an accidental effect – of little causal significance:

- Errors may be produced when two different data sets (e.g. death certificate and census data on occupation) are combined in order to calculate mortality rates for social classes.
- The failure of health inequalities to diminish in recent decades may be counterbalanced by the reduction in the proportion of the population in the poorest classes as a result of increased upward social mobility.

Recent developments

Following *The Black Report*'s own conclusions, research tended to favour the materialist/structural hypothesis. This was supported by the discovery of similar socio-economic differentials in health and mortality in European countries, as well as in the USA and Australia. Although the developing consensus acknowledged the other explanations, these were given a subsidiary role. Cultural influences could be at work, but any behavioural differences in sub-cultures were seen to be directly related to social classes. There was also some evidence for indirect health selection, via differences in nutrition and other behaviours and attitudes, though less for direct health selection. Longitudinal studies carried out on census data tended to diminish the importance of the artefact explanation.

More recently, *The Acheson Report* (Stationery Office 1998) brought the empirical findings up to date and discovered the worrying fact that social class inequalities are in fact increasing.

Conclusion

Each of the above theories has practical implications as to what needs to be done to reduce social class inequalities in health. Although recent research favours a combination of materialist and behavioural approaches, where healthy or unhealthy lifestyles are seen to be linked to people's social positions, Wilkinson's ideas (see Case study) suggest that if we reduce income inequality, whilst at the same time increase various forms of social security provision, then social class inequalities in health will diminish. Judge and Paterson (2001), however, have suggested that the most important strategy is for policies to reduce poverty, especially in families with children. The latter approach was strongly favoured by *The Acheson Report*.

Of course we should also be aware of the important role doctors can play. Acheson stressed the crucial role of the NHS at all levels for helping to reduce inequalities in health. For example, doctors can ensure that their patients are claiming the benefits to which they are entitled.

Case study

The Wilkinson controversy

Wilkinson's work (1998, Marmot and Wilkinson 1999) casts the inequalities debate in a new perspective. He did this by bringing the relational concept of relative deprivation into play. It was not so much the total amount of disposable income available to people in each social class that was important (as had been argued in the materialist explanation), but rather the scale of the differences between the social classes that was crucial (in other words we should focus on the relationships between the classes).

Large gaps between rich and poor in developed societies threatened social cohesion and produced high levels of social conflict leading to social distintegration. These were the mechanisms that lead through to the development of inequalities in health. His policy focus, therefore, stressed the need for societies to develop good social security provisions for their citizens.

Social class and health

- Mortality rates for all social classes have been falling over the last 100 years.
- However, the mortality rates for social class I have been decreasing faster than rates for social class V.
- Morbidity rates follow a similar pattern to mortality.
- The main explanations are: materialist, behavioural, social selection and artefactual.
- High rates of disparity between rich and poor in affluent countries may be a significant contributor to disparities in social-class mortality rates.
- Different explanations for the relationship between social class and health imply different health, social and economic policies.

Gender and health

Gender is one of the important divisions in society along with social class and ethnicity. Gender patterns from wider society are reflected in medicine. People working in the health services need to understand gender differences and their implications for health and health-service uptake in order to provide the most appropriate and acceptable care to patients.

Gender and sex

Social scientists make the distinction between sex and gender, whereby 'sex' refers to physical and biological differences and 'gender' refers to the social definitions of how women and men should behave under certain circumstances. Society 'prescribes' how the biological sex is transformed into the social gender. Thus biological men learn to behave in a male way and to carry out male tasks. The philosopher Simone de Beauvoir (1960) summarized this transformation in the phrase: 'One is not born, but rather becomes, a woman.' Every society produces norms, rules, expectations for each gender and these differ from place to place as well as over time. Consequently, what is regarded as male behaviour in one time and place can be seen as female in another. Thus society as a whole produces women and men.

■ Women live longer than men but are more likely to be ill. What explanations can you give for this paradox?

Difference in mortality and morbidity

Women in most countries live longer than men, with the exception of a small number of the least-developed countries (Fig. 1). Men are more likely to die, compared with women in the same age group, from the day they are born. Table 1 clearly shows some gender differences in Scottish mortality statistics. The perinatal mortality rate indicates that in any 1 year baby boys are more likely to die than girls. This pattern is the same for any other age group in Scotland and for other industrialized countries, and many developing countries.

Morbidity statistics for Scotland (Table 1) indicate that middle-aged women are more likely to visit their GP than men in this age group. However, men over 85 are more likely to visit their GP than women of that age.

Possible explanations for gender differences in health

Some of the gender differences in mortality, especially in babies and infants, are related to 'natural' differences in biological and genetic make-up. However, as boys grow up to become men, social causes of death, especially those related to lifestyle, become more important. Men are more likely to be exposed to a hazardous environment than women, and

■ Why are women more likely to be residents in mental institutions than men are?

many hazardous occupations in Britain are male dominated: e.g. mining, fishing, and construction work. Men are more likely to display more dangerous behaviour – to drink, to drive too fast, to use illegal drugs, or be involved in dangerous sports such as boxing or motor racing.

At the same time many diseases that do not in themselves kill but are often chronic and disabling affect more women than men. Approximately two-thirds of the disabled population in the UK are women, and a large proportion of that inequality is due to age difference (see below). However, not all differences between men and women can be traced back to social factors. Some of the difference between male and female mortality and morbidity in coronary heart disease can be linked to the contraceptive pill and hormones (Committee on Health Promotion 1996).

Health service use and gender

Women are not only more likely to be ill, but also more likely to use health services. Figure 2 illustrates that both poor and rich American women consult their doctor more often than men do. This pattern holds for other industrialized countries.

Women visit the doctor more often than men even if one ignores the consultations related to childbearing (Miles 1991), but the hospitalization rate is higher for men than for women, when maternity and gynaecological cases are excluded (Leeson and Gray 1978), except for mental illness (Table 1).

Differences in illness patterns of women and men will lead to different needs for health-care provision. Women live longer than men, so consequently a large proportion of the elderly are female. The overwhelming majority of hip-fracture patients are elderly people, hence the majority of patients with a hip fracture are female, and they are more likely to occupy a bed in an orthopaedic ward. Moreover, the uptake of health care is not only determined indirectly through morbidity, but also directly by social and cultural factors. Two main factors are highlighted below:

■ What is defined as illness in women is often a social definition instead of the purely scientific exercise of diagnosis and treatment. Childbirth, for example, helps to define women as being ill, because of their biological role.
■ Women consult family doctors more often than men do, not only for themselves but also for their children and elderly relatives.

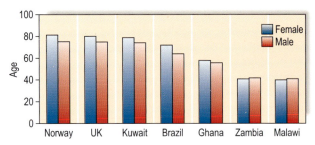

Fig. 1 **UN 2001 world population prospects 1950–2050. The 2000 revision.** (Source: Database of Department of Economics and Social Affairs, Population Division.)

Table1 **Selected mortality and morbidity rates for men and women, Scotland 1999**

		Measure	Female	Male
Mortality	Perinatal mortality rate	Rate[1]	6.7	8.4
	Under 1	Rate[2]	4.2	5.6
	15–19	Rate[2]	0.4	0.8
	45–49	Rate[2]	2.6	3.9
	85 and over	Rate[2]	181.9	211.6
	General practitioner consultation (2000)[2]			
	45–59		3.999	2.426
	85 and over		4.878	5.190
Morbidity	Mental illness: hospital inpatient admissions	Rate[3]	641	596
(per 100 000 population)	Mental illness: hospital inpatient residents	Rate[3]	154	168

1. Rates per 1000 total births including stillbirths and deaths up to 7 days after birth
2. Rates per 1000 population
3. Rates per 100 000 population
(Source: ISD Table A 5.1; E1.3; 29 from www.ISD/SCOTTISH. HEALTH. STATISTICS/SHS 2000

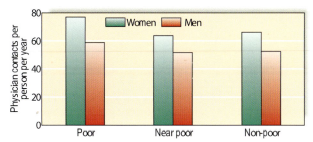

Fig. 2 **Physician contacts, according to sex and poverty status: USA 1991**. (National Center for Health Statistics 1995, Table 77. Poor persons are defined as below Bureau of Census poverty threshold. Near-poor persons have incomes to less than 200% of poverty. Non-poor have incomes of 200% or greater than poverty threshold.

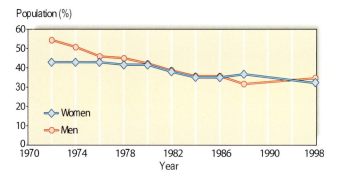

Fig. 3 **Smoking prevalence in Scotland among ages 16 and over**.

Case study

M. is an obstetrician who visits the family doctor because of sleeping problems. During the consultation the doctor asks him about factors that might have an influence on getting to sleep. He mentions the heavy work load in the maternity hospital, drinking a little too much in order to deal with stress and sleeplessness, the frequent quarrels with his partner for no apparent reason, having two noisy children (under 5 years) at home, and living a long distance away from elderly parents. Do you think the family doctor would advise this patient differently if you were told that obstetrician M. is a woman rather than a man?

The first explanation is related to the fact that all societies make assumptions about what is appropriate gender-related behaviour. This is often referred to as sexual stereotyping. One aspect of this in Western cultures is that female socialization makes it more acceptable for women to adopt the 'sick role'. One of the possible explanations is that women are less likely to be in full-time employment, therefore they are likely to lose less income than men when they take on a sick role. There is also evidence that doctors give different emphasis to the 'same' symptoms, according to gender. For example, men's 'back troubles' are regarded more seriously, being seen as directly caused by heavy work. Women's 'back problems' are often labelled as part of general gynaecological conditions. Similarly, mental health problems in women are seen to be internally caused, and thus subject to medical intervention, while in men these are seen as caused by external factors. In other words, men's problems are seen to be related to what they do, and women's problems are related to what they are.

Smoking

Smoking illustrates the importance of gender for the medical profession for two quite distinct reasons (see pp. 80–81). First, smoking is the most important cause of preventable death. Secondly, patterns in smoking prevalence between men and women have been changing over the past 3 decades. It also shows that differences between men and women in health behaviour, in this case smoking, are not static. Forty years ago it used to be 'normal' among men from all social classes to smoke, whilst only a small proportion of women smoked. Smoking prevalence among adults has fallen steadily since 1972. However, whilst the proportion of men who smoked regularly dropped, the proportion of female smokers increased in the same period. In the 1980s the proportion of women taking up smoking in their teenage years increased rapidly. Figure 3 indicates that smoking levels in Scotland have declined faster amongst men than women. In 1988 the proportion of Scottish women smoking was, for the first time ever, greater than that of men. The reason for this change has been sought in women's emancipation, advertising, and health promotion.

Furthermore, the incidence of lung cancer is increasing among women, and this is closely related to the social changes in smoking prevalence.

Gender and health

- At any age men are more likely to die, but women are more likely to be ill.
- Gender differences have a greater impact on health and health care than differences in biological sex.
- Women consult doctors more often than men do.
- Medical professionals have different expectations of and ways of dealing with male and female patients.

Ethnicity and health

It is important for health professionals to consider their roles in developing and delivering equitable and appropriate health services for all ethnic groups in their countries, as evidence indicates that such care is not as accessible to people in minority ethnic groups as it is to other groups.

Race, culture and ethnicity

In order to monitor whether equitable access to health care is achieved, the UK government requires NHS hospitals to record the ethnicity of all admitted patients. Ethnicity is also often collected as a variable in epidemiological research. However, defining the concept of ethnicity in relation to understandings of race and of culture is fraught with difficulty.

The concept of 'race' does not exist in any biologically meaningful way. There is more genetic variability within than between so-called 'racial groups', and over 99% of the genetic make-up of human beings is shared by all ethnic groups. Although there are clear differences in physical characteristics between people whose ancestry lies in different parts of the world (colour of eyes, skin or hair), these characteristics are of no major importance to health. Physical characteristics are only important when values are attached to them in a society, so that one group defines another group as 'different' and assumes them to have particular behavioural characteristics because of the way they look.

Culture is a set of shared beliefs, values and attitudes that guide behaviour. People identify themselves as members of a group on cultural grounds, they may share similar histories, language, religion, food, lifestyle and origins and this helps them define their ethnic group. We all have ethnic identities, whether we consider ourselves to be 'Scottish', 'English', 'Australian', 'Bangladeshi' or any combination that describes our national, cultural and social identities. Thus the concepts of 'race', culture and ethnicity are interrelated.

Measuring ethnicity

In the UK ethnicity is now measured by asking people to assign themselves to a category, as in the 2001 census in England. This approach attempts to capture the way people think of themselves in relation to colour of skin, continent of ancestral origin and 'cultural background'. Other questions included country of birth and religion, so that when analyzed, these data should help in the planning of services that are appropriate in relation to religious observance and diet.

Most recent estimates suggest that about 4 million people living in Britain consider that they are from a minority ethnic group. That is about 7.1% of the total population (Johnson 2003), between 40 and 50% of whom were born in Britain. Most people in minority ethnic groups live in cities, and some towns or metropolitan boroughs become known for local concentrations of people from particular ethnic origins.

Socio-economic inequalities between ethnic groups in Britain

Unemployment rates for most minority ethnic groups are considerably higher than those for whites, particularly amongst young people (see pp. 56–57). Although national data on average income are not routinely broken down by ethnic group, a survey by Leicester City Council in the

STOP THINK

- How might the various components of your ethnicity and culture relate to your own experience of health and illness?

mid-1990s showed evidence of lower incomes amongst people of Asian origin: the gross median weekly earnings of 'Asian' men and women were just 82% of the earnings of 'whites'. Similarly, whilst about 19% of the white population live in areas described as 'council estates and low income areas', about 40% of Black and Indian groups, and as many as 63% of Bangladeshi and Pakistani groups live in such areas (Johnson 2003). However, there remain significant differences in the socio-economic experiences of different groups of minority ethnic groups.

Diversity in health and disease

Patterns of health and disease are profoundly influenced by socio-economic, environmental, genetic and cultural factors (see pp. 40–41), and there are significant differences in patterns of disease between ethnic groups. However, the major health problems of ethic minority communities, and, therefore, priorities for health improvement and health care, are similar to the majority population (for example, cardiovascular disease and cancers). This is an important when using epidemiological information on ethnicity in the planning of health services (Kai and Bhopal 2003).

Table 1 shows that *comparing* deaths emphasizes differences. For example, liver cancer or tuberculosis stand out as much more common in men from the Indian sub-continent but they account for fewer deaths. Looking at *absolute number* of deaths, the major fatal diseases for the minority group are seen as similar to those of the population as a whole. Thus, while there are differences in experience of health between all ethnic groups, the major diseases of the majority population are also very important to minority ethnic groups.

The varied and complex patterns in the experience of health and illness between people in different ethnic groups do not have a single explanation. Genetic inheritance contributes to the aetiology of some diseases, e.g. the prevalence of sickle cell disorders in the UK is higher in people of African and Indian origins. However, lifestyle and cultural factors (especially smoking, diet and exercise), exposure to poor living circumstances and the stress of racism will also contribute. Explanations for differences in experience of health and illness that point out the impact of socio-economic inequalities and racism are used less often by researchers (who used to tend to stress cultural or genetic differences), but used more often by people in minority ethnic groups themselves.

Experience of racism and prejudice

In 1997, about 25% of white people said that they were prejudiced against people from minority ethnic groups, whilst between 20% and 33% of people from a range of minority ethnic groups reported being worried about being racially harassed (Coker 2002). This fear is not unfounded. Police figures show that reported racist incidents in London increased from 11 050 in the year ending March 1999 to 23 345 by March 2000 (Coker 2002).

'Racism' and 'institutional racism' have been defined:

> *'Racism' in general terms consists of conduct or words or practise which advantage or disadvantage people because of their colour, culture or ethnic origin. In its more subtle form it is as damaging as in its overt form.*

> *'Institutional Racism' consists of the collective failure of an organisation to provide an appropriate and professional service to people because of their colour, culture or ethnic origin.*
>
> (Macpherson, 1999)

Table 1 **Deaths and SMRs* in male immigrants from the Indian sub-continent (aged 20 years and over; total deaths = 4352)**							
By rank order of number of deaths				**By rank order of SMR**			
Cause	Number of deaths	% of total	SMR	Cause	Number of deaths	% of total	SMR
Ischaemic heart disease	1533	35.2	115	Homicide	21	0.5	341
Cerebrovascular disease	438	10.1	108	Liver and intrahepatic bile duct neoplasm	19	0.4	338
Bronchitis, emphysema and asthma	223	5.1	77	Tuberculosis	64	1.5	315
Neoplasm of the trachea, bronchus and lung	218	5.0	53	Diabetes mellitus	55	1.3	188
TOTAL	2412	55.4	–	TOTAL	159	3.7	–

Standardized mortality ratios, comparing with the male population of England and Wales, which was by definition 100.
(Source: Senior and Bhopal 1994, including data originally published by Marmot et al 1984; reproduced with permission of BMJ Publications)

Case study

Lack of services for sickle cell disease in the UK

Sickle cell disorders and thalassaemia are inherited disorders of the red blood cells that mainly (but not exclusively) affect black and ethnic minority groups. A similar number of people are affected by these illnesses as are affected by haemophilia and cystic fibrosis.

Services for sickle cell disease, although improving, are lagging behind the numbers of cases arising in the UK. Major obstacles to progress are the inadequate education of health-care professionals, disadvantage within the black community and institutionalized racism.

A consultant haematologist wrote in 1990:

I was hearing that not enough money goes to research on sickle cell. It's not a disease of the white people and they don't know much about it . . .

Debbie (17 years) wrote:

They know that I have got the disease but they don't really know too much about it, and I don't think, this is my personal view, I don't think they're interested because it's not a white man's disease, and I mean, from once it's not a white man's disease, and I can't see them really digging into this thing to get any knowledge out of it, because it is black people, and it's black people's problem. (quoted in Anionwu 1993)

Epidemiological studies that include perceptions of racism or prejudice are rare but a 3-year study in the general population in the Netherlands found statistically significant higher rates of 'delusional ideation' (a suggested precursor of psychotic disorder) amongst people who reported discrimination than those who did not (Janssen et al 2003).

Unequal and inappropriate provision of health care

For a range of reasons, some related to unwitting but institutional racism in health-care organizations, many health services are inappropriate to the needs of minority ethnic populations. For example, health services have been concentrated on issues that are seen by health professionals to be of special relevance to particular ethnic groups, whereas people themselves may not attach such significance to them. In Britain this led to health education on such issues as rickets or fertility control, whereas, until recently haemoglobinopathy services have been largely ignored (see Case study).

The other criticism of health services is that the methods by which health issues are brought to the attention of minority groups is often inappropriate, and interventions are, therefore, often unsuccessful. For example, recent policies to increase fruit and vegetable intake and decrease the proportion of fat in the diet all too frequently miss out foods often eaten by minority ethnic groups. Therefore, there is a risk that the health-education message does not reach (some) ethnic minority groups.

Ethnicity and health

- The concept of 'race' does not exist in any biologically meaningful way.
- Ethnicity is a complex concept consisting of the interplay between culture, history, language and so on. We all belong to an 'ethnic group'.
- Ethnic minority groups are at increased risk of being poor, principally through the effects of racism and negative discrimination.
- The major diseases and health problems of most minority ethnic groups are the same as for the general population (e.g. coronary heart disease, stroke, cancer).
- There is evidence of unequal and inappropriate provision of health services for people in ethnic minority groups.

Quality of life

There is no universally accepted definition of quality of life.

The World Health Organization (WHO) (1946) defined health as 'complete physical, mental and emotional well-being'. Health and health-related quality of life were no longer seen as being about only physical health and an absence of illness. In 1993, the WHO defined quality of life as 'individual's perceptions of their position of life in the context of the culture and value systems in which they live and in relation to their goals, standards and concerns' (WHO Division of mental health 1993). The definition includes six domains:

- physical health
- psychological state
- levels of independence
- social relationships
- environmental features
- spiritual concerns.

Similarly, the WHOQOL Group defined quality of life as 'an individual's perceptions of their position in life taken in the context of the culture and value systems where they live in relation to their goals, expectations, standards and concerns', and they subsequently developed a standardized measure, the WHOQOL (WHOQOL Group 1998). In contrast, Calman (1984) proposed that quality of life is the extent to which hopes and ambitions are matched by experience, and Bowling (1995b) suggested that it is the things people regard as important in their lives.

It would probably now be agreed that quality of life is a multidimensional dynamic concept that includes both positive and negative aspects of life.

Functional or subjective?

Quality of life used to be seen as an objective assessment of the person's functioning, whereas the current approach tries to measure quality of life as an individual's perceived health status or well-being. Quality of life is very much an individual construct (Fig. 1). Physical functioning might mean the ability to perform specific tasks or the activities of daily living and of mental functioning in performing cognitive tasks and social interactions. A person's own appraisal of their health status may be more influenced by the way that they perceive their relative health status and by other non-medical aspects of their lives. Health professionals may have a different perspective from the individual patient (Fig. 2).

Behavioural questions such as 'can you walk up stairs?' (functional quality of life) may be easier to answer than 'does your health interfere with your enjoyment of life?' (individual or subjective perspective of quality of life), but the latter may be regarded as being more important by the person. Subjective indices of quality of life correlate reliably with standard measures of depression and anxiety (Muldoon et al 1998). The expectations of medical treatment on quality of life may also differ between patients and health professionals.

There is a paradox in that patients who have significant health and functional problems do not necessarily have poor scores of quality of life. People with severe disabilities may report having a good quality of life despite having difficulties with activities of daily living and being socially isolated (Albrecht and Devlieger 1999).

Who should assess quality of life?

The perspectives of individuals, carers and health professionals may be very different. In a healthy state it is hard to imagine what life would be like if wheelchair bound, or visually impaired. We can gain some insight from novels or films, but there is a qualitative aspect to quality of life, which may not be captured by standardized scales. Like pain, quality of life may be best regarded as what patients tell us.

The patient-generated index (PGI) is an attempt to assess the extent to which patients' expectations are matched by reality (Ruta et al 1999). The SEIQoL was also devised to allow people to describe their lives in terms of factors that they consider important (McGee et al 1991). In patients with incurable cancer, family concerns were rated more important than health (Waldron et al 1999). There is no one correct measure and assessments need to be chosen carefully.

Quality of life is a dynamic construct and changes over time. People assess their health related quality of life by comparing their expectations with their experience. If expectations match experience there is no impact on quality of life, but if it is worse then there is an impact. Clinical trials of efficacy of therapy often require assessment of quality of life, and outcomes of therapy may depend on expectations (Alder 2002).

Quality of life in elderly people

In assessing quality of life in older people the medical model searches for a cure and the reduction or absence of symptoms and thereby an increase in the level of functioning. In contrast to this, the older person may be more concerned with issues of self-identity, and preservation of meaning in life. Brandstater and Greive (1994) see the gradual ageing process as leading to successive loss of control, and higher rates of depression (which may be associated with bereavement) and lower self-esteem (there is an emphasis on youth and beauty in Western society). They suggest that elderly people cope by moving through stages of assimilation, accommodation and using immunizing mechanisms. In assimilation people maintain current activities, goals and aspirations. For example, women might make strong efforts to maintain fitness by taking exercise, and use aids such as reading

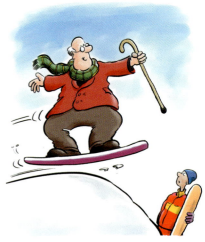

Fig. 1

glasses to achieve their goals. As the ageing process continues, they replace current goals and aspirations with new ones. They give up difficult goals or reduce their level of expectations about their level of performance.

Quality-adjusted life year

Health economists often use a utility or decision-theory approach to measuring quality of life The utility approach assesses the value that someone places on the consequences of different courses of action. For example, if chemotherapy would extend life but involve costs of treatment and side effects, how would this be valued against no treatment costs or side effects but a shorter life.

The quality-adjusted life year or QALY is a measure derived from a combination of mortality, morbidity and function, with quality-of-life value or utility with increased time of survival resulting from treatment. The Oregon experiment (see p. 153) is one of the best-known applications of this approach. Considerable reservations have been expressed about the applications of this approach, as it may differ between healthy people, patients and health professionals and does not take into account expectations, previous history or the time spent in ill health (Fallowfield 1990).

Improvement in quality of life will be the goal of both patients and health professionals and it is important to ensure that they understand each other's meaning when discussing treatment options.

STOP THINK
- What are the most important aspects of quality of life in your own lives now?
- What do you think they will be when you are 50, and when you are 80 years old?

Case study

Susan is 28 and has had a diagnosis of breast cancer. She is considering the effect of treatment options on her quality of life. She was anxious about feelings of mutilation and altered body image. She was aware that the physical effects of chemotherapy and radiotherapy might be nausea, vomiting and diarrhoea, tiredness and loss of libido. The hospital was 20 miles away and involved taking two buses. She was confused because she knew that radioactivity caused cancer and thought that the radiotherapy might be dangerous.

The medical and nursing staff discussed breast reconstruction, and how to cope with possible hair loss. She was reassured that tiredness was to be expected. She was offered help with travel expenses from a hospital fund. Leaflets explaining the procedures gave her more confidence in its safety and efficacy. She was encouraged by the survival rates in breast cancer as it had been caught at an early stage and her sister had now survived more than 5 years since her diagnosis of breast cancer. She made plans for the future and was redesigning her garden.

Consider the impact of psychosocial support on her quality of life

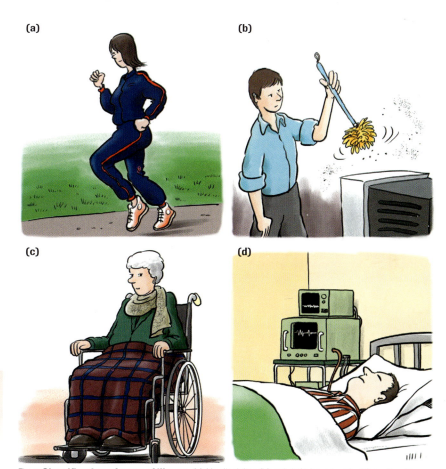

Fig. 2 **Classification of state of illness.** (a) No disability, (b) only light housework, (c) confined to wheelchair, (d) unconscious. (Source: adapted from Fallowfield 1990)

Quality of life

- Quality of life has many different definitions.
- Measures of functional quality of life may differ from a person's individual appraisal.
- QALY analyses require careful appraisal.

The media and health

The rôle of the media

The mass media are a rich source of information about all aspects of health. They are constantly presenting us with ideas about everything from the symptoms of disease or the risks of different behaviours to the validity of government health policy or the trustworthiness of the medical profession. That is why so much money is now spent on trying to affect media representations – through advertising, public relations activities, media advocacy and direct health-education initiatives. However, the role of the media is not straightforward. A direct impact may be evident when, for example, doctors are flooded with enquires after a particular health 'scare' or news about a 'miracle cure'. However, such responses are often very short term. People are certainly not naïve and unreflective media consumers, ready to absorb any message indiscriminately. If they were, then campaigns to encourage us to stop smoking or eat less fat would be more successful!

In fact, most research shows that people act as sophisticated audiences, choosing how to engage with media facts, images, stories, characters and plots, and how they relate these to their own lives (e.g. Philo and Henderson 1999). In addition, each media 'message' competes with ideas and information from other media, and broader cultural, sources. How we respond also depends on social and economic context, the ease with which we can change our behaviour and the ways in which any particular media representation relates to our self-image, aspirations, group identity and networks. Sometimes the same media representations can even generate diametrically opposed responses from different social groups. For example, the British soap opera, *Brookside*, included a storyline about a businesswoman, 'Susannah', successfully standing up to a man who complained about her breastfeeding in a café-bar. This storyline was welcomed by middle-class breastfeeding women, who felt inspired by the scene. Reactions were strikingly different among a group of young working-class women. Susannah's strength of will did not fit with these women's self-perceptions: '*You need to be confident which I'm not*'. Clearly, if breastfeeding in a café-bar might cause a scene and necessitate a robust defence then trying to do it in the local burger joint would be likely to be even more controversial. For these women the *Brookside* episode seemed to reinforce the fact that breastfeeding in public was ill advised, rather than encourage them to think of it as an option (Henderson et al 2000; see Case study).

- How do media representations influence how *you* think about your own health or how you respond to patients? Has the media influenced your images of the 'type' of person liable to engage in particular risk behaviours?
- If you were going to design a campaign to promote a health behaviour, what social factors would you take into account? How would you set about designing your message for a specific group? How would you pre-test it and on whom?

It is thus important for anyone working in health and medicine (whether, for example, as a medical researcher, a GP or a health promoter) not to assume they can easily predict how people will make sense of any information/representations. This is true, whether the information is delivered via the mass media, personal communication or health-promotion posters. It is also important to acknowledge the different levels at which influence may operate. Perhaps the mass media's most significant role may be in how they cultivate underlying, common-sense understandings of the world. Newspapers, television, radio, magazines and, indeed, cinema, both reflect and *promote* ideas about what is normal – whether this relates to body weight, smoking, or breastfeeding (see the case study below). The media can also promote stereotypes by, for example, portraying people with mental illness as violent, thus encouraging fear and stigma (Philo 1999). Fictional programmes may be particularly important in promoting emotional identification and can reach important new audiences. At the same time their power to provoke identification with particular characters and to convey forceful stories can mislead. The drama and human interest potential of stories about 'inherited' breast cancer, for example, generated many fictional TV representations and helped to raise its profile, but has also made many people overestimate the role of genetic risk factors (Henderson and Kitzinger 1999).

Health and social issues

Newspaper reports and both factual and fictional television may also offer 'scripts' for thinking and talking about social and health issues. When the media started to acknowledge incestuous sexual abuse during the 1980s, this allowed some children and adult survivors to talk about such abuse for the first time (Kitzinger 2001). The media breaching of taboos about bowel and testicular cancer have been similarly important. The media also played a vital role in putting AIDS

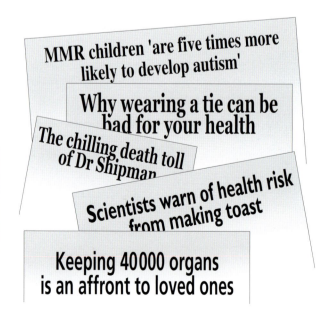

MMR children 'are five times more likely to develop autism'

Why wearing a tie can be bad for your health

The chilling death toll of Dr Shipman

Scientists warn of health risk from making toast

Keeping 40000 organs is an affront to loved ones

Fig. 1

and safer sex on the public agenda. However, the coverage has also been limited. One study of TV fiction found that, although young people were shown talking about sexual attraction and whether or not they wanted sex, condom use was never discussed, offering no 'scripts' and modelling of behaviour for young people (Batchelor and Kitzinger 1999). Another study revealed that the media's early voyeuristic fascination with the gaunt, sickly 'face of AIDS' encouraged people to think you could tell by looking who was infected (Kitzinger 1995). Sometimes a message can also be confusing because the producers/scriptwriters or health educators attempt to avoid explicit language. The term 'body fluids' often adopted in AIDS discussions allowed some people to believe that saliva was dangerous. The advice to use a condom unless you are '100% sure of your partner' backfired – associating condom use with a lack of trust (Miller et al 1998).

Medicine and the media

The medical profession is also acutely aware of how the profession as a whole is represented in factual and fictional media. Doctors may be still heroes in fiction, but intense public attention has also been given to the villains: the Alder Hey hospital scandal about the use of children's organs, for example, or the doctor turned mass-murderer, Dr Harold Shipman. The mass media also have a crucial role to play in the development of scientific and medical research. In the field of human genetic research, for example, public acceptability is increasingly important. The ground was prepared for changing legislation on stem cell research, for example, by intense media lobbying. Interestingly, the resulting coverage, although arguably 'balanced' around the 'rights of the embryo' debate, excluded wider social and political questions and gave little opportunity for explorations of ambivalance (Williams et al 2003).

Understanding how the media represent health and illness, medical practitioners, health policy and scientific research is important for medical students. In-depth research about media representations and audience responses suggests that the relationship with public attitudes, however, is more complex than might at first appear. It is important to go beyond personal impressions and anecdotes to take into account the diversity of media and of audiences, and to consider the implications of the associated research.

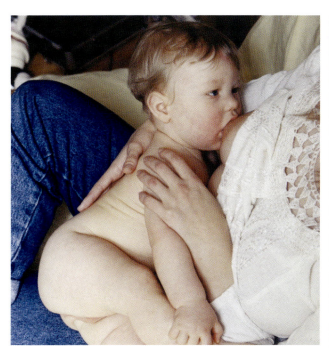

Fig. 2

Case study

Infant feeding in the media

A systematic content analysis of 1 month's UK press and television coverage showed that the overall pattern of coverage implies that breastfeeding is odd or problematic whereas bottle-feeding is largely normalized, associated with 'normal' families and represented as being problem-free.

- Breastfeeding is rarely shown. There was only one scene on TV of a baby on the breast and nine of a breast pump (not in use), but 170 scenes with babies' bottles or bottle-feeding.
- Babies' bottles have become a routine and iconic way of visually representing babyhood.
- Whereas a baby may be bottle-fed in a background scene on television, breastfeeding, where it does feature, is foregrounded as a focus for debate.
- Breastfeeding is used to characterize particular types of women, e.g. as middle-class 'earth mothers'.
- Bottle-feeding is used to symbolize positive male involvement in fatherhood.
- Problems with breastfeeding are highlighted, whereas difficulties with bottle-feeding are rarely mentioned. For example, there was only one reference to potential difficulties associated with bottle-feeding ('hassle' of bottle washing) but 42 references to problems attributed to breastfeeding (sore nipples, 'saggy' breasts, sleepless nights).
- Routine mass-media coverage rarely acknowledges the health implications of bottle-feeding. There was only one, oblique, reference within the entire sample to the potential disadvantages of formula milk compared to breast milk (Henderson et al 2000).

The media and health

The mass media can:
- Put new health issues on the public/policy agenda or help raise their profile
- Provoke debate about the ethics of scientific and medical developments
- Convey factual information and advice
- Promote or challenge stereotypes (e.g. about people with schizophrenia or about who is likely to contract HIV)
- Cultivate common sense understandings of health and illness and support ideas about what constitutes appropriate behaviours
- Play a key part in short term 'health scares'

However, media influence is not straightforward or all powerful
- There is a large gap between what people *know* and what we *do*
- Wider social issues are often more important than health messages on their own
- The impact of media representations vary depending on format (e.g. fictional versus factual programmes) and the type of narrative, vocabulary, images and associations which are used
- The impact will vary depending on how much the public trust the 'sources' of the story (e.g. government scientists)
- Different audiences may respond to the same programme or report quite differently depending on their identities and context of their own lives.

Social aspects of ageing

Definitions of ageing

There is a widespread view that ageing, especially during the later part of life, is an inevitable process of physical and psychological decline produced by biological change. In this 'biomedical' view, ageing is seen rather mechanistically as a result of the increase in life expectancy. The solutions proposed to the 'problem of ageing' tend, therefore, to be medical ones: if a 'cure' for ageing does not exist at the present time, then hopefully one will be discovered in the future. But ageing is more than a biomedical fact of life. It is a lifelong process involving an interaction between biological, psychological, and social factors which are in practice difficult to isolate. Therefore care for older people must involve these three dimensions.

Social scientists acknowledge biological ageing but highlight how our experiences of ageing must be understood in terms of the social environment. Thus, ageing can be described as a 'relational experience': that is, changes taking place in the body alter our relationships with other people. For example, a statutary retirement age of 65 changes people's status in personal and public spheres, but there is no biological reason for retirement to be set at 65. Ageing into old age is a gradual process that varies from individual to individual. There is no single or universal answer to the question: 'when does old age begin?'

Ageism

Ageism, or prejudice against people simply because they are old, may be indicative of fear of old age in contemporary society (Bytheway 1995). This fear is associated with the belief that chronological age results inevitably in mental and physical decline. Jerrome (1992) studied nine old people's clubs and three organizations for older people in a church community in England. She concluded that old age should be defined as a 'state of feeling and behaving' (p. 130) rather than a chronological state. She observed that older people work hard to cope with the ageing of their bodies and often turn physical ageing into a personal challenge. Participation in clubs for older people helps members to make sense of the ageing process as a journey through life. Involvement in club activities helps them explore the meaning of growing older and negotiate the point at which it is socially acceptable to acknowledge frailty or illness and withdraw from social activities. Talking about illness is not, therefore, a self-pitying preoccupation, but a social process through which older people come to understand changes in their roles and decide how they should behave as older people: 'One cannot be ill by oneself and know that one is ill' (p. 101), feelings and experiences have to be tested out with others.

The ageing body and the self

It is increasingly recognized in social gerontology that a better understanding of ageing as a personal experience grounded in social relationships requires more information about the relationships that older people experience in everyday life. Language, for example, has an important part to play in the ageing process. From a detailed study of the choice of words in conversations between younger and older women, Coupland and colleagues (1991) show how age identities are shaped in sequences of talk. References to ageing and old age by both younger and older women does not necessarily indicate the older women's experience of ageing, but reflects assumptions that older people are preoccupied with old age. Aspects of age-related speech include the disclosure of chronological age, references to time passing, and a self-association with the past and recognition of social change over time. Age-identity is found to be a fluid process that varies according to time, place and the people involved. Thus, older people's view of themselves as older persons is not fixed, but varies according to social context. Put simply, older people do not necessarily see themselves as 'old' in all circumstances.

Other evidence suggests that older people may retain an image of themselves as younger than they are. This leads to a disjunction between how people experience themselves and their body, so that the self may be experienced as a kind of 'ageless' or youthful prisoner

■ Consider the saying, 'You're only as old as you feel.' How does this relate to the old people you know, perhaps your grandparents or other relatives or family friends?

inside an ageing body. The ageing body and face act as a kind of mask disguising the inner sense of personal selfhood or identity (Hepworth 1995, Biggs 1999). The relationship between the body and the self is therefore complicated by perceptions of the body and the value placed upon it. People who value their youth and beauty may be much more unhappy with their bodies as they grow older than those who value the inner self more. People who value the inner self may find physical ageing less burdensome and an opportunity for personal growth and development. It is therefore important to find out how people perceive their bodies as they grow older as well as looking for information about biological change (see pp. 14–15).

Acknowledging that older people may not think of themselves as 'older' may help health-care professionals understand their feelings and behaviour. It also cautions us against stereotyping older patients.

Alzheimer's disease

Alzheimer's disease is not infrequently described as the loss of self. In their research with persons with Alzheimer's, Sabat and Harré (1992) divide the self into two parts: 'Self i' and 'Selves ii'. Self i is the 'personal singularity' indicated by the use of expressions such as 'I', 'me' and 'mine', which is made possible by the structure of language. The 'I' is the sense of personal identity we all possess. Selves ii is the social aspect of identity and this is made up of the ensemble of social selves that is displayed during our relationships with other people. Selves ii require the collaboration of other people in recognizing our various social identities. These are the selves that are socially presented: public expressions of a type of character drawn from a 'local repertoire' (p. 452). For example, we may present different identities as 'student' and 'son' or 'daughter'.

Sociological studies of dementia suggest that the process may be more than simple loss of capabilities due to physical changes. Kitwood (1997) developed a person-centred approach to understanding dementia. In answer to the question: 'Does personality change?' (p. 31), he suggests that the changes that are observable tend to result not only from biomedical factors, but are also related to loss of resources including social support for the self. Biomedical change is, therefore, aggravated by changes in the responses of other people to the sufferer when they withdraw the social support he or she needs to continue maintaining a social self. Thus, social support and interaction are also factors in the development and manifestation of dementia. Kitwood (1997) argued that 'those who are well-supported only very rarely suggest that their relative has acquired a different personality or "disappeared". Perhaps they have found ways of maintaining relationships and communication and can deal more accurately with their own feelings of loss and bewilderment.'

Ageing and social change

The expansion of the population aged > 50 years is increasingly recognized as one of the major demographic changes in contemporary society. Increased life expectancy and reductions in the birth rate are resulting in a situation where people aged over 50 years will no longer be a minority group in the population. This change will not necessarily result in an increased 'burden' of older people (Coleman et al 1993), because the evidence is that many older people continue to make an active contribution to social life. The role of grandparents within changing patterns of family life is a good example.

What is important is that this demographic change means that the traditional modes of the roles of older people in society (derived from a time when surviving older people were a minority) are no longer relevant. The experience of ageing is changing and becoming more diverse as societies become more complex, and new models and images of ageing have to be created. In, for example, the study of ageing in fiction it is suggested that contemporary novelists are developing new models of growing older which emphasize much more positive attitudes to later life. It is no longer acceptable to regard life after the age of 50 as a period of 'decline' into old age. Care provision is not just a matter of looking after the body, but must, therefore, change to ensure the continuity of personal identity and individual independence in later life.

Case study

The writer Linda Grant (1998) provides a detailed and moving account of the effects of Alzheimer's disease on the 'self' of her mother Rose (who suffered from Alzheimer's) and on herself. She discusses in vivid detail Rose's gradually developing sense of confusion as a threat to her mother's sense of identity. Rose sometimes seemed to be aware of the changes taking place in her ability to control her presentation of self on the occasions when she would show she was 'ashamed, embarrassed and afraid of (the) response (of other people). She had cut herself off because she could no longer manage the skills she needed to be in company . . . ' "I cringe inside when someone tells me I'm repeating myself," she said once, in a rare acknowledgment . . . ' (p. 130)

Eventually Rose is taken into care and conversations with the carer responsible persuaded Grant that individuals do not have a fixed identity that is constant through their lives, but throughout their lives experience a range of selves.

Social aspects of ageing

- Biological ageing always occurs in a particular social environment.
- Ageing is a relational process.
- Physical and mental decline are not inevitable in later life.
- As people grow older they work to maintain their own sense of personal identity.
- People may experience the self as 'younger' than the body.
- Alzheimer's disease does not necessarily mean the loss of self.
- The increase in the population of people aged > 50 years does not mean that they are a 'burden' on society.
- As society becomes more complex, new models of ageing and old age are emerging to replace traditional beliefs and attitudes.

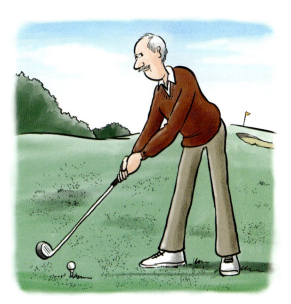

Fig. 1 **The experience of ageing is changing and new images of ageing must be created.**

Housing, homelessness and health

Housing affects health directly and indirectly. Lack of adequate housing causes both mental and physical ill health. It can make existing illness and health problems worse, and can delay recovery from illness. Lack of adequate housing has detrimental social and economic consequences, which reduce people's opportunities to protect and promote their own health. Energy-inefficient housing causes fuel poverty and is detrimental to the environment and this has consequences for the health of the whole population.

Housing and health

In Victorian Britain, concerns about housing conditions causing ill health led to programmes of slum clearance. This commitment to improving public health by changing harmful social conditions contributed to the decline in infectious diseases and increases in life expectancy (see pp. 40–41).

The 1950s and 1960s saw growth in public sector housing. The focus on quantity rather than quality brought problems such as dampness, lack of sound insulation and privacy, as well as social isolation. Research evidence emerged during the 1970s and 1980s showing the negative health impact of these 'new' housing problems, but health policy focused on individual behaviour as the cause of ill health rather than social conditions such as housing.

The late 1980s and 1990s saw a decline in the availability of affordable housing and a rise in the numbers of homeless people who were roofless or in temporary accommodation. In the early 21st century concerns about energy efficiency, the environment and fuel poverty have begun to reinforce the centrality of housing to public health once more.

Homelessness and health

The term homelessness is used to describe people who are 'roofless' and living on the streets and those living in temporary accommodation. People who are homeless are exposed to extreme environmental hazards such as damp, cold and noise as well as overcrowding, risk of violence, risk of accidental injury, poor hygiene and poor access to health services. Figure 1

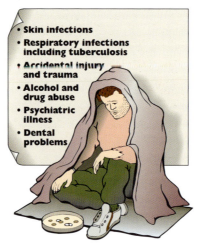

- Skin infections
- Respiratory infections including tuberculosis
- Accidental injury and trauma
- Alcohol and drug abuse
- Psychiatric illness
- Dental problems

Fig. 1 **Illnesses associated with homelessness.**

shows the main illnesses associated with homelessness.

Housed but homeless

Social policy currently distinguishes between people who have permanent accommodation and the homeless. A definition of homelessness based on the 'lack of a right of access to own secure and minimally adequate housing space' (Bramley et al 1987) would mean that people are seen as homeless if permanently housed in accommodation that is harmful to health or deprives them of resources that are necessary to maintain or protect health.

The health impact
How does lack of adequate housing affect health?

The housing environment can affect health both directly and indirectly (Table 1).

The direct effects of lack of adequate housing can be explained using a medical model whereby specific aspects of the environment have physical effects that lead to specific symptoms or illness.

Another model of illness is the 'general susceptibility model,' in which aspects of the environment act as stressors that make people more susceptible to illness. Specific features of the environment are not linked to specific illness as they are in the medical model. This model takes some account of the indirect effects of housing on health.

In both models researchers have to rule out the possibility that

associations between housing and health occur as a result of other factors. The two most common 'artefact' explanations that have to be ruled out are those of 'confounding factors' and 'downward drift' (see Table 2). If researchers have data on other social conditions and past health and housing history, statistical techniques can be used to take account of these factors and assess the independent contribution of housing to health.

A third model that can be used to understand the health impact of housing is a socio-economic model. This holistic model recognizes that it is important to understand the experience of living in inadequate housing, the impact on daily life and the compound effects of different aspects of inadequate housing and other conditions of social deprivation.

Work on the energy efficiency of housing has drawn attention to the fact that people with low incomes are more likely to live in poorly constructed, least energy-efficient housing – they

Table 1 **Lack of adequate housing: effects on health**
Direct effects
■ Exposure to physiological effects of the environment or harmful agents fostered by environmental conditions.
Indirect effects
■ Exposure to poor living conditions in childhood may have consequences for health in later life
■ Causes stress or discomfort, which increases general susceptibility to physical illness and emotional problems
■ Exacerbates or delays recovery from existing health problems
■ Undermines social relationships
■ Makes it difficult or stressful to get on with the tasks of daily life
■ Makes it difficult to access other resources which are necessary to sustain or promote health
■ Can drain other household resources, including income, that protect and improve health
■ Impacts on energy effciency and the environment, which in turn impacts on public health.

Table 2 **Key problems in establishing the links between lack of adequate housing and ill health**
Confounding factors
Lack of adequate housing is frequently associated with other factors which are known to cause ill health, such as unemployment or low income
Downward drift
People in poor health 'drift' into poor housing or homelessness because of the consequences of ill health

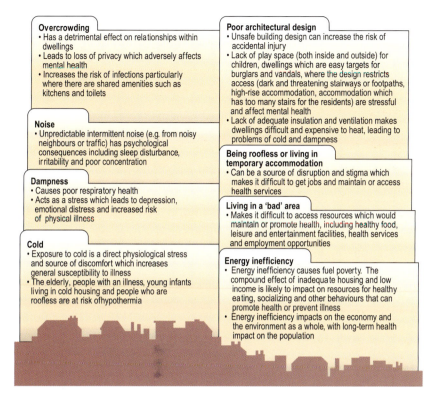

Fig. 2 **Features of inadequate housing which are detrimental to health.**

The contents of Fig. 2 boxes:

Overcrowding
- Has a detrimental effect on relationships within dwellings
- Leads to loss of privacy which adversely affects mental health
- Increases the risk of infections particularly where there are shared amenities such as kitchens and toilets

Noise
- Unpredictable intermittent noise (e.g. from noisy neighbours or traffic) has psychological consequences including sleep disturbance, irritability and poor concentration

Dampness
- Causes poor respiratory health
- Acts as a stress which leads to depression, emotional distress and increased risk of physical illness

Cold
- Exposure to cold is a direct physiological stress and source of discomfort which increases general susceptibility to illness
- The elderly, people with an illness, young infants living in cold housing and people who are roofless are at risk of hypothermia

Poor architectural design
- Unsafe building design can increase the risk of accidental injury
- Lack of play space (both inside and outside) for children, dwellings which are easy targets for burglars and vandals, where the design restricts access (dark and threatening stairways or footpaths, high-rise accommodation, accommodation which has too many stairs for the residents) are stressful and affect mental health
- Lack of adequate insulation and ventilation makes dwellings difficult and expensive to heat, leading to problems of cold and dampness

Being roofless or living in temporary accommodation
- Can be a source of disruption and stigma which makes it difficult to get jobs and maintain or access health services

Living in a 'bad' area
- Makes it difficult to access resources which would maintain or promote health, including healthy food, leisure and entertainment facilities, health services and employment opportunities

Energy inefficiency
- Energy inefficiency causes fuel poverty. The compound effect of inadequate housing and low income is likely to impact on resources for healthy eating, socializing and other behaviours that can promote health or prevent illness
- Energy inefficiency impacts on the economy and the environment as a whole, with long-term health impact on the population

live in fuel poverty. A greater proportion of lower incomes is spent on energy and this may still not alleviate the problems of cold and dampness. Poor housing is seen to compound the problems of living on a low income rather than low income being seen as a potential confounding factor in the relationship between housing and health.

Case study

The direct effects of dampness on health

A study in Britain (Platt et al 1989) looked at whether toxic fungal air spores which are present in damp and mouldy houses could explain the association between dampness and respiratory symptoms. The study involved the collection of health information from around 800 respondents. Measures of the internal housing environment were then taken by an independent team of surveyors who were 'blind' to the results of the health survey.

Reporting of respiratory symptoms was higher when the levels of damp and air spore counts were higher, indicating a 'dose-response relationship'. The health survey asked about other factors which might influence respiratory health such as smoking, ownership of pets and the use of indoor appliances as well as other social factors known to be associated with poor health. The relationship between respiratory symptoms, dampness and air spore count remained after all other possible explanatory factors were statistically ruled out.

Indirect effects of dampness on health

Dampness can lead to overcrowding when occupants avoid using a damp room. Dampness and mould cause damage to property and add to the financial burden of those on low income. Keeping the house clean can be difficult, and visible mould and the smell of dampness may lead to embarrassment about inviting friends and family in. Concerns about the impact of dampness on the health of children can be an additional stress.

STOP THINK
- For a family with young children living in damp and over-crowded conditions, what are the possible consequences for the health service of housing-related illness? What are the possible costs to the health service of inadequate housing?

A range of factors associated with housing have been shown to cause physical illness and discomfort as well as depression and emotional distress (Fig. 2).

It's very noisy being right by the motorway but we couldn't open the windows anyway because of all the break-ins. The walls are running with damp and there's mould on our walls, our clothes and shoes. It's freezing cold most of the time and in winter we all huddle into the one room. The kids are always sick and I'm at my wits' end. (Hunt 1997).

Working in the home

There are fitness standards for formal work environments such as offices (see pp 56-57), but not for domestic housing. People who are not in formal employment may spend substantial amounts of time in housing environments which would not meet the minimum occupational health standards. Carrying out 'housework' such as child care, cleaning and cooking is particularly stressful in poor conditions.

Housing and health services

Health professionals must consider the extent to which patients' illness or distress are the result of their living conditions. Health professionals are sometimes asked to comment formally on this in assessments of medical priority for rehousing or assessments for community care (see pp. 146–47). The moves to day-case interventions and early discharge from hospital make it even more important that health professionals know about patients' housing conditions and ensure that poor living conditions do not exacerbate illness or prejudice recovery.

Housing, homelessness and health

- The housing environment affects health directly and indirectly.
- Overcrowding, noise, dampness, cold, poor design and poor neighbourhood are detrimental to health.
- Being housed does not necessarily imply having a home.
- 'Housework' is often carried out in conditions that would not satisfy 'Health and Safety at Work' standards.
- Provision of adequate, affordable housing is an important component of a policy for health.

Work and health

The United Nations Declaration of Human Rights states that 'Everyone has the right to work'. Does this imply that work is 'good' for us and for our health? Is all work good for us? Table 1 summarizes some of the characteristics of work which have been identified as important for health. The other side of this picture is that the absence of these criteria can lead to ill health and injury. World Health Organization statistics tell us that 1 million people worldwide die each year from work-related accidents and disease. The 'right to work' is, therefore, complemented by the United Nations International Labour Organization's (ILO) commitment to 'adequate protection for the life and health of workers in all occupations'.

The world of work is changing as we enter the 21st century. The health of working people will be affected by these changes which include: increased use of IT; increase in small businesses; falling trade union membership; more women and older people in the workforce; intensification of work; 24-hour society (e.g. call centres); increased demand for flexibility; more temporary/short-term contracts; growing inequality in skill levels; downsizing; privatization of state-owned industries. Globalization of industry is accelerating and can lead to the export of health and safety risks from the developed to the developing world. The ILO estimates that the fatal injury rate for established market economies is 5 per 100 000 workers whilst that for Asia reaches 23 per 100 000 workers.

Income and health

Economic growth and the creation of national wealth has enabled many people to enjoy higher standards of living than their grandparents or their parents. However, inequalities in income and wealth contribute to poorer health of people on lower incomes (see pp. 42–43).

Environment at work

Discovering accurate information regarding the extent of work-related ill health and injury is difficult. In the UK there is systematic under-reporting. The government accepts that less than half of non-fatal incidents reportable by law to the Health and Safety Executive are in fact reported (HSE 2000a). As well as official reporting mechanisms, data comes from a number of sources including voluntary reporting schemes by occupational physicians and regular Labour Force surveys at both UK and European levels. The latter indicate that about 2m people in the UK are suffering from work-related ill health and that 27% of European workers consider their health to be at risk from their work.

Accidents

Accidents at work account for less than 5% of all accidental deaths in the UK, but this rises to 20% in adults. Work-related fatalities rose in the latter 1990s, dropping slightly in 2002 to stand at 249. The rate of major-injury accidents rose in the years 1999–2001.

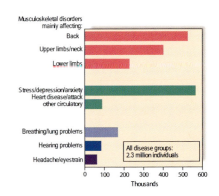

Fig. 1 **Prevalence of self-reported, work-related ill health and injury in the GB workforce.** (Source: www.hse.gov.uk/statistics/pdf/swi3p5.pdf/)

Concern about the failure to reduce these statistics has resulted in the launch of a major new government strategy, *Revitalising Health and Safety* (HSE 2000a). Its targets include a 10% reduction in fatal and major injuries by 2010. It is important to recognize that risk of accidents is not uniform, but is concentrated in certain industries, e.g. construction, and among certain groups of workers, for example young workers, who are at 37% higher risk of injury.

Occupational ill health

A less visible but more extensive problem is that of work-related ill health and disease (Fig. 1), with attributable deaths running at well over 10 times that caused by work accidents. This includes a wide range of conditions including back and other musculoskeletal problems, occupational cancers, respiratory conditions such as asthma and bronchitis, work-related dermatitis and a variety of physical and psychological conditions related to workplace stress. Although some of the traditional diseases related to heavy industry are on the decline, for example bladder

Table 1 **Characteristics of 'healthy' jobs**	
Pay and Conditions	Good wages/benefits
	Security
Physical environment	Protection from physical, chemical, biological hazards
Demands	Neither too much nor too little work. Not excessive hours
	Clarity of role and no conflicting demands
	Minimal unsocial hours or shiftwork
	Minimum conflict between demands of home and work
Skills	Ability to use skills and be creative
	Opportunity to develop new skills
Control	Ability to control how you work
	Participation in decision-making
	Ability to organize independently
Support	Collaboration and collective effort
	Good communication
	Good relationships with colleagues and supervisors
	Being valued and respected
	Equality of treatment

Case study

Clare, a young textile worker, went to her GP complaining of episodes of dizziness and fainting. Her symptoms were worse during the working week and improved when away from work. This pattern suggested that her ill health might be the result of chemical exposure at work. She was referred to an occupational physician, who confirmed that this was the likely cause. The chemical was probably formaldehyde, a chemical used to pretreat permanent press garments. It was recommended that exposure levels be limited as far as possible. After communication between her GP, the occupational physician and Clare's employer, her employer agreed to improvements in ventilation and in the chemical process involved, and Clare's symptoms subsequently disappeared.

cancer caused by chemicals used in the rubber industry, others are becoming more prominent, for example occupational asthma caused by exposure to wide range of substances including latex in disposable gloves, and stress-related conditions.

Responsibility for health at work

There is an inherent conflict for employers in the implementation of a healthy and safe environment. Creating such an environment can be costly in terms of both time and money. What they do not often take into account is the cost of *not* taking action, including sickness absence, increased turnover, compensation costs, damage to morale and industrial relations, as well as, of course, the personal cost to the individual worker. Employees too may be caught in an economic conflict and may ignore health and safety, for example, in situations where pay is related to speed or levels of production.

The law places the responsibility for workplace health firmly with the employer, although employees too have duties to take care of themselves and others and to follow health and safety rules. Most accidents are systems failures. Two independent studies found that in only about 18% and 11% of cases respectively was the employee responsible for the accident and even in these cases part of the cause may be lack of training, low morale or pressure of work.

Tackling occupational health and safety: prevention through risk assessment

Throughout Europe, and increasingly internationally, the accepted place to start in addressing workplace health protection is risk assessment. In the UK this principle is now enshrined in the Health and Safety at Work Act 1974 through its many sets of regulations. It entails:

- pro-active, detailed consideration of the work environment and all work tasks; identification of hazards (something with the potential to do harm)
- assessment of levels of risk (the likelihood of harm occurring) and severity (how serious the harm would be)
- planning and implementation of action to eliminate hazards or reduce risk
- monitoring to ensure the effectiveness of that action.

By definition, risk assessment:

- is a management responsibility
- must be carried out by a 'competent' person
- should involve consultation with the workforce.

One of the key groups in effective risk assessment and reduction are occupational health physicians, nurses and other occupational health professionals. However, HSE figures indicate that two-thirds of working people in the UK have no access to occupational health expertise and support,

a failure recognized in another government strategy, *Securing Health Together* (HSE 2000b), with the major aim of reducing work-related ill health by 20% by 2010. The UK situation compares badly with Europe, where in some Nordic countries coverage nears 100%.

Stress at work

Stress is now the second largest cause of work-related ill health and sickness absence in Europe, next only to back and other musculoskeletal conditions. Research has shown that failure to provide the elements listed in Table 1 can result in work-related stress (Cox 2000). Evidence of the link between stress and ill health is growing. Research shows that job insecurity leads to increased self-reported ill health and clinical symptoms, with those at the lowest levels of the company being worst affected. The introduction of new technology can lead to psychological distress, particularly among lower-paid, less-skilled and older workers. There is clear evidence of links between stress and coronary heart disease but conflicting evidence about which stress factors are most implicated. Overtime work is associated with high blood pressure. It is known that stress can suppress the immune system (Platt et al 1999).

It is now accepted that organizational solutions (primary prevention) aimed at addressing the causes of stress are more effective than interventions targeted at individual coping skills (secondary prevention) or counselling (tertiary prevention), although the best employers will provide all three. Factors that potentially lead to stress are now included in those which employers must risk assess.

Work–life balance

A problem reported by workers throughout Europe is the difficulty in achieving a healthy balance between work and life outside work. This is exacerbated in the UK by the longest working hours in Europe. Women bear the brunt of this. Even when working full time, women still carry much higher levels of responsibility for the home, including care of children and other dependents. On the other hand, there is now clear evidence that financial and physical well-being are strongly linked to paid employment. Domestic labour can be routine, boring, unpaid and undervalued. However, when women choose to enter paid employment they are consistently paid less than men, which means that childcare costs take a proportionately higher percentage of their income. There is now some pressure on employers to consider the introduction of 'family friendly' policies to address this issue, for example 'term-time' working, job shares and subsidized childcare.

STOP THINK ■ When making diagnoses and considering causes of ill health, it is important for doctors to think and ask about work as well as biological and social factors. Did you know that approximately 8% of patient-visits to GPs are about work-related conditions? Higher numbers will be suffering from some form of condition caused or made worse by work.

> ### Work and health
>
> - Official figures for occupational death, injury and disease underestimate the total amount of occupational ill health.
> - It is crucial in occupational health as well as any other health field to prioritize prevention.
> - Worldwide trends in employment have important implications for occupational health and safety.
> - High-demand and low-control jobs create stress, which can cause ill health.
> - One major issue facing all workers but particularly women is finding a balance between demands at work and at home.

Unemployment and health

As we move into the era of what has been called 'liquid' capitalism, we are witnessing increased part-time employment, more flexible work patterns and more self-employment. At the same time unemployment over the life-course will become a more common experience for a sizeable section of the population. Unemployment will be especially high for young men (Luck et al 2000). There will be more chronic unemployment and more workless households. Medical professionals will increasingly be faced with having to deal with the possible health effects of unemployment (Wadsworth et al 1999).

The evidence

Psychological morbidity

An important series of studies on psychological well-being was carried out by Warr (1978) and colleagues on different sub-groups of the unemployed. An index of present life satisfaction was found to be strongly negatively associated with unemployment for both redundant steelworkers and men attending unemployment benefit offices. On the other hand, a measure of constant self-esteem yielded no differences between managers with or without a job.

A similar pattern emerged for measures of positive well-being, where a person was asked if he/she had experienced positive events in the past few weeks. Positive effect in recent weeks among redundant steelworkers was clearly associated with their employment status at the time of interview. Indicators of negative well-being, where the interviewees were asked if they had experienced negative events – for example, feelings of loneliness – in the past few weeks, showed the clearest overall relationship, with significant differences between employed and unemployed respondents in every case.

These studies also threw light on some of the factors that moderated the negative impact of unemployment:

- People who were committed to their work and who became redundant were found to be particularly disadvantaged.
- Age and length of unemployment were likely to be intercor-related, and so older people were less likely to become re-employed and were more likely to be sick. The middle-aged unemployed, in fact, were found to have the lowest well-being scores.
- Although they found differences between the sexes, with men having higher rates of psychological morbidity than women, this was thought to be related to personal commit-ment to their work. When the variable of personal work involvement was held constant, the sexes were equally affected.

A recent study by Weich and Lewis (1998) on 7726 adults drawn from the British household panel study found that unemployment was associated with the maintenance of episodes of most common mental disorders.

Physical morbidity

Any cross-sectional analysis comparing groups of employed workers with unemployed men and women shows that

Table 1 **Trends in death rates/100 000 persons by employment status and social class among men aged 36–64. 1971 cohort, England and Wales**

Social class	Follow-up period			
	1976–81c[+]	1981c[+]–85	1986–91c[+]	1991c[+]–95
Employed				
Non-manual	3361	2518	2178	1642
Manual	4105	3281	3281	2455
Unemployed				
Non-manual	4689	3980	2500	2889
Manual	5917	4505	6059	4113

+ 1981/91 refers to day before census day in the first time period and census day onwards in the following time period. Adapted from Harding et al 1999.

employed people are healthier despite occupational hazards. These studies also give us some interesting pointers towards the health condition of the long-term unemployed (for more than 1 year), among whom there are likely to be far more health problems than among the short-term unemployed. Such studies cannot, however, tell us whether these effects are specifically caused by unemployment. Selection processes operate; individuals may have become unemployed because they had health problems to begin with. It is also difficult to separate out the direct effect of unemployment from any indirect effect of poverty, bad housing conditions, geographical location and social class. Although most research produces correlations between unemployment and health, the establishment of causality requires studies over time, looking at workers before termination of their employment and following them through and after redundancy.

An important American longitudinal study looked at 100 men who lost their job and 74 controls who did not as a result of two factories closing. The study followed the cohort from pre-closure to 2 years post closure. The controls were found to be healthier than the terminees. Myocardial infarction was at the expected level, but the risk of coronary heart disease had increased among the terminees. Research by Beale and Nethercott (1985) on a factory closure in south-west England found increased consultation rates with GPs and increased referral rates to hospital among redundant workers and members of their families compared with controls.

Recent work by Wadsworth et al (1999) looked at a longer time-frame, focused on younger age groups, and considered the effects of today's increasingly fluid labour market. They concluded that 'prolonged unemployment early in the working life of this population of young men was likely to have a persisting effect' on their future health.

Mortality

Death rates have been found to rise in times of economic depression; unemployed people have higher death rates than the employed; and death rates rise with the increasing duration of unemployment. A British study (Moser et al 1984) looked at 5861 men aged 15–64 years who were waiting to take up a job or were seeking work in the week before the 1971 census. The standardized mortality ratio for 1971–1981 for men aged 15–64 years at death who were seeking work in 1971 was 136. It was particularly high among those under 54 years, reaching over 200 in those aged 35–44 years. The causes of death that predominated among the unemployed were malignant

Case study

The personal effect of unemployment

CM: is an unemployed 28 year old and lives with his partner in obvious conditions of hardship.

CM: *I could do better. I could pack up the fags with an effort of will. I think I could stop drinking. But there is a kind of need there as well. When I go for a drink, I don't really feel like it's enjoyment. I feel its a need to get pissed, a need to get stoned. . . . It's like a downward spiral you are on. . . . because you kind of feel shit that you have got no money so you try to look for a release or escape from that and then because it costs you money to do that so you end up on this downward spiral. . . . There is also a big tension because I know quite a bit about health and diet. It was always an interest of mine. The impact of the way you lived on your health and stuff. So I do feel a total idiot sometimes that I smoke, because I know all the stuff and I never wanted to see myself as a 'smoker'. I wanted to be healthier than that. . . . People say you drink and smoke and take drugs and it is seen that you do that because you like to have fun, but it is not about that at all. They are missing the point totally. It is a form of escapism if you like. . . . You do sort of push things aside. Like you numb your brain with certain chemicals and things and that is the escapist aspect of it. You try and escape it. It is about numbing yourself.*

(From A. Dolan, PhD Thesis, University of Warwick 2003)

neoplasms (particularly lung cancer), accidents, poisonings and violence (particularly suicide). These findings have been corroborated by findings from the British Regional Heart Study (Morris et al 1994), which, after controlling for social class and health at time of entry into the study, found that unemployed men aged 40–59 years were 1.7 times more likely to have died after 5-year follow-up than men who were not unemployed during that time. The most recent study by Harding et al (1999), analyzing data from the Office for National Statistics Longitudinal Study, found that from 1976 to 1995 mortality among the unemployed was higher, within each class grouping, than among the employed (Table 1). As Drever and Whitehead (1997) state: 'Losing his job doubles the chances of a middle-aged man dying within the next five years.'

Mechanisms

Recent research has been able to capitalize on the volume of work carried out in the 1980s and gives more attention to the mechanisms that cause ill health. In order to understand the relationships between unemployment and ill health and mortality, four mechanisms are important (see Fig. 1):

- the role of relative poverty
- social isolation and the role of self-esteem
- health-related behaviour
- the effect that a spell of unemployment has on subsequent employment patterns.

■ Social scientists are now predicting rapidly increasing trends towards flexibility in the world's labour markets (Westergaard et al 1989). They also believe that detrimental health effects will be particularly bad for the younger person (Lewis and Sloggett 1998).
■ What do you think?

Both the work of Wadsworth et al (1999) and Weich and Lewis (1998) stress the interplay between unemployment itself and linked financial elements. Psychological health is seen to be affected by financial problems that increase the frequency of stressful life events. Mental health is also affected by decreasing social activity and participation, and diminishing social support. Although alternative social networks may eventually be formed, these may involve groups who have withdrawn from the norms and values of mainstream society. They may, thus, be more likely to indulge in health-damaging behaviours: tobacco and alcohol use, drug taking and bad diet. In terms of physical health the 'stress pathway', involving physiological changes (for example, raised cholesterol and lowered immunity), is believed to be the main mechanism. The importance of relative rather than just absolute disadvantage has also been highlighted in the recent literature (see pp. 42–43, 46–47).

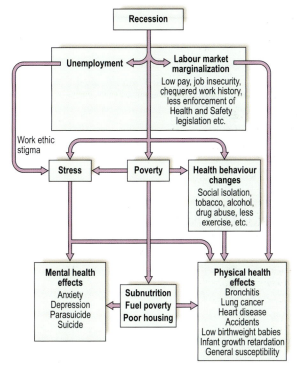

Fig. 1 **How might unemployment lead to poor health?** (Source: Smith 1987)

Unemployment and health

- All cross-sectional studies show the employed to be in better health than the unemployed. Longitudinal studies strongly suggest that the contrast is caused by unemployment rather than by selection within the labour market.
- The main causes of mortality among the unemployed are malignant neoplasms (particularly lung cancer), accidents, poisonings and violence (particularly suicide).
- Relative poverty, social isolation and the lack of self-esteem, and damaging health-related behaviours are the major factors associated with the production of ill effects among the unemployed.

Labelling and stigma

Labelling and stigma are terms used to describe negative evaluations made by individuals or groups about other individuals or groups. The terms are significant for medical practitioners for two reasons. First, negative labels are not infrequently applied by the public at large to people with particular diseases such as epilepsy or schizophrenia. Second, medical practitioners act as important labellers in much of what they do.

Doctors and labelling

A psychiatrist has a pivotal role in diagnosing mental illness. When such a diagnosis is made it may result in institutional care. General practitioners sign sick notes and declare people unfit to work. A chest physician may be called upon to assess the degree of loss of lung function in a man with asbestos-related illness who is making an insurance claim against his former employer. In each of these three examples the medical diagnosis is also an important social label. The medical diagnosis is a biological or medical explanation of some underlying pathology in the body or mind. However, that diagnosis has social effects that go well beyond biology and may have profound social consequences for the person so labelled.

Social reaction

The behaviour of people at large may be strongly influenced by medical labels. For example, knowing that someone has epilepsy, or has been a patient in a psychiatric hospital, can strongly affect the way others respond to him/her. They are responding not just to the biological pathology, but to what they regard as its social significance. When the social significance of the label carries a strongly negative quality, this is referred to as stigma. The two terms – labelling and stigma – are not interchangeable because certain labels are highly positive. However, in the context of medical work, it is the negative attributions by self or others that are of particular significance.

The case study shows that an important distinction needs to be made between the presence of some deviation from normality – the

---

Case study

Negative labels applied to self: the case of coronary heart disease

A middle aged man has begun to experience the early symptoms of angina. He does not know what the pains are and he merely assumes they are caused by his playing vigorous games of cricket with his grandson. So long as he believes his pains are harmless, he will do nothing to alter his behaviour; indeed he continues to smoke and to drink alcohol as he has done for the last 40 years. A biological abnormality is present that could be medically detected but has not been. Therefore, it has had no social consequence for the man or his family.

However, let us assume this man goes for a routine insurance medical because he wants to alter his pension plan. He describes his symptoms and the doctor suspects heart disease. Following investigation, coronary heart disease is diagnosed. The medical label is applied and treatment can begin. But let us also imagine how the man feels. He is now a patient who thinks of himself as a cardiac case. He is very frightened. He immediately stops smoking. He also gives up drinking and goes onto a low-fat diet. He becomes extremely concerned about over-exertion and gives up playing cricket with his grandson. His wife also becomes anxious and discourages him from digging the garden and insists that he sit in an armchair at home. Finally, he is unable to get additional insurance and alter his pension. We can see that this man's life has been transformed, even though biologically speaking his angina is no worse now than it was before he had his medical check-up. However, his own behaviour, that of his wife and, indeed, that of his insurance company have all changed as a consequence of the medical label.

---

presence of unrecognized coronary heart disease, and the social reaction to the diagnosis – the change in the man's behaviour and the response of his wife and the insurance company. Sociologists have called this distinction *primary* and *secondary deviation* (Lemert 1951). Primary deviation is some kind of physical or social difference of an individual or a group. Secondary deviation is the response of self and others to the public recognition – the label – of that difference.

This idea of primary and secondary deviation was originally developed in the context of crime by Edwin Lemert (1951). He noted that many people commit crimes. He also noted that for the vast majority of people this is only a brief excursion into things like petty shoplifting or speeding in their car. The point was that these activities did not lead to a life of crime. Indeed, the vast majority of people who have at one time or another transgressed the law actually regard themselves as morally upright citizens. For most people, in other words, their lawbreaking has no long-term effects because it is not detected and it is not punished. Their lawbreaking is primary deviation since a deviant act has been committed. Secondary deviation occurs if and when the general public, the courts and the police respond to an individual as a criminal and that person's whole life

gets caught up in that social role.

There are many examples of this process. People who are HIV positive will look no different from the way they did before they acquired their positive status (see pp. 106–107). However, once they themselves have the knowledge that they are HIV positive, their whole life may change. They may ruminate on their own mortality and perhaps alter their sexual conduct. If their HIV status becomes publicly known, or they choose to disclose it to others, then this in turn may alter the behaviour of others to the person doing the disclosing. It is not just patients with HIV or CHD who may experience the social consequences of illness. Insurance companies and employers, for example, frequently enquire into the health status of prospective customers/employees and effectively refuse to do business or employ people on the basis of the diagnosis. It is not so much that companies or employers do not have reason to protect their interests, it is rather that in so doing, they may produce profound social and psychological consequences among those whom they refuse to do business with and to employ.

Stigma

The term stigma is most usually associated with the work of Erving Goffman (1968a), who was particularly

■ What are likely to be the primary and secondary deviations as a consequence of screening for disease? **Note:** no screening test is 100% accurate.

interested in the public humiliations and social disgrace that may happen to people where highly negative labels are applied. He made the distinction between *discreditable* and *discrediting* stigma. A discreditable stigma is one that is not known about by the world at large. Only the person with the stigmatizing condition and a few close intimates will know about it. A discrediting stigma, on the other hand, is one that cannot be hidden from other people because it is obvious and visible. People respond to the stigma rather than to the person (Fig. 1).

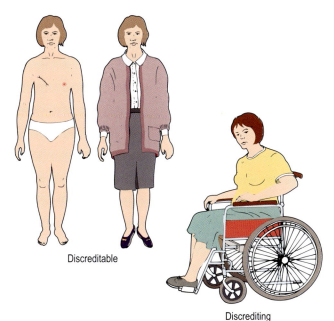

Discreditable

Discrediting

Fig. 1 **Discreditable and discrediting stigma.**

■ Not all medical conditions carry negative labels. Patients with the common cold, chickenpox, measles, and influenza, or who fracture their legs playing soccer, do not generally attract stigmatizing labels, and the social response of the general public is usually unremarkable. Indeed, such illnesses may attract sympathy. Why do these illnesses attract sympathy?

■ Problems such as alcoholism, schizophrenia, syphilis, HIV/AIDS, and epilepsy, however, frequently do attract highly negative labels. What is the reason for these conditions attracting negative labels?

■ Will smoking-related diseases, and diseases related to poor diet and lack of exercise, come to carry stigmatizing labels in years to come?

■ What are the implications of the existence of groups of illnesses that are stigmatized for the provision of care?

A good example of a discreditable stigma is a patient who has had a mastectomy or an ileostomy (see pp. 114–115). To people in the street such patients look quite normal when they are fully clothed. Apart from their closest intimates, their doctor and the few other people they might wish to inform, theirs is a hidden stigma. Other people do not react to it because they do not know about it. The person with a mastectomy or an ileostomy may go to great lengths to conceal it – say by not going to a swimming pool and never getting undressed in front of strangers. The existence of their mastectomy or ileostomy has an important effect on their own behaviour, but not the behaviour of others (Kelly 1991).

In contrast, someone with an amputation, or who is in a wheelchair, or who has lost an eye, does not have the option of concealing these things from others and people respond on the basis of the visible difference rather than the person (Fig. 1). What this means is that for some disabilities and disease conditions, the person has much less control over the publicly available information about them than is the case in other disabilities and diseases. As that information may be the basis of judgements, both positive and negative, and these judgements can have profound social and psychological effects, they are important medical issues.

Felt stigma and enacted stigma

A distinction that is sometimes made is between *enacted stigma* and *felt stigma*. Enacted stigma is the real experience of prejudice, discrimination and disadvantage as the consequence of a particular condition, say epilepsy. However, the research shows, at least in the case of epilepsy, that such frank negative stigmatization and labelling is thankfully relatively rare (Scambler and Hopkins 1986). However, it is the fear that such discrimination might occur – which is defined as felt stigma – that can be so worrying. This is why the degree to which people feel able to be in control of information about themselves is so important. In epilepsy, for example, the worry may stem from the fact that the disease is not well controlled, and the concern is about having a seizure in public.

Labelling and stigma

■ Labelling refers to the social response of individuals and groups to physical, psychological or social differences in others.
■ Medical diagnoses are an extremely important example of labels, and doctors are key people in some labelling processes.
■ Not all labels are negative, but some medical ones certainly are.
■ Primary deviation refers to the fact of biological, physical or social difference.
■ Secondary deviation refers to the social response of the individual and others to the difference.
■ Stigma is a particularly negative form of labelling.
■ The fear of stigmatization is a very powerful force affecting people's behaviour.

What is prevention?

The goals of prevention are to preserve and promote good health in society by preventing disease and minimizing its consequences. It is useful to distinguish between three types of prevention, usually referred to as primary, secondary and tertiary prevention. The distinction between these three types of prevention is that each has a different goal. Have a look at Table 1 before you read on.

Primary prevention: disease incidence

The incidence of disease is measured in terms of the number of new cases of disease occurring in society, usually during a specified time period, such as 1 year. Primary prevention can be undertaken whenever the cause of disease has been identified.

Perhaps the best-known form of medical intervention in primary prevention is mass immunization. Over the years, immunization has been introduced against poliomyelitis, tuberculosis, measles and many other diseases. However, since it usually takes several years of medical research before a virus is identified and a vaccine developed, the impact of immunization on disease incidence is sometimes very small. Poliomyelitis immunization is probably one of the few medical interventions to have had a demonstrable primary prevention effect in the last century (Fig. 1).

Health education (e.g. advice to use condoms during sex) and public health measures that help people avoid contact with viruses and bacteria may be particularly valuable early interventions.

The major causes of death in developed countries today are diseases of the circulatory system and neoplasms (see pp. 40–41). These diseases have been linked to particular behaviours, such as smoking cigarettes. Figure 2 shows that smokers' life expectancy during the last century has increased only half as much as that of non-smokers, a remarkable finding given the improvements in nutrition and sanitation that have occurred during the same period. In developed countries primary prevention efforts have been particularly concerned with health education regarding personal behaviours (see pp. 68–69).

Secondary prevention: disease prevalence

Prevalence is defined as the number of people who have a particular disease at any one time. Clearly, if diseases are left untreated and new cases are occurring all the time, the prevalence of a disease will increase. Although doctors are continually involved in secondary prevention, from time to time campaigns are mounted to increase the likelihood of doctors detecting particular diseases. For example, skin cancer may go unrecognized by patients and doctors unless specific efforts are made to identify it during consultations. Some forms of secondary prevention, such as screening for relatively rare diseases such as cervical cancer, require the participation of practically all women in society if those with the disease are to be detected and the screening programme is to prove cost-effective. Efforts to persuade people to take part may, therefore, be seen by some as efforts to compel people to participate in secondary prevention programmes, and doctors delivering these services need to be aware of the anxieties people have about screening tests (see pp. 64–65).

Tertiary prevention: adverse consequences of disease

As a result of increased life expectancy there is increasing concern for the care of people who survive treatment of, for example, heart disease, cancer or stroke. This means ensuring that patients experience the best possible health for the longest possible period of time following diagnosis. Tertiary prevention is concerned with a wider range of health indices than either primary or secondary prevention. For instance, tertiary preventive interventions might have as their goals the reduction of disability and promotion of psychological well-being.

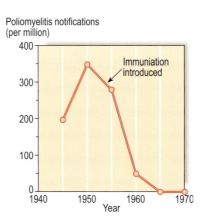

Fig. 1 **Poliomyelitis notifications before and after introduction of immunization: England and Wales** (adapted from McKeown 1979)

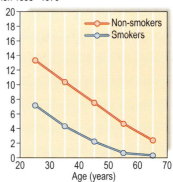

Fig. 2 **Increase in expectation of life of men 1838–1970** (adapted from McKeown 1979)

Table 1 **Goals of prevention**			
Type of prevention	**Distal goal**	**Proximal goal**	**Behavioural goal**
Primary prevention	**Prevent new cases of disease**		
	Prevent new cases of AIDS	Prevent infection with HIV	Use of condoms during sexual intercourse
Secondary prevention	**Reduce number of people with disease at a given time**		
	Reduce cases of cervical cancer	Identify cervical cancer early and treat effectively	Uptake of test to detect cancer and pre-cancer Uptake of treatment
Tertiary prevention	**Minimize consequences of disease or impairment**		
	Minimize disability in children with cerebral palsy	Identify disability	Uptake and maintenance of skills training

Table 2 **Levels of intervention to achieve behavioural change: fat in the diet**		
Level of intervention	**Example of intervention**	**Behavioural changes**
Governmental/societal	Legislation requiring manufacturers to specify the fat content of products on packaging	Agricultural policies to restrict animal fattening Research investment to develop low-fat food products Department of Health incentives to doctors to undertake prevention
Social/environmental	Mass-media health education	Provision of low-fat choices in schools/ worksite canteens
Individual	Screening by doctors to assess risk and provide motivation and healthy-eating advice	Rehabilitation programmes by nurses and doctors to promote diet change, e.g following heart attacks Food and cookery demonstrations and workshops in community centres School health education to provide motivation and skills

Exercise and rehabilitation programmes may be provided in medical settings and during follow-up care to enable stroke survivors to walk and acquire control over a range of movements (see pp. 116–117).

Chronic conditions that are genetically acquired or acquired during childhood or early adulthood are also a focus of tertiary prevention. These conditions cannot be cured, but much can be done to minimize the extent to which they result in disability or distress. A person with asthma can exercise control over his or her condition by using medication effectively and practising behavioural strategies to avoid attacks.

Levels of intervention

The success of prevention depends to a great extent upon the ability of the health-care system and health-care professionals to deliver preventive interventions to people who believe themselves to be in good health, and on the extent to which people take up interventions and are motivated and able to comply with behavioural recommendations. In order to bring about behavioural change, it is important to acknowledge the cultural and social influences that govern behaviour (see pp. 72–73).

Strategies to change behaviour occur at many different levels (see Table 2). Action by governments is important in facilitating health-related behavioural change, among both doctors and patients. For instance, in 1990 the British government changed the general practitioner contract in order to encourage greater participation in preventive health care. One target for change was in primary and secondary prevention of heart disease. GPs were offered financial inducements to encourage them to screen patients with respect to their diet, smoking habits, exercise and blood cholesterol levels, and to offer appropriate treatments or behavioural-change clinics to help people to modify their lifestyle. Governments may also seek to prevent heart disease by imposing taxes on cigarettes to limit their consumption or passing legislation that ensures that the fat content of food is clearly marked on labels so that people are able to make informed choices about their diet.

A second level of change concerns attempts to modify the social environment or commonly held views about health and health-related behaviours. People will be unable to change their diet if they have limited access to fruit and vegetables in local shops or works canteens. Community-and organizational-level interventions can do a great deal to assist individual behavioural change. People are very much influenced in their behaviour by what they see or believe others do, and by what they think will be approved or disapproved of by others (see pp. 54–55).

At an individual level, health-care professionals are directly involved in communicating to patients what preventive strategies they might use and advising them on how to implement these strategies. Doctors' advice to patients can be very effective in motivating people to change. Many preventive behaviours require people to acquire new skills and confidence in their ability to control or promote their own health. It is on the development and delivery of effective behaviour-change strategies that much of primary and tertiary prevention depends (see pp. 70–71).

Dilemmas and problems in prevention

For many years, prevention has been seen to be the province of a specialty known as public health medicine. A shift towards prevention requires that all health professionals acquire new skills in the effective communication of health-education messages and behaviour-change strategies.

Some forms of prevention rely upon the participation of everyone in society in order to make them cost-effective. For example, infectious disease control depends, to a large extent, on what is known in epidemiology as herd immunity. These considerations may have led some to question how we distinguish between education, persuasion and compulsion. Other forms of prevention that are now becoming available rely on the detection of fetal abnormalities. The introduction of genetic screening has raised concerns about the ethics of parental choice and society's view of those with genetic disorders (see also pp. 66–67).

STOP THINK

- How might you go about making a case for spending money on prevention?
- What ethical issues are associated with preventive programmes to (a) immunize all children, (b) screen all women for cervical cancer, (c) ban worksite smoking, and (d) conduct genetic tests for fetal abnormalities?
- What skills do doctors require in order to practise preventive medicine effectively?

What is prevention?

- Primary prevention refers to the prevention of disease incidence.
- Secondary prevention refers to the prevention of disease prevalence.
- Tertiary prevention refers to the prevention of disease impact.
- Preventive efforts occur at many levels: the governmental or societal policy level, the social or environmental level and the individual level.

Health screening

Wilson & Junger criterea

Health screening is potentially very valuable as part of preventive medicine. For those who screen positively there is the possibility of early diagnosis or early identification of risk with the resulting benefits of early medical intervention. Those who screen negatively are likely to benefit from reassurance. However, the usefulness of health screening may be limited if the uptake rate is low or if no benefits are obtained by patients found to be positive on screening. In addition, there may be disadvantages to patients if the techniques simply serve to increase their anxiety.

Procedures have been developed for screening patients for disease (e.g. phenylketonuria, breast cancer), for precursors of disease (e.g. cervical cytology, HIV test and tests for chromosome abnormality) or for risk factors for disease (e.g. smoking, poor diet, hypertension).

Screening: process and results

Usually those found to be positive will go on to have further tests which will determine whether the first result was a true or false positive. Since no screening test is perfect, there will always be a number of false positives and false negatives and the number will depend on the sensitivity and specificity of the test. The four possible outcomes of screening are shown in Figure 1.

Uptake of screening

No test achieves 100% uptake by the relevant population. Doctors may fail to offer the test and patients may not accept it if offered. While the reasons for patients declining a test have been investigated in some detail, research suggests that doctors may not offer a test even when it would be appropriate, perhaps when the doctor thinks the test is ineffective or believes the patients would not take the

appropriate actions (e.g. change diet, adopt safer sex procedures), or simply forgets to offer the test. If a test is not offered, the patient will be unable to make an informed decision.

Those offered a test may refuse to take it because it is incompatible with their health beliefs (see pp. 146–147), for instance, they may not think they are susceptible to the condition being tested. For example, women were more likely to have amniocentesis if they thought they were likely to have a Down's baby; and uptake was related to *perceived* risk, but not to *actual* risk as indicated by the maternal age. Patients may also decide not to have a test, for example, when a pregnant woman declines tests on her fetus because she would not consider termination of pregnancy.

Adverse effects for those tested

Patients show high levels of anxiety when being screened and awaiting results. Informing the patient that the test is negative lowers anxiety more effectively than telling them to assume the result was normal if they hear nothing more. However, even communicating a negative result can have adverse effects. A *true negative* result can be harmful if the individual overgeneralizes the reassurance; pregnant women screened negative for spina bifida and Down's syndrome frequently believe the tests showed that their babies would be normal. A *false negative* result can be harmful if it prevents the patient from receiving appropriate treatment or advice on lifestyle; a false negative HIV test might result in the patient putting others at risk by sexual transmission and remove the motivation to adopt safer sexual practices.

Patients testing positive

Following a positive screening-test result, there are further stages of tests, results and medical management. Each of these involves further social and behavioural processes, as shown in Figure 2.

When the initial test result is positive or ambiguous but is followed by a clear negative result, i.e. the patient has received an initial *false positive* or invalid result, patients may

continue to be anxious long after being told the negative result.

If the result is a true positive, patients' reactions will tend to vary with the implications of the results, depending on the seriousness of the condition and the available preventive or curative medical treatment. Nevertheless, there may be unexpected reactions. For example, individuals found to be positive for genetic disease such as Huntington's chorea or polyposis have reported feeling relieved, perhaps because their uncertainty was reduced.

When screening identifies people at risk of disease, there may be adverse effects of labelling the individual and it has been found that they may respond *as if they are ill* rather than just at risk (pp. 60–61). Studies of people shown on screening to have hypertension have found that they subsequently show higher levels of distress, report more symptoms, take more time off work, and participate less in social activities. The level of distress is affected by the way in which the diagnosis is communicated. For example, those informed that they were hypertensive and given leaflets describing hypertension as 'the silent killer' were more anxious months later than those fully informed that it was a risk factor and reassured about management (Rudd et al 1986).

Implications of a positive result

For some test results, such as Huntington's chorea, the result carries no specific implications for action in a clinical context, although the recipient may choose to make relevant plans for the future. For other tests, such as genetic tests with a probabilistic rather than certain result, there may be continued uncertainty and further clinical monitoring will be required. For yet others, such as hypertension, appropriate medical management may reduce the likelihood or severity of the condition.

Other positive results may require the recipient to make critical decisions (such as whether to terminate a pregnancy) or to consider changes in behaviour and lifestyle (such as reducing fat intake or practising safer sex). While there is ample evidence that many people will make these

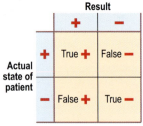

Fig. 1 **Four possible outcomes of a screening test.**

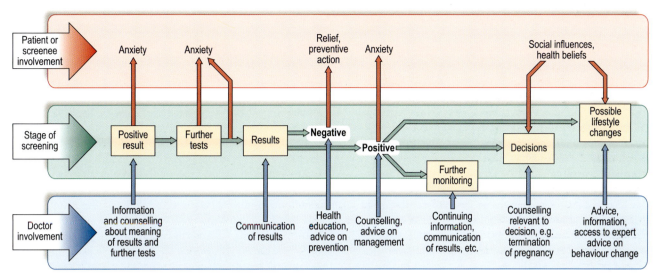

Fig. 2 **Schematic outline of health screening and the social and behavioural factors involved — the process following a positive result.**

changes successfully, a substantial number of people will attempt to change and fail. The overall success of the screening programme may be limited by failures to change behaviours in those screening positive.

The role of doctors

Doctors may play key roles at every stage (see Fig. 2 and list below). The results of screening, both in terms of successful detection and management of clinical conditions and in terms of the potential adverse effects for those tested, depend on the doctors' behaviours. The role of doctors in screening includes:

- offering screening: inviting the individual to attend without raising unnecessary fears
- counselling about screening: giving information about procedures, potential benefits and limitations, and checking comprehension, thereby enabling the individual to reach an informed decision
- providing health education: before screening, e.g. for serum cholesterol or HIV; after positive screening, e.g. for risk factors for cardiovascular disease
- communicating results that may be complex: providing enough information to enable patients to understand; achieving a balance between raising unnecessary anxiety and giving inappropriate reassurance
- advising on decisions following positive results: giving information to enable informed choice and consent
- clinical management: varies depending on the type of screening
- assisting individuals to make necessary lifestyle changes: e.g. smoking, diet, exercise, medication, safer sex, repeated screening or monitoring.

STOP THINK

- Think of one area of health screening, such as in pregnancy, for genetic disease, or for cardiovascular risk factors. Follow the flow charts in Figure 2 and consider what adverse effects might arise at each stage. How might doctors minimize these adverse effects?

Case study

Mrs Green had been alarmed to be recalled for further tests after blood tests suggested something might be wrong with her baby. She had taken a long time to conceive and this was a much-wanted child. Although she thought the pregnancy might already show, she felt she could not tell her friends at work until she got the result of the amniocentesis and could be sure the baby was all right. After the amniocentesis, the obstetrician said there was nothing to worry about as the test result was normal. However, Mrs Green continued to be concerned – why had the original test been positive? Surely that indicated something was wrong, after all 'There's no smoke without fire' – if one test was positive and one was normal, how could the doctors be sure which one was right? Her continuing anxiety led her to be on the lookout for signs that things were going wrong even after the birth of her normal healthy baby.

Health screening

- For any screening test, a substantial number of those offered the test do not accept – a result of poor information, social influences or, in some cases, good decisions.
- Screening may have adverse effects, especially raised anxiety, which may persist even when the result is normal.
- The way in which results are communicated can affect the impact of the results on the individual.
- Those being screened require information and counselling before and after screening.
- For some tests, those being screened may need health education and advice on behaviour and lifestyle change.
- People do not always succeed in making lifestyle changes without further professional assistance.

The social implications of the new genetics

Developments in molecular genetics have major implications for society and individuals, doctors and patients. The knowledge and techniques which have arisen from the development of recombinant DNA are likely to affect profoundly how we think about and deal with health, risks to health, disease and illness (Cunningham-Burley and Boulton 2000, Pilnick 2002). The search for genetic components to a range of diseases, behaviours and traits is well underway.

The new genetics touches the social, cultural, ethical and personal realms as well as the biological, and has implications for some of the fundamental principles that guide research and clinical practice – confidentiality, autonomy, informed consent and individual choice. The new genetics promises great improvements in health, and increased control and choice for individuals, especially in relation to reproduction. Many scientists, clinicians and others take the social and ethical implications seriously and contribute to the important debate about how this knowledge may be used (Nuffield Council on Bioethics 1993).

Genetic testing

The genes for many single-gene disorders have been identified, and genetic components in common multifactorial conditions are now being researched. Testing for a range of genetic diseases (e.g. for late-onset dominant conditions or for carrier status for single-gene recessive disorders) is now available in many industrialized countries. Experience gained in the introduction of existing genetic-testing programmes provides a good illustration of the social, cultural and ethical issues involved, and may help shape the application of scientific development in the future.

Predictive testing: Huntington's disease

Huntington's disease is an autosomal dominant condition. All those who inherit the gene will develop the disorder; it is of late adult onset, fatal and untreatable. Definitive testing is now available that can identify those who will develop the disease. At first glance, the provision of predictive testing within families known to be at risk of Huntington's disease may seem to be desirable, not least because an individual who has been identified as inheriting the gene may wish to control their own reproduction. It can be anticipated that any testing brings with it specific concerns about the rights of individuals to know or not know their genetic status, the rights of other family members to information and the psychological impact of a positive result. However, the experience of introducing predictive testing for Huntington's disease has thrown up other pertinent issues, and few individuals have actually come forward for testing. Those who have fall into three different groups:

■ Those who want to be tested in order to plan their lives or avoid passing the gene on to children.
■ Those who want to obtain an early diagnosis (they are already suspecting symptoms).
■ Those who want to establish that they are free from the disease (they are past the age when they would be likely to develop symptoms).

Several reasons have been identified to explain why people have not come forward for testing. Firstly, a positive test result would have implications for their existing children, some of whom may have inherited the disorder. Secondly, there is no effective treatment for the disease, so testing may not bring any medical benefits. Thirdly, some people were worried about the loss of health insurance. Lastly, some felt that the completion of their own childbearing removed any reason to have the test. It has also been found that both positive and negative results can cause distress to individuals and their families. Those found to be free of the disease may experience survivor guilt. The certainty provided through testing is not always welcomed. Families have lived with uncertainty in terms of the risk status of its members, and this uncertainty forms a crucial part of identity and experience (Richards 1993). The experience of introducing testing for Huntington's disease suggests that the information is not always desired by those at risk, and that an individual's right to refuse to be tested must be preserved. The situation is even more uncertain in relation to genetic susceptibility for disease. The case study identifies some dilemmas relating to testing for susceptibility for breast cancer (see also Hallowell 2000).

Carrier testing for recessive disorders: beta-thalassaemia

Beta-thalassaemia is an inherited blood disorder. If both parents are carriers of the trait, there is a one in four chance of passing the disease on to their child, while carriers themselves remain free from the disease. The disease can be fatal without proper treatment, and the treatment is complex. Knowledge of carrier status makes possible greater reproductive choice, particularly the use of prenatal diagnosis and the abortion of affected fetuses where this is personally and culturally acceptable. In Cyprus, where the trait is common, the orthodox church insists that people are aware of their carrier status for beta-thalassaemia when they marry. Where both partners are carriers, the couple then use prenatal diagnosis and

> ## Case study
>
> Susan is 32 years old and has two young daughters. Her mother died from breast cancer at the age of 56 years. She thinks that other female relatives may have had breast cancer. Susan had not really given her risk of breast cancer much thought and certainly viewed herself as a healthy person. However, when her older sister was diagnosed, she began to think it might be 'in the family'. She had read that susceptibility genes had been identified (BRCA1 and 2) for some familial breast cancers and that the test was available to those at risk. She wondered whether this could explain her family history and what the consequences of that would mean. Would she want to be tested? How would she discuss this with her sister? What might happen to her – would she have to have both her breasts removed or would she just have regular check-ups? After worrying about all these things for several weeks, she decided to see her GP. On the basis of her family history, the GP referred her to a clinical geneticist.

abortion to avoid the birth of an affected child. Abortion is accepted on these grounds, but not on others. This programme has virtually eliminated the births of children with beta-thalassaemia in Cyprus.

Screening for carrier status can raise a range of other issues too. For example, screening for sickle cell trait in the USA demonstrated that stigma can be attached to carrier status, leading to further discrimination of black people (see pp. 46–47). Additionally, where people do not perceive themselves to be at risk, because they have little direct knowledge of the disease being detected through carrier testing, uptake has been low, for example, with testing for cystic fibrosis carrier status in parts of the UK (Marteau and Anionwu 1996).

Understanding susceptibility to common diseases

Most diseases are multifactorial in aetiology, involving the interaction of many genes with each other and with the environment. Research may lead to tests to identify genetic susceptibility to a range of common diseases in individuals. One major research investment in the UK is Biobank UK, where healthy volunteers aged between 45 and 69 years will contribute genetic, lifestyle and medical histories to a database. This will then be further investigated and analyzed in order to promote a better understanding of common disorders and to develop appropriate treatments.

Population screening for susceptibility to disease could be beneficial where treatment or lifestyle modification improves health outcome. With the development of pharmacogenetics, treatments may become better suited to an individual's genotype. However, population screening raises concerns (Clarke 1995, Willis 2002). Firstly, screening whole populations in order to identify individuals with genetic susceptibility to common diseases is commercially attractive to those corporations developing tests and treatments. Secondly, like other forms of screening, those not considered at high risk may view themselves as invulnerable to disease, while those at high risk may not necessarily be helped, especially if lifestyle modification is difficult or treatment options limited. Thirdly, population screening may lead to a view that genes determine health. The geneticization of disease may result in a neglect of other solutions to the problem of ill health, such as social and environmental interventions.

Limits to the use of genetic technology and genetic explanations for disease

Two general issues are relevant to the application of knowledge gained from research into the genetic components of diseases and behaviours: eugenics and individual choice.

Eugenics

Concerns about eugenic control of populations are sometimes raised. The identification of genes implicated in disease can quickly lead to the availability of tests, such as those for Huntington's disease and beta-thalassaemia outlined above. Where such testing aims to provide people with the information to make informed decisions (e.g. greater choice in relation to reproduction in order not to pass on the disease to their children), this can mean aborting affected fetuses. The elimination of disease in this way may add to the stigma and discrimination currently experienced by disabled people in our society, and may affect the resources available for their care. Concerns also relate to the potential increase in the number of tests available and, therefore, the range of diseases that may be deemed serious enough for interventions of this kind.

Individual choice

Many of the concerns expressed about eugenics are muted by the presence of individual choice in democratic societies. The rights of individuals to choose whether to be tested and whether to abort affected fetuses are considered paramount: there should be no coercion to make a particular decision. While the preservation of individual choice is important, it is also crucial to recognize that decisions are not made in a social vacuum. There are many constraints on individuals that can make one choice more favoured than another. There may be subtle rather than overt pressures to conform to what is expected to be the obvious or right decision, or people may not have sufficient information with which to make informed decisions. Where there are inequalities, discrimination and concerns about the costs of care, the extent of choice available to individuals is culturally and socially restrained.

Practical application

Those involved in health care should be aware of the effects on individual patients and on society more generally. Within consultations, it will be important to discuss social and ethical issues with patients, and consider the context within which decisions are made. It is also important for doctors to work towards ensuring that the possible negative outcomes of genetics (e.g. increased discrimination, stigma and inequality) are minimized. This can be achieved through self-regulation, through engaging in open and public discussion, and through actively promoting regulation and control of those institutions whose functioning is likely to be directly influenced by genetic research and its application – insurance, employment and health-care provision.

- Will research into the genetic basis of disease lead to geneticization, where other causes are ignored?
- How can we avoid the stigma and discrimination that those with genetic disease may face?
- What sort of information will help informed decision-making for patients?

The social implications of the new genetics

- Research into the genetic basis for disease can quickly lead to applications in clinical practice, but we need to be sure of the ethical and social consequences.
- Genetic testing raises important social and ethical issues for individuals, doctors and society, and these need to be discussed and debated openly.
- Decisions taken by patients and doctors should be understood within their social, cultural and economic context; these may vary across cultures and social groups.

Changing people's beliefs and attitudes

Often we can change people's behaviour by changing their environment. Changing the consequences of action by changing the law or the ease with which people can act affects what they do. For example, making condoms, dental care or medication easy to access and inexpensive is crucial to health promotion. We may also be able to change behaviours by changing how they think about the world (i.e. their 'cognitions', see pp. 146–147).

The health belief model (HBM) can be applied to increase the proportion of emergency patients who attend follow-up appointments (see pp. 92–93). Champion (1994) evaluated another intervention based on the HBM. This time the aim was to increase mammography attendance amongst women over 35 years old. A randomized controlled trial was used to compare four conditions: 1) a no-intervention control group; 2) an information-giving intervention, 3) an individual counselling intervention designed to change HBM-specified beliefs and 4) a combination intervention designed to provide information and change health beliefs. Controlling for attendance levels prior to intervention, the results indicated that only the combination intervention had a significantly greater post-intervention adherence rate than the control group. This group were almost four times more likely to be adherent to attendance guidelines. This suggests that both information provision and belief change are required to maximize

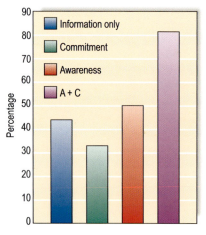

Fig. 1 **Cognitive dissonance and health promotion. Percentage buying condoms.** (Source: Stone et al 1994).

mammography adherence. The belief change interventions resulted in greater perceived seriousness, greater benefits and reduced barriers but not increased susceptibility.

Contradictions and change

Festinger (1957) and others have observed that people tend to seek consistency in their beliefs. Festinger's cognitive dissonance theory proposes that being aware of two inconsistent cognitions (e.g. beliefs or attitudes) causes an aversive psychological state, which we are motivated to eliminate through cognitive change. For example, being aware that smoking makes one susceptible to serious illnesses and that one is a smoker may facilitate cognitive change.

An experiment by Stone et al. (1994) shows the relevance of cognitive dissonance theory to health promotion. In this study participants were randomly allocated to four conditions: 1) receiving information about condom use (information only); 2) receiving information and giving a talk promoting condom use that might be used in health education in schools (commitment); 3) being made aware of past failures to use condoms by recalling these failures (awareness), and 4) a combination of the commitment and awareness conditions. All participants were then given an opportunity to buy condoms. Figure 1 shows that generating commitment and making participants aware of their own past failures led to greater condom purchase than the other three strategies. Participants in the combined condition (4) would have found it difficult to change the belief that condom use was worthwhile, because they had been persuaded to promote the importance of condom use. Yet they could not change their awareness of their own past failures to use condoms. In these circumstances, cognitive dissonance theory predicts that they would seek to reduce their cognitive dissonance by distancing themselves from their past failures. Affirming the intention to use condoms in the future, and regarding themselves as different from the person who failed to use condoms in the past, resolves the cognitive contradiction created by the 'hypocrisy'

condition. Hence many more people in this group (82% versus 50% in the awareness condition) took the opportunity to buy condoms. This study also emphasizes that providing people with information alone may not be enough to motivate them to take action (only 44% bought condoms in the information only condition).

In the experiment described above the researchers made it easy for participants to buy condoms. However, perceived control over action is not always high. For example, a smoker may not find it easy to distance herself from her smoking past and so may not resolve to give up. Instead, she may resolve her dissonance by changing her beliefs about susceptibility to future illness. She may, for example, convince herself that her genetic make-up will protect her from the risks of smoking or, alternatively, that other risks mean that she will die prematurely whether or not she smokes (see pp. 84–85). Thus it is critical to take account of perceived barriers and perceived control when attempting to make people to change their behaviour (see pp. 146–147). In some cases this may mean that people have to learn new skills before they can change their behaviour. For example, how to cook tasty meals with vegetables, how to relax without smoking or drinking alcohol, or how to discuss condom use with a partner.

How people process persuasive messages

The way in which people are persuaded by a message designed to change their beliefs or attitudes can also affect the extent to which they remain persuaded and the impact that such persuasion has on their behaviour. Petty and Cacioppo (1986) argued that people put more or less cognitive effort into the way in which they process persuasive messages. They called this 'cognitive elaboration' and their model is known as the 'elaboration likelihood model' (ELM). When people think about the content of a message, and consider and evaluate the arguments put forward in terms of what they already know, this is known as 'central route' processing (involving cognitive elaboration). Persuasion by this route is most likely to lead to longer-term changes in

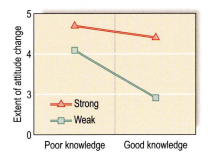

Fig. 2 **Prior knowledge and the effect of argument strength on persuasion.** (Source: Wood et al 1985).

attitudes and to influence action. However, people may not always be able or willing to devote the cognitive resources necessary for central route processing. In this case, they may make decisions about persuasive messages without properly understanding and evaluating the arguments. For instance, when people are under time pressure, or do not understand what's being said, or think that the issue is not especially relevant to them, they may be persuaded without central route processing. They may decide on the basis of what they feel about the message or use simple rules such as 'expertise = accuracy', i.e. she's an expert so that must be right, or 'consensus = correctness', i.e. if so many people agree they must be right (Chaiken 1980). This kind of cognitive processing is called 'peripheral route' processing. When people are persuaded in this way the apparent belief changes may not be sustained because underlying knowledge and beliefs have not been related to the new information.

If we want to persuade people of health-promotion messages (see pp. 74–75) we need to ensure that they have the opportunity and motivation to engage in central route processing. One barrier to understanding messages is a lack of knowledge. If we cannot understand a message we cannot engage in central route processing (see pp. 92–93). Peripheral route processing also makes it more likely that people will be persuaded by weak arguments because they are not evaluating the arguments, whereas those who use central route processing will be able to dismiss weak arguments. We can see this effect in data from an experiment by Wood et al (1985). They compared the impact of messages containing weak and strong arguments on people who had either good or poor prior knowledge. Figure 2 shows that those with good knowledge changed their attitudes in response to the strong arguments, but were not persuaded by weak arguments. By contrast, those with poor knowledge, who we can assume were engaged in peripheral route processing, showed almost as much attitude change in response to weak as strong arguments.

Encouraging people to take greater responsibility for their health is an important aim for health services. This will be facilitated when people develop good knowledge. For example, knowledge of how their body works, what symptoms mean and how medication has its effect. Presenting well-informed people with well-argued messages that appear relevant to them, in a manner that allows them to concentrate on and revisit presented information, will enhance cognitive processing and persuasion. Persuading people of a new position and then contrasting this with their current behaviour can generate cognitive dissonance and

thereby motivate change. However, behaviour change is only likely to follow from attitudinal and motivational change when people have confidence in their ability to change and can do so in a supported and graded manner. Where this is not possible people may reject health promotion messages and reaffirm attitudes associated with health risk behaviours (see pp. 24–25 and pp. 70–71).

■ Imagine you want to persuade an over-weight patient to take more exercise. What would you say to her? What cognitive processes might you think about in deciding what to say? Why might giving this person free membership of a gym fail to increase the amount she exercised?

Case study

Henry has been intending to stop smoking for a number of years and had stopped for a day or two on a few occasions. He now feels he cannot stop because it makes him feel so bad. Henry is reluctantly persuaded to go to a smoking-cessation clinic. They offer him nicotine patches and teach him simple relaxation procedures. They point out that this will help him give up without feeling as bad as he did on previous occasions. They also demonstrate to him that, although he thinks that smoking makes him feel better and more relaxed, the continual nicotine withdrawal actually has a negative effect on his mood that he is continually trying to compensate. Explaining how nicotine affects him helps Henry understand why he has found it so difficult to give up, and the patches and relaxation techniques bolster his confidence that he can quit. The clinic staff also emphasize how bad he is likely to feel if he does contract lung cancer, and help him acknowledge that he is worried about becoming ever more unfit. They talk through what he sees as the main barriers to giving up and plan out what he might do in the first couple of weeks to overcome these various difficulties. In Henry's case this includes going to the non-smoking coffee room during breaks at work and not going to the pub for 2 weeks. They pair Henry up with another person who is trying to quit and talk to him about what he will say to his partner about quitting. They also provide Henry with a contract that asks him to specify his reasons for (or advantages of) quitting and the day on which he will start his quit attempt. Henry begins his quit attempt the next day.

Changing people's beliefs and attitudes

■ Cognitive dissonance theory proposes that being aware of two inconsistent cognitions causes an aversive psychological state, which we are motivated to eliminate.

■ Attitude change may be prompted by cognitive dissonance but if behaviour change is thought to be difficult people may reject health-promotion messages rather than change their intentions.

■ People may process persuasive messages using the central or peripheral route. Central route processing is more likely to lead to enduring attitude change and action.

■ Providing information alone is unlikely to change behaviour, but knowledge is important to central route processing of health-relevant messages.

Helping people to act on their intentions

The theory of planned behaviour (pp. 146–147) highlights intention as an important cognitive antecedent of action. Strength of intention is a good indicator of how motivated a person is to act and how much effort they will put into trying to enact their intention. If someone does not intend to change their behaviour they are unlikely to do so. For example, across a series of studies of health-related behaviours, Sheeran (2002) found that only 7% of those who did not intend to act subsequently did so. Thus, if a patient leaves a consultation without intending to pick up a prescription and then take prescribed medication as directed, she is very unlikely to do so. Consequently, the first step in health promotion (whether encouraging exercise, smoking cessation or adherence to medication regimens) is persuading people to *decide* to change, that is, motivating them to intend to act.

Even when people intend to change they do not always succeed. Sometimes this is because they have diminished control. For example, approximately half of all smokers intend to quit over the next year but only about 30% of them try and only about 2% succeed. In this case both pharmaceutical (e.g. nicotine patches) and behavioural interventions (e.g. support groups) can help translate quitting intentions into action (Fiore et al 1996).

Even when there are no issues of dependency, people often fail to act on their intentions. Across studies of screening attendance, exercise and condom use Sheeran (2002) found that 47% of intenders failed to act on their intentions. This has been called the 'intention–behaviour gap' and has prompted psychologists to investigate cognitive processes that make it more likely that people will act on their intentions. Increased self-efficacy, anticipated regret and task analysis have been found to increase the likelihood that people act on their intentions (Fig. 1).

We have seen that perceived control or self-efficacy is important (pp. 146–147). If we lack prerequisite skills then we may fail in our attempt and abandon our intention. However, even when we just lack confidence this low

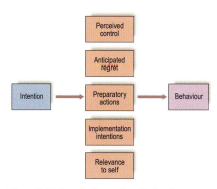

Fig. 1 **Bridging the intention–behaviour gap.**

perceived self-efficacy may result in reduced effort or poorer performance. Consequently, it is helpful to focus on past successes, the ease with which others like oneself accomplish tasks and small steps towards a goal when learning a new skill or trying to change an established behaviour. For example, Fisher and Johnston (1996) manipulated self-efficacy by inviting chronic pain patients to reflect on past experiences of high or low control and found that this manipulation altered levels of self-efficacy which, in turn, accounted for different performances on a lifting task. Those who had focused on past success were more successful at the task.

Anticipated regret can also prompt people to act on their intentions rather than remaining inactive. Regret is a powerful negative emotion that people want to avoid. Consequently, making future regret salient can help people maintain and enact intentions. In a series of studies, Abraham & Sheeran (2003) found that people with higher anticipated regret were more likely to sustain their intentions to exercise over time and to take more exercise as a result. Even amongst those with strong intentions to exercise, people with high levels of anticipated regret exercised more often than those with low levels of anticipated regret. Thus prompting people to think about the regret they will feel if they do not seize opportunities to act can help them bridge the intention–behaviour gap.

Health-related intentions may also require planning and preparatory actions. For example, one may need to acquire condoms before using them or obtain sportswear before

exercising. Thus planning a sequence of actions focusing on achievable steps that lead towards an intended outcome can facilitate the enactment of intentions. Studies have found that such task analysis can enhance perceived control. Stock and Cervone (1990) report that dividing a complex task into a series of sub-goals led to higher self-efficacy at task outset and heightened self-efficacy and satisfaction at the point of sub-task completion. This also resulted in greater overall task persistence. Consequently, helping people plan out a sequence of steps involved in what they intend to do can help promote the enactment of intentions.

People often explain why they did not do the things they intended by saying that they forgot, were too busy or did not get round to them. This usually means that they had more important or more pressing intentions which took priority over the intention that was not enacted. Thus, the intention behaviour gap is partially created by competing intentions. We intend to do many things but only act on a proportion of our intentions. Consequently, if we can prioritize any particular intention we increase the likelihood of acting on it. Linking intentions to particular environmental contexts and to one's representation of oneself can boost their priority.

Gollwitzer (1999) has shown that turning an intention into an 'implementation intention', which specifies when and where we will act, facilitates the translation of intentions into action. For example, resolving to take one's medication in the bathroom, immediately after a morning shower, or to go swimming at the local pool at 2.00pm on Friday afternoons makes it more likely that one will act rather than just intending to act. Implementation intentions enable aspects of our environment to prompt intended actions so giving them priority in that context at that particular time. For example, once an implementation intention is made to take medication in the bathroom after a morning shower, stepping out of the shower can be enough to prompt taking the medication. Without the implementation intention, a genuine intention to take medication may be postponed and then forgotten in the midst of other morning priorities. Thus by helping people to identify a time and place when they will undertake particular actions we make it more likely that they will translate their intentions into behaviour. Implementation intention formation has been shown to have this effect for a variety of health-related behaviours such as breast self examination (Orbell et al 1997, see Research Case study box), taking vitamins, attending screening and rehabilitation after surgery (Sheeran 2002).

Whether we translate intentions into action also depends on the relevance of intentions to our self representation. If a person sees herself as the type of person to whom exercise is important then she is more likely to act on an intention to begin running or swim regularly than someone who sees exercise as less relevant to who they are. If an intended action seems peripheral to our sense of self then that intention may be more likely to change over time as it is overridden by intentions more relevant to the self. Thus if someone decides to take exercise to please their partner they are less likely to take action than someone who decides they will exercise because they want to feel fit. Similarly, someone who decides to take medication to please their doctor may be less likely to succeed than someone who decides to do so because they believe the medication is important to their health. Feeling 'I want to do that' (as opposed to 'I should do that') can help prioritize an intention. Therefore, if an intention can be anchored in a person's self image or seen to serve another goal that is very important to that person (see Fig. 2) it is more likely to maintain priority in competition with other intentions. Thus achieving concordance with a patient (see pp. 92–93) is likely to involve linking new health-related intentions to the patient's view of themselves and their important goals.

When encouraging people to change their behaviour it is crucial to focus realistic intentions. When people intend to do things for which they lack the skills to initiate, or things that are difficult within their environment, they are not likely to succeed. Behaviour change must begin with things

we can achieve. Hence walking from home may be a more realistic approach to initiating exercise than joining a gym or resolving to travel to a public pool that takes time to get to. Once a small change is established further change may be easier to initiate. Even when people's intentions are realistic there are a variety of ways in which we can facilitate the translation of intentions into action: enhancing confidence or self-efficacy; highlighting anticipated regret; realistic task analysis and planning; implementation intention formation; and linking intentions to important goals.

- Imagine a patient who tells you that she always intends to take her preventive medication but never seems to manage it. What would you ask her? What might you say to help her take her medication?

Research Case study

Orbell et al (1997) promoted implementation intention formation in relation to breast self-examination (BSE) in a survey of women on a university campus. Women were asked about past BSE and their intentions to perform BSE in the next month. Intervention questionnaires were randomly distributed to half the sample. These questionnaires informed women that:

You are more likely to carry out your intention to perform BSE if you make a decision about when and where you will do so. Many women find it most convenient to perform BSE at the start of the morning or last thing at night, in the bath or shower, or while they are getting dressed in their bedroom or bathroom. Others like to do it in bed before they go to sleep or prior to getting up. Decide now where and when you will perform BSE in the next month and make a commitment to do so.

This text was absent from the control questionnaires. Women in the control and intervention groups did not differ in intention to perform BSE or experience of BSE. However, a follow-up questionnaire 1 month later found that 64% of women in the intervention had performed BSE while only 14% in the control group had done so. All of the intervention group women who had intended to perform BSE (in the first questionnaire) did so but only 53% of control group women who had intended to perform BSE did so over the month.

This study demonstrates how deciding when and where you will perform an intended action makes it more likely that you will act on your intention.

Helping people to act on their intentions

- The intention–behaviour gap may be partially bridged by enhancing perceived control and by making anticipated regret salient.
- Planning out a series of preparatory actions leading to a health goal may also make it more likely that people act on their intentions.
- Specifying when and where one will undertake a particular action makes it less likely that it will be forgotten or postponed in the specified context.
- Linking a new intention to a person's sense of themselves or to their important goals increases the likelihood they will act on that intention.

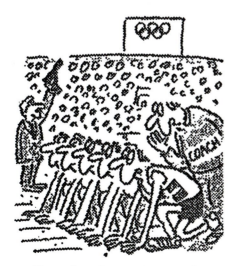

'Psst, there's someone at the finishing line who's interested in buying your house'

Fig. 2 **Linking intentions to pre-existing self-relevant goals can increase the likelihood of action.** Copyright The Daily Telegraph 2001. Reproduced with permission.

The social context of behavioural change

Few would dispute that good health is a worthy goal for individuals and for states/governments to pursue. In most industrialized countries, government health-education bodies promote healthy, and discourage unhealthy, behaviour. The emphasis on the individual's responsibility to make good health choices is evident in the messages that these authorities promulgate. We could sum up this idea in the recent Scottish slogan: 'You can save a life: your own.' However, individuals operate within a social context and we need to take this into account when considering behaviour change.

This spread looks at two ways in which behaviour change can be seen in a social context. First, the social context in which individuals come to alter their behaviour; second, the role society plays in influencing citizens' health behaviour.

The social context of individual behaviour change

There is clear evidence that behaviour such as smoking, eating large quantities of animal fats and failing to exercise is detrimental to health. Lay people are aware of this (health warnings are printed on the sides of cigarette cartons, for instance) and it seems only 'common sense' that people will make sensible decisions to change their behaviour on the basis of such information. So why do people often fail to do so?

You will see that the health belief model and the theory of planned behaviour (pp. 146–147) endorse the assumption that the individual will, indeed, think rationally about costs and benefits before engaging in particular behaviour. Both models have developed theoretically over the years and have been shown to have good predictive power in certain health domains. However, to the extent that they forefront the role of a person's cognitions (e.g. perceived susceptibility to disease) in influencing their intentions and hence behaviour, they are heirs to early research in persuasion, where it was believed that influencing behaviour was simply a matter of targeting people's thoughts (attitudes/beliefs), on the basis that attitudes cause behaviour in a fairly unproblematic way. Pioneer health promoters therefore assumed that information, once disseminated, would be sufficient to alter beliefs and hence behaviour: they were wrong!

Interestingly, advertising companies had long recognized that the most successful of campaigns will usually be effective in altering the consumption habits of only a small percentage of the targeted audience. Originally, health-education initiatives probably had too high expectations of behaviour change and, importantly, (unlike advertising campaigns designed to, say, switch the consumer's allegiance to another brand of soap powder) they were often aimed at altering behaviour that was *pleasurable*, such as smoking, and therefore of considerable consequence to people. Further, in some cultural contexts, hazardous behaviour may be valued and engaged in precisely because of the associated risk, e.g. a type of cigarette marketed under the brand name 'Death Cigarettes' has sold successfully (Bunton and Burrows 1995). A person's established behaviour may also become habitual (automatic; independent of conscious thought). As there is evidence that such a person is less likely to attend to information relating to his/her habit, persuasion is even more problematic as a behaviour-change strategy. If a habit is addictive as well, persuasion becomes only one element in a

battery of potential interventions and supports for behaviour change. Particularly important here would be the availability of appropriate alternative activities (see Case study).

Investigating 'unhealthy' behaviour

A classic study that illustrated the importance of investigating the social context of a behaviour such as smoking was that by Hilary Graham (1984). Graham argued that caring for children and managing the financial and organizational burdens of domestic life may be so stressful that smoking behaviour can be conceptualized as a coping strategy. One of her respondents, for instance, said:

> *After lunch, I'll clear away and wash up and put the telly on for Stevie (her son). I'll have a sit down on the sofa, with a cigarette . . . It's lovely, it's the one time in the day I really enjoy and I know Stevie won't disturb me. I couldn't stop, I just couldn't. It keeps me calm. It's me [sic] one relaxation is smoking.* (Graham 2000)

Here, smoking fills a critical role for the carer in that it *enables* her to be a more effective mother. Graham termed this phenomenon 'the responsibility of irresponsible behaviour'. Note that nicotine does, indeed, act neuropharmacologically to reduce stress (File et al 2001).

Studies like Graham's give us some indication of how behavioural change is constrained by social circumstances and hint at some of the reasons behind social class differences in health behaviour (and outcomes), e.g. why working-class mothers (with fewer material resources) may find it harder to give up smoking than middle-class mothers

---

Case study

Mrs Berry, a 29-year-old mother of three young children, visited her GP, Dr Hall, for advice about how to give up smoking as she was very worried about its effects on her own health and that of her children. Mrs Berry's anxiety was magnified by knowing breaking the habit would be difficult; smoking helped her remain calm and cope with the difficulties of raising children on a low income, as well as providing one of her few pleasures. Dr Hall told her that giving up was simply a question of will power, though she could try nicotine patches. Later that month, Mrs Berry hurried to the surgery with her youngest child, who had inserted a foreign body (nasturtium seed) up his nose. Dr Stephens, who dealt with the child, noticed how stressed Mrs Berry was, and enquired after her health. In the supportive atmosphere of Dr Stephens' surgery, Mrs Berry admitted that her attempts to stop smoking had been disastrous. Dr Stephens, a mother herself, realized that the main priority was finding an alternative way for Mrs Berry to achieve a sense of calm and control. Knowing that the area in which the Berrys lived was lacking in resources for families, she suggested that Mrs Berry identify other mothers who might be interested in forming an action group to lobby for some kind of recreational/playgroup facility. This seemed a daunting task, but once Mrs Berry started organizing and campaigning, her sense of agency and self-confidence increased and her need to smoke diminished. The facility the local authority eventually established provided an effective way for mothers to achieve an 'island of calm' from their children and social interaction with other adults, thus making some aspects of the task of quitting smoking a little easier (see Stead et al 2001).

(see pp. 42–43). It would be difficult, indeed, to get an idea of the sheer *complexity* of the role played by smoking in Graham's respondent's life by looking solely at psychological factors, such as her attitude towards quitting the habit.

The social context of mass behaviour change

Mass education campaigns directed at people's attitudes may have limited success in changing behaviour. Sometimes the state targets the actual behaviour by introducing sanctions: just as we might privately decide to deny ourselves a chocolate bar if we fail to complete an assignment on time, the state might implement external incentives – perhaps legal penalties – if we do not conform to a particular behaviour.

Car seat-belt legislation is a good example of this strategy: after failing to persuade people to wear seat-belts, the Swedish government made it compulsory for front-seat passengers in private cars to do so. Seat-belt use increased from 30 to 85% (Fhanér and Hane 1979). Note that rates of adherence to legislation of this kind varies across nations, reflecting the influence of wider culture.

Many people would probably agree that it would be unacceptable for the state to legislate directly to forbid practices such as smoking or drinking – except perhaps in public places (though taxation may be used to discourage them). In these cases, persuasive health-promotion campaigns aimed at our views and beliefs are the alternative.

But can you save your own life?

The UK government's current approach to health education represents us as having responsibility for our health and the freedom to choose a healthy lifestyle.

There are some problems with these ideas. Dentistry, for example, is becoming increasingly privatized, so the poor may be unable to afford oral health no matter how strongly they value it. The classic Alameda County study in California (Berkman and Breslow 1983) demonstrated that even after taking into account the influence of all known behavioural risk factors, there were still substantial differences in morbidity and mortality between high- and low-income families. Material and environmental conditions also play significant roles in generating health inequalities (Acheson 1998, Graham 2000). Poor people are more likely e.g. to live close to factories and major roads that generate air-borne pollution, which encourages respiratory problems; these may be exacerbated by mould spores arising from damp, under-heated housing (see pp. 54–55).

Addressing these issues must be the responsibility of government and industry, and the potential financial costs are enormous. Clearly governments have conflicting interests: while wishing to promote their citizens' health, they must also generate wealth by supporting industrial development but in doing so produce the pollution and dangerous work conditions that make some of us ill. So, while the state-endorsed message, 'look after your own health', is a liberal sentiment in that it allows individuals control over their lives, it also serves to *deflect attention* from the role material and environmental factors play in illness causation. It can therefore be seen as a politically expedient

message. A sociologist (Prior 1995) has likened the use of such individualistic (behavioural) explanations of ill health to explaining variations in the homicide rate in Northern Ireland in terms of personal shortcomings, such as failing to belt one's flak jacket. It is as absurd to ignore cultural/political factors in explaining illness.

In addition, the UK government, for example, receives vast revenues from the sale of tobacco and alcohol, and it is perhaps not surprising that it allows companies producing such products to advertise themselves, e.g. by sponsoring sports events. The 'look after your own health' ideal has also spawned a burgeoning health industry; we are enjoined to purchase every conceivable 'health' product from yogurt to gym memberships! The overall context in which we play out our behaviour is thus determined ultimately by political and economic considerations, and, therefore, can only be influenced by collective action.

The role of health professionals

Health professionals are high-status repositories of knowledge about the lives of lay people and can operate as powerful influences on individuals (e.g. by advising patients to alter their behaviour), on local government (e.g. by supporting community self-help groups) and on national government (e.g. by recommending a reduction in the amount of alcohol that drivers may legally consume).

- If a person fails to take responsibility for their health should they be denied (or have to pay for) certain medical treatments?
- Should governments/health professionals only have the power to attempt to change behaviour by informational means or, as in the case of water fluoridation, should they be able to introduce sweeping changes to our lives for our own good?

The social context of behavioural change

- Financial constraints mean that treatment decisions in the NHS trust you work for are being reviewed. The needs of non-smoking patients requiring high-cost cardiac surgery might in future be prioritized over those of heavy smokers. Would you support such a strategy?
- The social context of behavioural change can refer to the background to an individual's efforts to stop a deleterious (or start a beneficial) behaviour or to the overall societal influences upon how we behave and think.
- Individuals' behaviour is not always best understood by accessing the beliefs and attitudes. Attempts to effect mass behaviour change are often more successful if behaviour itself is targeted (e.g. legal sanctions for failure to conform are introduced).

  The idea that individuals can exercise choice over their health status can deflect attention from environmental/material explanations of health inequalities.
- Health professionals have the power to help individuals and groups to change their behaviour.
- Trying to influence behaviour always has ethical implications.

What are the objectives of health promotion?

The World Health Organization defines health both as the absence of disease and as a positive sense of well-being. Thus, the objectives of health promotion are:

- to prevent disease
- to promote health in the sense of well-being.

The two are related. For example, the management of chronic pain can involve the patient maintaining as full and positive a life as possible – maximum well-being, which, in turn may reduce pain experience.

Health promotion is relevant to almost all areas of medicine. Most attention is on diseases that have a substantial lifestyle component (Table 1).

Tones and Tilford (1994) have suggested three philosophies of health promotion: social engineering, individual prevention and individual empowerment.

Table 1 **Main areas for health promotion**
Smoking
Diet and weight
Contraception and HIV prevention
Blood pressure monitoring
Screening for cancers
Alcohol and substance abuse
Responsible medication use
Child care
Exercise.

Social engineering

Social engineering assumes that ill health is caused by social phenomena such as poverty, poor living conditions, lack of education, inappropriate cultural norms and inadequate health care. Objectives should be to improve living standards, change norms and improve health-care access. Social engineering can be effective: for example, in Southern India for cultural reasons birth control was often not used, but increasing women's literacy there also made them more likely to adopt and encourage birth control. Unfortunately, mass social engineering is often expensive and it can also be criticized for imposing change against some people's will or without consultation. For example, some people are opposed to the fluoridation of water, despite the dental benefits.

Individual prevention

This school of thought believes that health is strongly influenced by the behaviour and conditions of individuals and can, therefore, be improved by changing the individuals' health behaviours by education, advertising, specific physical interventions, such as seat belts, or making the holes in salt cellars smaller, and special medical treatment and screening. This approach fits with much medical thinking, which tends to be oriented towards treating individual patients. The most common form probably being the provision of leaflets informing patients about lifestyle factors (Fig. 1). Unfortunately, individualistic prevention involving education alone is rarely effective (see pp. 68–69; 70–71). Also, there can be an element of patient-blaming in individual health promotion. This may be inappropriate because in most diseases addressed by health promotion, such as cardiovascular disease, the patient's behaviour is only one causal factor among many.

Individual empowerment

Individual empowerment involves giving people the means to take responsibility for their health and to change their social conditions. Empowerment can be effective, but people may choose not to make health their priority. In health-care provision there is an increasing emphasis on empowering individual patients to make their own informed choices about their health and their medical treatment. This requires that patients become educated about health, disease and treatment so that they can make informed decisions. When patients are not fully educated, there are ethical issues involved in medical professionals deciding which health-related decisions the patient has a right to make. Most would agree that patients are free to choose their own diet, but few would allow a patient to decide which anaesthetic they would prefer. The difference is in the level of knowledge and expertise involved in making the decision and in the risks involved. Another difficulty is that much health promotion claims to be empowering, while strongly encouraging people to make the 'correct' health decision. What does one do, for example, with someone who chooses to smoke and risk dying early? Many health-care practitioners find it difficult to respect such a decision, although patients' rights to refuse any and all treatment – even unto death – have been upheld in court.

The practice of health promotion

Health-care practitioners can provide patients with information via leaflets (Fig. 1), other written sources, such as self-help books (e.g. Heather and Robinson 1996), computer systems and other media such as posters or multi-media displays in waiting areas, or serve to facilitate social change, for example, by pressing for improved housing conditions. But health-care practitioners probably do most health promotion via personal contact. The doctor's attitude and approach to patients can also promote health. A paternalistic pill-

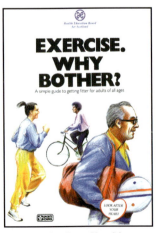
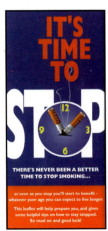
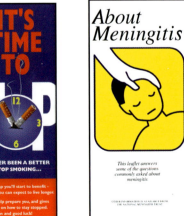

Fig. 1 **A selection of health-promotion leaflets found in a GP's surgery.**

■ What is the difference between health education and health promotion?
■ When might giving patients leaflets about their condition not affect their behaviour?
■ What steps might a doctor take to ensure that leaflets were effective?
■ Health information is sometimes seen by patients as patronizing and unrealistic. Why might this be so?

pusher is liable to develop patients who believe in quick medical repairs for their ailments, rather than prevention. A doctor with better communication skills may listen to patients and discuss how they should deal with their health problems. This may help inform and empower patients on health issues (see pp. 88–89; pp. 94–95).

Many consultations provide scope for opportunistic health promotion, where the doctor promotes health in a consultation concerning something else. Two examples would be the following: a patient with a head injury from falling may also have an alcohol problem and the doctor should take the opportunity to enquire about this; and a patient over 40 years of age attending their GP these days is likely to have their blood pressure monitored, whatever the presenting problem.

A related way of promoting health is to take detailed histories of health behaviours and social circumstances. Until recently health behaviours were rarely recorded. Accurate histories allow patient behaviours to be followed up on subsequent visits.

Primary care also provides specific facilities, programmes and clinics for different health behaviours. It is often appropriate to offer patients available aids for behaviour change. These range from simply monitoring change, for example by weighing the patient on each visit, to prescriptions, for instance for nicotine gum or patches for heavily dependent smokers, to advisory leaflets. Many health centres now also have access to dieticians, specialist nurses and psychologists to help with a range of health behaviours.

Minimal intervention

If doctors systematically ask all patients about their smoking or drinking and simply suggest to the smokers that they stop, or the drinkers that they cut down, without providing further intervention, then this has a small but significant impact on behaviour. About 5% more smokers quit than a control group (Pieterse et al 2001) and over 15% more drinkers reduce their alcohol intake to safer levels (Raistrick et al 1999, p. 168). Although effects are modest, minimal intervention is quick, cheap and not subject to the problems of successfully recruiting and retaining patients in more intensive interventions. Indeed, more intensive interventions do not always have larger effects.

Avoid fear messages

It is commonly believed that the best way to change people's behaviour is to warn them of its frightening consequences. The doctor would spell out the risks of coronary heart disease, cancers, AIDS and other diseases. Fear can be a powerful motive for changing behaviour, but fear messages can easily 'misfire' because their impact depends upon a number of complex factors (Ruiter et al 2001). Greater objective risk of

Case study

Andrea is a married woman aged 48 years. She is severely obese, with high normal blood pressure (140/95). She is moderately active, given her obesity. Andrea attended because she wanted help to lose weight. In what follows the GP expresses concern about her smoking, but does not risk alienating the patient by pushing the issue.

GP: '*So you take about five or six drinks a week. That's well within the safe limits and I don't think it will be having much effect on your weight. Do you smoke?*'
Andrea: (Laughs) '*Yeah, I've always got something in my mouth.*'
GP: '*How many a day?*'
Andrea: '*About 40.*'
GP: '*That's quite a lot. Have you ever thought of quitting?*'
Andrea: '*One thing at a time, doctor. I don't need to put on more weight.*'
GP: '*Actually, your smoking is worse for your health than your weight problem. I would like to see you try and stop.*'
Andrea: '*I'd rather get this fat off first.*'
GP: '*OK. Would you like to make an appointment with our dietician? I'll talk to you about smoking again in a few months.*'

harm (or greater fear) do not necessarily lead to greater behaviour change or compliance with medical advice.

Arousing fear can inhibit appropriate behaviour change, rather than facilitating it. Fear can lead patients, particularly those who perceive themselves at risk, to fail to attend properly to the relevant information. Patients may try to reduce fear by avoiding thinking about it, or may minimize the dangers, to reduce cognitive dissonance (see pp. 68–69). This may result in their rejecting the doctor as a credible source of information on the topic, or avoiding the entire issue. It is important also to emphasize the positive aspects of behaviour change, to increase patients' motivation to protect themselves from risk and develop a workable plan of action (see pp. 70–71).

Mass-media fear campaigns remain popular. 'Shocking' approaches to topics such as child abuse, drunk driving, drug overdose or lung cancer attract publicity and debate, but generally, the people most impressed by such campaigns are those least at risk. Such campaigns may raise awareness of issues, but they do not change behaviour by themselves.

What are the objectives of health promotion?

■ The objectives of health promotion are to prevent disease and promote health.
■ Objectives can be achieved by social engineering, individual prevention, empowerment.
■ The doctor can promote health by:

– information provision
– facilitating social change
– setting an example
– communicating effectively with patients
– including health behaviours in history-taking
– recommending healthy behaviours
– providing support for behaviour change.

(http://www.cochrane.org/cochrane/revabstr/ab001292.htm)

Illegal drug use

Over the last 40 years, illegal drug use has become common in many countries, particularly amongst younger people, and this has created extensive concern. The UK has one of the highest drug-use prevalence rates in the world and Figure 1 shows the most widely used types of drug. Some forms of drug use, such as cannabis smoking, are ceasing to be unusual or deviant in the UK, and many illegal drug users, particularly the more moderate ones, probably suffer few problems, just like many alcohol drinkers. This is no reason for complacency, for as prevalence has increased, drug-related problems have increased and diversified. Whereas 15 years ago drug services mostly saw heroin or cocaine users, these days people who seek help for drug-related problems commonly include people whose primary problems are one (or more) of the following:

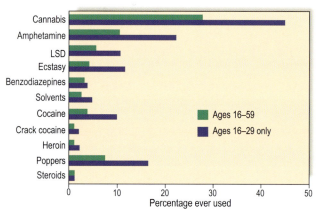

Fig. 1 **Illegal drug use in the UK.** (Source: Adopted from British Crime Survey 2000)

■ Cannabis abuse or dependence (see Box 1), usually with alcohol and occasional use of other drugs. Because cannabis is the most prevalent illegal substance, there are more people dependent on cannabis than on all other drugs combined (Dennis et al 2002).

■ Heroin or opiate abuse or dependence, sometimes combined with benzodiazepines and other drugs, and typically involving drug injection (e.g. Neale 2002).

■ Cocaine or crack cocaine abuse or dependence. The likelihood and severity of cocaine dependence has sometimes been overstated (Ditton and Hammersley 1996). Yet, cocaine is becoming even more prevalent, which will lead to more widespread problems.

■ Amphetamine abuse or dependence (e.g. Klee and Morris 1997).

■ Psychotic or delusional symptoms related to drug use. This is more likely for people with pre-existing mental disorders and is most commonly found with amphetamines or cocaine (Farrell et al 2002), although it can also occur with cannabis or hallucinogens such as LSD. People already vulnerable to schizophrenia may have symptoms triggered or worsened by illicit drugs.

■ Overdose, most commonly on opiates, alcohol or benzo-diazepines, or mixtures of such drugs.

■ Ecstasy-related deaths are not overdoses but have a different aetiology, which is not yet entirely clear, though it includes hyperthermia (overheating) (see Burgess et al 2000).

People who seek help for drug problems often have other psychological, social and physical health problems, which may also need attention (for detail see for example, Dennis et al 2002, Farrell et al 2002, Klee and Morris 1997, Neale 2002, Orford 2000).

Treatment

A complication for treatment is that drug users seeking help include some who are doing so mainly because of the concern of other people. Many drug users have mixed feelings about use, which they enjoy and find beneficial in some way, and can sometimes fail to recognize the development of a problem as quickly as others do. Techniques for motivational enhancement (Miller and Rollnick 1991) can be particularly important to get users to consider frankly the costs and benefits of use.

Treating drug dependence is difficult, it can take a decade before a drug-dependent person stops, during which time they typically have repeated involvement with health and other services. They will usually have tried to stop or moderate their use several times, by several methods, relapsing each time. Relapse management is an important component of any competent anti-drug treatment. Users should also be provided with the information and means to minimize the harm their drug use causes. Information also benefits users who are not dependent (see Table 2). For opiate users, methadone or buprenorphine maintenance can allow users to stabilize their lifestyles and reduce the problems related to a criminal, drug-injecting lifestyle. Substitute prescribing is not yet available for other drugs.

No single treatment works best. A good relationship between the therapist and the patient is very important and it is best to see treatment as enabling clients to change

Table 1 **Situations where drug users may require special treatment**	
Situation	**Special problems**
Obstetrics	Maintenance or reduction of prescribing and counselling may be required to minimize harm to mother and fetus
Surgery	May show high tolerance to anaesthetics and sedatives
	May be HIV positive
General practice	Can be disruptive and deceptive
	May require specialized support services
Internal medicine	May fake pain to obtain painkillers
	May continue to use drugs that interact with their prescribed medicines
Infectious diseases	HIV, hepatitis
Casualty	Overdose, injuries through accidents while intoxicated, violence related to the drugs trade

Table 2 **Harm-minimization strategies for drug injectors.** (Adapted from Department of Health 1991 Drug Misuse and Dependence)	
Education	Hazards of injecting (especially equipment-sharing)
	Safer sex
	Getting sterile equipment and condoms
	Cleaning equipment
	Avoiding overdose
	First aid
Direct action	Hepatitis B immunization
	Provision of sterile injecting equipment and condoms
	HIV testing (with counselling)
	Substitution of oral methadone

Box 1 Diagnosing drug problems

The DSM-IV (American Psychiatric Association 2000) recognizes two forms of drug problems:

Drug abuse: Involves use over at least 12 months, with repeated problems interpersonally, or in social roles such as education or work, or legal problems, or dangerous behaviour linked to use and significant concern about those problems, but without dependence.

Drug dependence: Can additionally involve unsuccessful attempts to quit, classic signs of 'addiction', such as increased tolerance (taking higher doses over time) and withdrawal symptoms, spending excessive time seeking and taking drugs, and having difficulty controlling intake.

All drugs, including cannabis, can cause dependence, but none inevitably do so (see Orford 2000, Hammersley and Reid, 2002).

For people under 18, abuse or dependence may not be clearly diagnosed and it may be better to simply describe them as having drug problems (Newcomb 1995).

themselves (pp. 130–131). Detoxifying users humanely is only the beginning of treatment. Cognitive-behavioural approaches (pp. 134–135) can help, particularly in changing negative drug-related behaviours, such as harmful injecting practices (see Platt et al 1991, for review). Motivational interviewing is also widely used to help clients ready themselves to make change and prepare for the difficulties and possible relapses that will follow (Miller and Rollnick, 1991). Involving the client's relatives in family or systemic therapy can also be helpful, particularly for younger drug users. The 'Minnesota model' of treatment using a '12-steps' approach (pp. 78) and focusing on abstinence can also work. However, when treatment is evaluated properly, only about 20–30% of those treated will quit or reduce drug use and stay that way for 6 months or more. Alleged higher success rates tend to be due to biased selection of patients or weak measures of outcome (Miller and Sanchez-Craig 1996). Treatment is more difficult when the client has little social support, a chaotic lifestyle and also has other major psychological, health or social problems. Not only are the effects of treatment modest, but most substance users modify or quit use without treatment; however, encouragingly, recovery rates from substance-use disorders are higher than from most other mental health disorders (see Orford 2000).

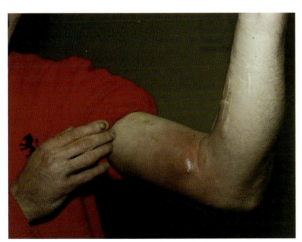

Fig. 2 **Damage to arm by use of injectable drugs.**

Case study

Mike is a 23-year-old drug injector with a history of criminal convictions and drug *misuse* going back to age 14 years. Two years previously he had been discharged from a residential detoxification programme for using drugs. He told the GP that he was now highly motivated by having a steady partner and a newly born daughter, but cannot give up heroin. The GP prescribed methadone and established a good relationship with Mike. With the prescription his general health improved and his previously hostile approach to NHS staff decreased. He was also referred for dental treatment because of numerous caries due to neglect and a sugary diet, the pain of these previously being concealed by high doses of drugs. Unfortunately, 6 months later Mike was arrested for burglary. He denied involvement and the GP testified in writing on his behalf, but as a persistent offender he was nonetheless convicted and sentenced to 2 years. In prison his maintenance regime was replaced by a rapid reduction of methadone dose. Mike was unable to manage and began to inject again occasionally, sharing a syringe. As a result he contracted hepatitis C. On release he was determined to stop injecting. However, his GP was now reluctant to prescribe methadone as Mike had not used opiates regularly in prison. This, and a serious quarrel with his partner, led Mike to resume heavy drug use and crime for some months. He returned to the GP requiring treatment for a large abscess (see Fig. 2). He is now back on methadone, requires regular monitoring for liver damage from hepatitis C and has re-established a relationship with his family, although he no longer lives with his daughter's mother.

■ Do doctors push drugs? Some doctors see prescribing methadone as selling addicts drugs to keep them quiet and feel that this is immoral. Others feel that the practical benefits of methadone outweigh the moral issue. Another issue is the prescription of minor tranquillizers to make anxious, stressed or emotional patients feel better. Where is the line between taking a drug to feel better and taking a drug for fun? Should doctors encourage people to use drugs to feel better?

Illegal drug use

■ Illegal drug use is quite common.

■ Much illegal drug use is not a medical problem, but most drugs do cause occasional acute problems, even deaths.

■ There are a number of different common patterns of drug problem.

■ The dependent drug user may take a long time and repeated attempts to stop. Prior to stopping he or she may benefit from help with:

– harm reduction, including substitute prescribing, such as methadone for heroin, or advice on safe injecting

– general medical care

– life problems as well as drug dependence.

Alcohol problems

Alcohol is the most widely used recreational drug in the Western world. While many users come to no harm, its use can cause medical, psychological and social problems. The management of alcohol should be a major public health and public policy issue (Raistrick et al 1999; Edwards 2000).

The medicalization of alcohol problems

In the 18th and 19th centuries alcohol was generally regarded as a wholesome foodstuff. Excessive drinking was seen as a vice rather than a medical problem, although the main medical effects of alcohol had already been noted. For example, in Britain there was particular concern about the working classes abusing gin, and drinking levels were much higher than today. Between about 1850 and the late 1950s alcoholism came to be considered a disease caused by some biological reaction to alcohol. This reaction was supposed to be permanent, so the only palliative treatment for alcoholism was permanent abstinence. Still widely believed, this idea is faulty:

- Many problem drinkers come to harm from drinking but are not alcoholics.
- Even dependent drinkers have some control over their drinking. Some, not all, people with severe alcohol problems can moderate their drinking to problem-free levels, often without help (see Heather and Robinson 1983).
- Some very heavy drinkers survive unchanged for 30 years or more (Valliant 2003).

Alcoholics Anonymous emphasizes abstinence (see below), as do some professional treatments. Other treatments include monitored detoxification for severely dependent drinkers, counselling to enable the patient find methods of coping other than drinking, or therapeutic communities where patients stay off alcohol and undertake group therapy. Given a choice, some patients opt for abstinence and some for moderating their drinking. Occasional relapses to heavy drinking are common, even amongst those trying to abstain, and patients are taught to expect and cope with this. Controlled follow-up studies suggest that approximately 80% of people treated for alcohol dependence by any method have relapsed within 2 years. Alleged better rates tend to be due to bias (for example, treatment programmes that only admit people who have virtually stopped drinking already) or poorly controlled research (see Miller and Sanchez-Craig 1996).

The 12-steps approach

Alcoholics Anonymous (AA) (http://www.alcoholics-anonymous.org/) consists of groups of recovering alcoholics who provide mutual support and aim at complete abstinence from alcohol. The philosophy is the famous 12-steps approach, which requires that the alcoholic surrender to a higher power (or God), admit their wrongs and try to rectify them (pp. 138–139). People who benefit more from this approach have religious or spiritual feelings, accept abstinence as a goal and were heavily dependent. AA has less to offer people who are not dependent. Doctors often suggest AA as a supplement to treatment. There are also professional residential programmes that offer a 12-steps approach, sometimes called the Minnesota model treatment.

Drinking problems

Even quite moderate drinking increases morbidity (Table 1) and mortality. Consequently, the BMA recommended safe limits of three to four standard drinks per day for men and two to three for women. A standard drink is 1/2 pint of beer, a small glass of wine, or a standard measure of spirits. Some countries set the safe limit at as little as one or two units per day. However, many people, especially young men, drink above these limits (Fig. 1).

At the legal limit for driving (UK: 80 mg alcohol in 100 ml blood), reactions are slowed by about 20% and thought is impaired. People who are drunk may generally behave in risky, anti-social or foolish ways without adequately considering their actions. This causes some of alcohol's pleasurable effects – people are more likely to dance, flirt, or converse. Unfortunately, drunkenness also contributes to quarrels, violence, disorder, suicide, fires, road-traffic accidents, other accidents, child abuse and other problems (see Raistrick et al 1999, Chapter 4). It is also quite easy to overdose on alcohol, which can kill through respiratory depression.

Controlling the nation's consumption

Increasing the price of alcohol by taxation can reduce national consumption, which in turn reduces alcohol-related problems (Raistrick et al 1999, Chapter 6). Alcohol advertising in the mass media may influence children, but it has little effect on consumption levels (Raistrick et al 1999, Chapter 8). However, the portrayal of alcohol in TV programming and writing is predominantly positive (or

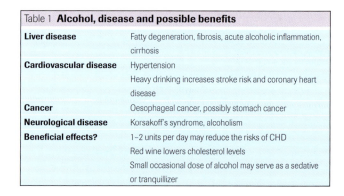

Table 1	Alcohol, disease and possible benefits
Liver disease	Fatty degeneration, fibrosis, acute alcoholic inflammation, cirrhosis
Cardiovascular disease	Hypertension
	Heavy drinking increases stroke risk and coronary heart disease
Cancer	Oesophageal cancer, possibly stomach cancer
Neurological disease	Korsakoff's syndrome, alcoholism
Beneficial effects?	1–2 units per day may reduce the risks of CHD
	Red wine lowers cholesterol levels
	Small occasional dose of alcohol may serve as a sedative or tranquillizer

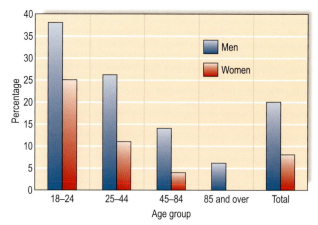

Fig. 1 **Percentage drinking above safe limits – note that some of all age groups drink heavily.** (Source: Lader and Meltzer 2001)

melodramatically negative) and there is scope for using mass media more skilfully to promote safer drinking. Other approaches try to change the way people drink by:

1. education about safe levels and risks. This may have helped change society's attitude to drunk-driving.
2. continued control over where, when and by whom alcohol may be consumed, with licensing laws. For example, decreasing under-age drinking may require a reduction in tolerance of violations of existing law.
3. manipulation of the physical and social settings where drinking problems are common. For example, the banning of alcohol on football trains and at football grounds to prevent disorder.

A major barrier to such changes is a widespread indifference to and minimization of alcohol problems. The health professional's role is, in part, to raise the profile of alcohol-related problems, by routinely taking alcohol histories and treating alcohol use as a priority health-care issue.

■ Some medical students and doctors drink excessively. Could you, or your colleagues, benefit from cutting down? How might you go about this? Doctors often drink as part of medical school culture, to 'cope' with stress and to relax, although drinking can end up worsening the stress and their work can be affected by drinking or hangovers. What other methods of coping might be more constructive? Would any changes to your school's culture help?

The role of medicine

■ To be aware of the contribution that alcohol can make to illness and injury in general practice and hospital specialities (see Table 1 and Box 1).
■ To counter the drinks industry's promotion of its products.
■ To press for better controls on the sale and pricing of alcohol.
■ To routinely ask patients about their drinking and relate this to illness and disease.
■ To advise patients of safe drinking levels and suggest that they adopt these levels.
■ To monitor patient's drinking, and praise and encourage reduced drinking.
■ To serve as a role model by drinking moderately, within safe limits.
■ To be aware of and refer to local specialized alcohol-treatment services.

Case study

Minimal intervention with a heavy drinker

Ralph is 35 years old and a travelling salesman. He presented with frequent abdominal pains, which he attributed to stress. From examination and tests there was no evidence of physical abnormality and non-specific gastritis was diagnosed. When Ralph attended the GP again to discuss the test results the GP asked him to go through the previous 7 days and list all the alcohol he had consumed (a retrospective drinking diary). Ralph was drinking over 50 units of alcohol a week – about two pints (four units) or equivalent at lunchtime and a further two in the evening to relax.

GP: *'You don't drink that much a day, but it's steady. Now the recommended safe limit for men is 21 units a week – that's about ten and a half pints of beer a week'.*

Ralph: *'Is that all? How much did I get through last week then?'*

GP: *'A bit too much, 58 units. I think that your stomach pains are made worse by your drinking. I'd like you to stop for a week or so and see what happens to your pain'.*

Ralph: *'I can't give up drinking! It goes with the job. A lot of my clients wouldn't stand for it if I didn't have a couple with them'.*

GP: *'I'm not suggesting you give up for ever, just for a week to see what happens, then maybe try and cut down a bit. Try not to drink every day, or have some soft drinks sometimes, or low-alcohol beer'.*

Ralph: *'That's going to be hard, but I guess I have to, don't I, doctor, if it's affecting my stomach and that?'*

GP: *'Yes. Come back and see after you've stopped for your week. If you want to know more about cutting down then there's a good book, 'Let's Drink to your Health''* (Heather and Robinson 1996).

Ralph now has the advice of the doctor as a motive for cutting down and can also use his health as an excuse when he feels social pressure to drink.

Box 1 Alcohol in medical practice

Alcohol abuse can play a role in:

■ Depression.
■ Anxiety and other psychiatric problems.
■ Problems of the digestive system.
■ Cardiovascular problems.
■ Neurological problems, apparent dementia and headaches.
■ Abuse of other drugs and medicines.
■ Family problems.
■ Falls and accidents.
■ Obesity.
■ Insensitivity to anaesthetics and pain relief.

Alcohol problems

■ Alcohol is often involved in many other health, psychological and social problems.
■ Alcohol use should be a routine part of history-taking.
■ Some people require treatment for dependence.
■ Others require advice to moderate their drinking.
■ Drinking beyond two to three drinks per day, 14 a week (women) or 21 a week (men) is not unusual, but it endangers long-term health.
■ Society tends to be complacent about the health risks of alcohol.

http://www.alcoholconcern.org.uk/

Smoking, tobacco control and doctors

The global picture

Smoking is the single most important cause of premature mortality and morbidity in industrialized countries, and is an increasing cause of death and disease in developing countries. Cigarettes kill half of lifetime users. Half of these deaths are under 70 years. Those dying before 70 lose on average 23 years of life. In 2000, tobacco killed over 4.2 million people. Half of these deaths were in developing countries. WHO estimates that by 2030 deaths will have more than doubled to 10 million; 7 million of these in developing countries (Mackay and Eriksen 2002). Death rates are higher in men than women as men have a longer history of widespread smoking. In countries such as the UK and USA, where women have smoked for several decades, the gap is closing rapidly.

The costs of smoking in the UK

Smoking affects health throughout the life course. 120 000 people in the UK are killed by smoking each year: one-fifth of all deaths (ASH 2001a). Most die from lung cancer, chronic obstructive lung disease (bronchitis and emphysema) or coronary heart disease. Smoking is also a risk factor for other cancers (mouth, larynx, liver, bladder, cervix), strokes, miscarriage, cot death, infertility, impotence, osteoporosis and many other diseases. Breathing in other people's smoke, environmental tobacco smoke (ETS), increases non-smokers' risks of developing lung cancer and heart disease by 25%. Children are particularly vulnerable, with ETS increasing their risk for diseases such as pneumonia, bronchitis, glue ear and worsening asthma.

The NHS spends £1.5 billion a year treating diseases caused by smoking. This includes 265 000 hospital admissions, 8 million GP consultations and over 7 million prescriptions (ASH 2001a). Other costs to the state include sickness/invalidity benefits, widows' pensions and social security benefits for dependants. British industry loses 34 million working days each year from smoking-related sick leave.

Smoking and inequalities

Cigarette smoking in the UK has declined significantly since the peak in the 1970s. This decline has been faster in men than women, and in more-affluent than poorer groups. Smoking is now a major cause of inequalities in health. In Scotland it accounts for at least two-thirds of the excess deaths due to inequalities in health. The more disadvantaged you are, the more likely you are to start smoking and the less likely you are to quit. In 2000, people in the unskilled manual socio-economic group (37%) had more than twice the smoking rate of those in the professional group (16%) (ASH 2001b).

The tobacco industry

Tobacco companies are in the business of making profits. They need to recruit young smokers to replace the 50% of their adult customers who die from using their product. They also need to keep their customers smoking as long as possible, by reducing motivation to quit and maintaining nicotine addiction. They achieve this through manipulating the marketing mix to appeal to different smokers and expanding their markets to developing countries (see Box 1).

Box 1 **The tobacco companies marketing mix**

Promotion: Tobacco companies fight advertising bans, delay their implementation and try to find loopholes. They maximize their promotions wherever they can, finding new ways to reach consumers. They cultivate powerful allies and 'do good works' to achieve a more acceptable public face.
Product: Tailoring the product for different groups, e.g. 'light' cigarettes for women, cigarettes acceptable to young people's palates, which have enough nicotine to be addictive.
Price: Producing a range of products at different prices, supporting smuggling, fighting increases in tax.
Place: Ensuring that cigarettes and smoking are ubiquitous, normal, and accessible, e.g. through vending machines, fighting no-smoking policies.

A tobacco-control strategy

Based on evidence from around the world, there is an international consensus on what action is needed.

- **A total ban on tobacco advertising and promotion**
  Tobacco companies argue that they do not target young people, rather that they encourage adult smokers to smoke their brand. Research studies and the companies' own confidential documents show that this is not the case. Banning tobacco promotion reduces smoking. Over 30 countries have introduced bans. Bans must include direct advertising and sponsorship, and indirect promotion such as putting cigarette brand names on other products, e.g. clothes (brandstretching) and paying for cigarette brands to appear in films (product placement). They should cover all types of media (see Fig. 1) and the internet.
- **Regular increases in taxation on tobacco**
  The level of smoking is highly related to price. The cheaper the price of cigarettes the higher the level of consumption. For every 1% increase in the real price of cigarettes there is

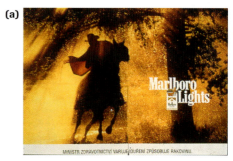

(a)

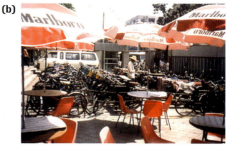

(b)

Fig. 1 **Examples of promotions for Marlboro – the most successful international cigarette brand. (a) Czech Republic, (b) China.**
(Source: personal communication)

Case study

The Massachusetts tobacco-control programme

In 1992 voters in Massachusetts agreed that 25 cents be added to the cost of a pack of cigarettes, with the extra revenue to be used to reduce smoking. Since 1993 Massachusetts has spent about $39 m a year on its tobacco-control programme – $6.50 for each person in the state. This is the highest per capita expenditure on tobacco control in the world. The programme is designed to increase quitting, reduce uptake, and reduce exposure to ETS. It includes:

- *Mass-media campaigns*: to inform the public about the dangers of smoking and ETS. Over 100 advertisements have been produced.
- *Services*: local cessation services, youth leadership programmes, telephone counselling, and educational materials.
- *Promotion of local policies*: funds local tobacco-control policies, e.g. smoking in public places, illegal sales to children.

The data in the figure show a significant reduction in smoking in Massachusetts compared to little change in the rest of the USA (with the exception of California, which has a similar programme). The Massachusetts experience shows that a strongly implemented, well-funded, comprehensive control programme can reduce a population's health risks from tobacco.

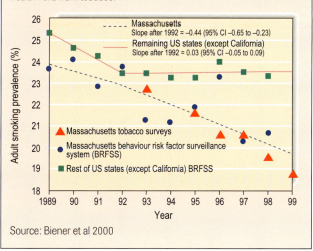

Source: Biener et al 2000

a 0.5% decline in adult consumption. The decline is even higher in young people. Tobacco tax can be used (hypothecated) to pay for other elements of the tobacco-control strategy, and to address factors (e.g. poverty) that make it difficult for smokers to quit.

Prohibition on sales to children

Even in countries such as the UK, where it is illegal to sell cigarettes to under 16s, surveys show that young smokers have little problem buying cigarettes. Laws need to be enforced. Cigarette vending machines should not be accessible to young people.

Firm, large health warnings on cigarette packets

These are particularly important in developing countries, where there is little awareness of the health effects of smoking. They should also include visual images, which can be powerful, especially where there are low literacy levels.

No-smoking policies

People have the right to breathe smoke-free air – where they work, study, shop, go for entertainment and live. As well as reducing exposure to ETS, no-smoking policies increase smokers' motivations to quit and reduce relapse rates.

Health education

This would address prevention and cessation. For example, young people need to be aware of the health effects, and

how quickly you become addicted even at low levels of smoking, and have the motivation and skills not to start.

Cessation support

Two-thirds of smokers want to quit. While most quit on their own, cessation support greatly increases success rates. This could include mass-media campaigns, telephone quit-lines, group support, one-to-one support, and providing pharmacotherapy, such as nicotine replacement therapy (NRT) and/or bupropion (Zyban).

Research and evaluation

In order to develop more effective approaches. In particular, in relation to disadvantage, gender and ethnicity.

- Around two-thirds of teenagers will try at least one cigarette, but less than half of these will become regular smokers. Thinking about yourself what were the factors that influenced you whether or not (a) to take your first cigarette and (b) to continue to smoke?

Doctors and smoking cessation

Helping people to stop smoking is one of the most cost-effective interventions that doctors can take. For example, the cost of smoking-cessation advice ranges from £212 to £873 per life-year gained compared to the cost of prescribing statins (cholesterol-lowering drugs), which is between £5400 and £13 300 per life-year gained (ASH 2002). Research shows that doctors giving a few minutes brief advice increases smoking-cessation rates in patients (Raw et al 1999).

National evidence-based cessation guidelines have been produced for doctors and other health professionals on how they can be most effective in helping patients quit (Raw et al 1999, HEBS/ASH Scotland 2001). In this approach the level of support is matched to patients' level of motivation to quit, tobacco use and nicotine addiction. This ranges from offering brief advice to providing NRT and/or bupropion (which doubles quit rates) to referring patients to cessation services. Since 1999 the government has provided health authorities and health boards with extra funds to set up local cessation services (Secretary of State for Health 1999).

Smoking, tobacco control and doctors

- Global deaths from tobacco are increasing rapidly and young people continue to take up smoking.
- Smoking in the UK is highly associated with disadvantage and is a major cause of inequalities in health.
- The tobacco industry needs to keep recruiting young people to replace smokers who quit or are killed by tobacco.
- Reducing smoking requires comprehensive action to ban tobacco promotion, increase prices, reduce access to young people, increase health education and cessation support.
- Doctors have an important role to play in supporting both patients to quit smoking and wider action by the government and other agencies.

ASH London: www.ash.org.uk; ASH Scotland: www.ashscotland.org.uk; Doctors and Tobacco – Tobacco Control Resource Centre: www.tobacco-control.org

Eating, body shape and health

Although a large proportion of the world's population suffer from malnutrition, a growing proportion suffers from overeating. We might expect that something as basic as the regulation of feeding would pose no problems for a species as advanced as ourselves. Yet problems associated with eating are the cause of a growing number of health-related conditions. Problems with eating are the product of over-abundance of palatable food and reduced exercise on the one hand, and unrealistic ideals about body shape on the other. The system responsible for appetite regulation is unable to cope adequately with these pressures. Most urgent is the increase in obesity in Western society. Obesity has well-documented health risks, including heart disease (see p. 104), diabetes (see pp. 122–123), high blood pressure and stroke. Of particular concern is the increase in childhood obesity, resulting in a range of health-related complications (Ebbeling et al 2002). Obesity also has psychological effects, with increased depression, feelings of ugliness and low self-esteem. Consequently, many overweight individuals diet to lose weight. However, disorders of eating associated with attempts to diet are also increasing, and the modern clinician is faced with the conundrum of how to promote healthy eating amongst people who are underweight through excessive dieting and how to help overweight individuals lose weight (see Case study).

Assessing weight status

The body mass index (BMI: Table 1) assesses weight status, and helps identify people who are outside the normal weight range. BMI figures are not definitive measures of health. The BMI of many elite athletes is above the 'normal' range, but their 'excess' is muscle rather than fat. In general, however, BMI remains a good approximation of weight status.

The perfect body

The ideal body shape portrayed in magazines has changed markedly over time, and anyone looking at pictures of women used as models in art across the ages will see remarkable changes in physique. Today the figure portrayed as

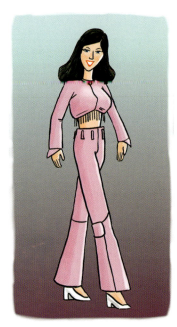

Fig. **1 A woman with a figure the same as popular dolls like this one would have a BMI of 16.6.**

ideal, that is, excessively thin and athletic, but often with enhanced breast size, is unattainable for the vast majority of women. Even the dolls idolized by young girls have a BMI in the anorexic range (see Fig. 1), coupled with a bust size that could only be obtained through surgery. While the ideal has got thinner, the average body size has increased, so the disparity between ideal and actual body shapes has grown. The result is widespread dissatisfaction with body shape, and it is perhaps no coincidence that levels of depression in women have risen in parallel with these concerns (Hankin and Abramson 1999). Men, too, are increasingly concerned with body shape, although eating disorders for men are concentrated in professions where weight is an issue (e.g. ballet dancing, jockeys and some athletes) and in homosexual men, who appear more sensitive to societal pressures (Carlat et al 1997; see pp. 50–51).

Table 1 **BMI calculation and classification**	
BMI = weight (kg)/(height (m))2	
BMI	**Classification**
<18.5	Underweight
18.5–24.9	Normal
25.0–29.9	Overweight
30.0–34.9	Mildly obese
35.0–39.9	Moderate obesity
40.0 +	Severe obesity

Dangers of undereating

The idea that healthy, often academically gifted, and likeable girls should refuse to consume sufficient food to maintain a normal body weight has baffled clinicians since anorexia nervosa was formally defined in 1873. Descriptions of the disorder pre-date that time, challenging the common view that anorexia nervosa is the modern dieting disease. Anorexia is associated with excessive dieting and a morbid pre-occupation with body shape, to the point where the sufferer refuses to consume adequate food to sustain a normal body size (see Mehler 2001). It remains a rare disorder, affecting 1/1000 even in the most at-risk groups (high-achieving middle-class girls aged 12–16). Claims that anorexia has become more frequent are hard to verify because of changes to diagnostic criteria, but many psychologists see the full disorder as the tip of an iceberg of women (and increasingly men) whose lives are controlled by attempts to diet. The causes of anorexia nervosa remain unclear, but there is evidence of some genetic predisposition (see Gorwood et al 1998). Mortality is high, and the disorder is very hard to treat.

Dangers of dieting

Guides to dieting feature heavily in 'the media' and few people in Western society have not at some time tried to restrict their eating. The increased prevalence of obesity indicates that these attempts rarely work, even though many diets result in initial rapid weight loss.

One consequence of frequent failed attempts to diet is the phenomenon of weight cycling, where a 'positive energy balance', defined as energy intake in excess of expenditure, results in weight gain, which leads to short-term dieting and consequent weight loss only for weight to be regained and the cycle continued. Research suggests that this pattern itself has adverse effects on health: weight cycling increases blood pressure more than sustained overweight, and other illnesses (see Foster et al 1997). Health professionals recommend people who are not obese maintain a stable weight to minimize these risks.

STOP THINK What are the consequences for health and psychological well-being of:

- being constantly overweight?
- cycling between overweight and normal weight?
- being underweight?
- alternately binge eating and dieting?

Binge eating: cause or consequence of dieting?

The defining feature of binge eating is the consumption of a much larger amount of food in a given time than is normal. Binge eating can be associated with obesity and a sub-type of anorexia nervosa, but is best known in the specific disorder bulimia nervosa (Table 2). Here, the sufferer has a regular behaviour pattern of dieting followed by periods of excessive eating. Binging is followed by attempts to counteract the anticipated consequences of the binge on bodyweight, by self-induced vomiting, use of purgatives or excessive exercise and dieting. The classic psychological model of binge eating was to see it as a secondary consequence of dieting. Accordingly, binge eating was characterized as compensation for the lack of food intake during dieting by overeating when the ability to maintain dieting broke down. The corollary of this is that binge eating should be seen only in people who are currently attempting to restrict their intake. However, sufferers from binge-eating disorder present the behavioural manifestations of binge eating but score low on measures of 'dieting' (see Dingemans et al 2002). This suggests that the tendency to binge eat may be a characteristic of certain individuals, but since unrestricted binge eating will lead to weight gain, binge eating itself may lead to attempts to diet. Dieting may then exacerbate the tendency to binge, and so lead progressively to bulimic behaviour. Thus binging and dieting are inter-related, but one may not inevitably lead to the other (see Polivy and Herman 2002).

Promoting a healthy lifestyle

The increase in obesity and eating disorders in Western society has occurred during a period when other aspects of eating have altered. Most notable has been the increase in use of 'fast foods' and pre-prepared meals at the expense of fresh produce. These types of foods often have high energy density, and high fat and salt content. With obesity and eating disorders both increasing in incidence, and dieting itself having potential harmful effects on health, how should society tackle these issues? Some see dieting as a necessary evil, since lack of dietary restraint in the face of plentiful high-energy food and low levels of exercise leads to obesity. Most health-care professionals concur that promotion of a healthy lifestyle, including healthy eating together with increased energy expenditure, is preferable. Indeed, many clinicians now routinely prescribe exercise as a component of their treatment for obesity, and although poor compliance can render this intervention ineffective, specific exercise programmes coupled with a life-long commitment for obese patients to achieve reasonable energy expenditure through exercise are recognized as the most effective alternative to drug-based therapy for obesity (McKinnis 2000). Obesity is, to some extent, a social problem related to our increasingly sedentary lifestyle, including convenience shopping and the replacement of walking and cycling by the use of the car. Only major changes in society, such as reducing the availability of high-fat food, designing amenities in ways to promote exercise, and increasing the opportunity for and safety of walking and cycling in urban situations, will ultimately solve the dual problems of obesity and disordered eating.

Case study

The problem of treating overweight
This description was provided by a GP during a discussion on eating disorders.

A family (parents in their early 30s, daughter aged 14) were seen during a routine 'well family' surgery. The daughter was in perfect health, but both parents were overweight and so were advised to increase their levels of exercise, and reduce their fat intake. One year later, both parents were still overweight but the daughter has lost considerable weight as a consequence of excessive dieting and is now diagnosed as having anorexia nervosa.

The critical point is that the GP had no intention of drawing the girl's attention to her own weight. However, adolescent girls have a heightened awareness of issues relating to body shape, and awareness of this sensitivity is crucial when communicating health advice.

Eating, body shape and health

- Being obese has serious consequences for physical and mental health.
- Anorexia nervosa has a high mortality rate.
- Repeatedly gaining and losing weight (weight cycling) has more health risks than remaining mildly overweight.
- The ideal body shape depicted by society is unattainable for most people.
- Binge eating can be found in obesity, anorexia nervosa and bulimia nervosa.

NIDDK's site on weight loss and control:
http://www.niddk.nih.gov/health/nutrit/nutrit.htm, The Eating Disorders Association: http://www.edauk.com/; The American Obesity Association: http://www.obesity.org/

Table 2 Clinical diagnoses associated with binge eating	
Characteristics	**Clinical diagnosis**
Binge eating with no dieting	Binge-eating disorder, often leading to obesity
Binge eating with dieting, excessive exercise, self-induced vomiting or use of purgatives. But no excessive loss of weight	Bulimia nervosa
Binge eating with dieting, excessive exercise, self-induced vomiting or use of purgatives, resulting in excessive loss of weight	Anorexia nervosa, purging sub-type

Perceptions of risk and risk-taking behaviours

The identification of risk factors for disease is important for prevention of ill health. We know that social factors are implicated in the patterning of ill health. However, there is also increasing emphasis on the importance of lifestyle and the role of health-related behaviours for certain diseases. These behaviours can be termed risk-taking behaviours, because of the known risk they pose for an individual's health. In recent years there has been a growing emphasis on an individual's responsibility for their own health and the promotion of behaviour change to reduce an individual's risk of disease and ill health (pp. 68–69).

This has brought with it an emphasis on self-control, on moderation in behaviour, and on the provision of information to inform people of the risks to health attendant with certain lifestyles. Individuals' potential for control over lifestyle and health is limited by the social circumstances that shape people's lives (pp. 42–43). Understanding people's own perceptions of risk and the contexts within which their risk-taking behaviours occur is important for doctors and others who may be assessing a patient's risk of disease and encouraging a more healthy lifestyle.

Perceptions of risk

Ignorance is often considered to be a major barrier to following lifestyle advice, although there is much evidence to suggest that the lay public are well aware of the publicized risks to health, such as the relationship between smoking and lung cancer or the range of risk factors associated with heart disease. In fact, research suggests that knowledge itself is not a powerful predictor of behaviour.

People may view a range of risks very differently. For example, salmonella infection from egg consumption was viewed as very risky when this was highlighted in the media, although the chances of infection were small. However, the longer-term risks of cholesterol and heart disease were not viewed in the same way. These different perceptions of risk may influence behaviour in different ways, with reactive lifestyle changes around egg consumption

occurring quickly, but modification of diet to prevent heart disease being much harder to achieve.

People have a tendency to believe that their chances of experiencing a negative event, including illness, are less than average, but higher than average for a positive event. This is called 'unrealistic optimism' or 'optimistic bias' (Weinstein 1982). Factors regarded by an individual as decreasing their risk include both personal actions (for example, engaging in preventive health behaviours or seeking appropriate help) and psychological attributes such as personality, values held, likes and dislikes (for example, being the type of person who does not let things get them down, or being 'health conscious'). These are both associated with perceived controllability of the event. Environmental or hereditary factors are not perceived in the same way. The predominant characteristics affecting optimistic bias are: the belief that if the problem has not yet appeared, there will be an exemption from future risk, that the problem is perceived as preventable through individual action, that the hazard is perceived as infrequent and that there is a lack of experience with the hazard (Weinstein 1987). Some research has suggested that people nonetheless overestimate their absolute risk of a disease, such as breast cancer, and also overestimate the chances of surviving 5 years after diagnosis, of the cancer being curable and the chances of cancer being detected by mammogram (Clarke et al 2000). However, in relation to perceived risk of disease, although people overestimate their own risk, they do this to a lesser extent than they do for others. In other words, they still retain an optimistic bias about themselves relative to similar others.

Optimistic bias may result in weakened intentions to prevent future ill health. However, in some cases, optimistic bias (in relation to control) may strengthen intentions to take preventive action because optimistic bias enhances self-efficacy (pp. 146–147) and belief in the controllability of negative events (Weinstein and Lyon 1999). For example, someone might overestimate

their ability to make lifestyle changes (such as giving up smoking or taking up exercise) but also overestimate the extent to which changes will reduce their risk of disease (e.g. eating less high-fat food will not remove the risk of heart disease). There is also some evidence that unrealistic optimism is associated with positive well-being. The relative importance of the positive or negative aspects of optimistic bias will depend very much on the nature of the health problem – compare a patient recovering from a heart attack, for example, with an intravenous drug user. It is important to understand risk perception as individuals are unlikely to engage in health-protective behaviours unless they perceive themselves to be susceptible (Petrie et al 1996, Weinstein 1984).

Differences between lay and expert perceptions of risk in relation to health can be better understood when lay knowledge is viewed in the context people's lives and experience. It is important that lay perceptions of risk are not just seen as wrong or based on ignorance, but rather as embedded in particular social and cultural circumstances, as examined in the following example.

Example 1: lay understanding of heart disease

A large, in-depth study of people living in South Wales investigated lay explanations of heart disease. This research took place during a large campaign to prevent heart disease (Davison et al 1991). The results showed that people had their own explanations for the causes of heart disease, which drew on, yet differed from, the publicized lifestyle risks. In this 'lay epidemiology', people drew on a range of knowledge and experience to explain who was a 'candidate' for heart disease (Table 1). This included lifestyle factors, heredity, social environment such as work, physical environment such as climate, and a degree of randomness attributed to luck and chance.

This demonstrates that people understand the risks associated with heart disease and draw on risk factors beyond those just associated with lifestyle. However, people are also well aware, from their personal

Table 1   People who may be identified as coronary candidates
Fat people; people who don't take exercise and are unfit
Red-faced people; people with a grey pallor
Smokers
People with a heart problem in the family
Heavy drinkers
People who eat excessive amounts of rich, fatty foods
Worriers (by nature); bad-tempered, pessimistic or negative people
People who are under stress from:
– work
– family life
– financial difficulty
– unemployment/retirement
– bereavement
– gambling
People who suffer strain through:
– hard manual labour
– conditions of work/home
– excessive leisure exercise
– overindulgence (sex, dancing, drugs, lack of sleep, etc.).
(Source: Davison et al 1991)

Case study

Young people and smoking

In a qualitative study of young people's perceptions of smoking, Allbutt et al (1995) found that those studied were well aware of the risks associated with smoking: indeed, some had direct experience of its effects within their own families. However, both smokers and non-smokers discussed the positive aspects of smoking, such as the image, weight loss or relaxation. These are some of the things they said: *'It felt good, I felt big.' 'It relaxes you, that's why I like it.' 'If you've got a drink or a cigarette it's easier to talk to somebody because you can do something with your hands if you're not talking to them.' 'It helps me when I'm stressed.'*

Smoking itself was experienced as an activity that took place within a group, where friendship is important. These positive aspects encourage risk-taking behaviour. Attempts to prevent young people smoking should go beyond the provision of relevant information, and acknowledge the meaning that the behaviour has for them, in the context of their own lives.

observations, that those at high risk of getting heart disease do not always suffer from it, and that sometimes those at low risk do. People know that predicting who will get ill is difficult in multifactorial conditions. Any attempt to oversimplify this with an emphasis on risk-taking behaviours is likely to be sceptically received, as lay people's own experience and knowledge tells them that the process is more complicated and less certain than such an emphasis implies.

Risk-taking behaviour

Just as it is important to understand lay perceptions of risk, risk-taking behaviour must also be examined in the context of individuals' lives. Risk-taking behaviours often do not take place in isolation, but in interaction with others. This can explain why some people indulge in behaviours that are considered to be, even by themselves, detrimental to health. The following example will help to demonstrate the importance of social context in understanding risk-taking behaviour: it considers the practice of unsafe commercial sex between men. The case study focuses on young people and smoking.

Example 2: unsafe commercial sex between men

A study by Bloor et al (1992) of the risk-taking behaviours of male prostitutes in Glasgow, Scotland, demonstrated the importance of social interaction and social relations in determining behaviour. All but one of the ten male prostitutes they contacted were practising unsafe commercial sex. However, these same prostitutes knew that this behaviour

was risky, especially in terms of HIV transmission, and also knew that they were vulnerable to infection. It was the social circumstances surrounding male prostitution that led to the practice of unsafe sex. Unlike much female prostitution, where negotiation of fee and terms is established by the prostitute at the start of the encounter, the male prostitutes studied were subjected to client control – they themselves had little say over what should happen. This situation can partly be explained by the covert and stigmatized nature of the activity: it is neither legal nor socially sanctioned.

Practical applications

Recognition of the social context of risk, in terms of both perceptions of risk and risk-taking behaviours, is important for doctors as they become involved in public health and health promotion and in dealing with individual patients. Doctors should try to elicit people's own explanations and treat these as reasonable and based on experience. This should lead to greater understanding and empathy between doctor and patient (pp. 92–93). Similarly, account must be taken of the circumstances within which people live and how this may influence their behaviour. Doctors should not promote 'victim blaming', where those who engage in behaviours considered damaging to their health are deemed to be irresponsible. Often such behaviour can be considered a rational response to poor social conditions, or the only choice in a situation where the individual has little control.

STOP THINK

- Why might knowledge of risk factors for ill health not influence an individual's behaviour?
- In what ways are individuals constrained in their actions?
- Think of some 'unhealthy behaviours' that you engage in. Now think about some others that your friends engage in? What explanations can you think of for both your own and your friends' behaviours?

Perceptions of risk and risk-taking behaviours

- The concept of a risk factor for disease is important for both professionals and the lay public.
- Risk perceptions and risk-taking behaviours are part of a wider social context including both social conditions and social interactions.
- These may constrain the choices that individuals can make; risk-taking behaviours should be seen, at least in part, as socially determined.
- Promoting healthy behaviours means more than encouraging individuals to change. People's own risk perceptions must be understood.

Deciding to consult

Understanding why people do or do not consult is important because some doctors feel frustrated and angry about 'inappropriate or trivial' consultations, and some patients feel frustrated and angry about doctors whom they perceive as uninterested in their problems. Both sets of feelings influence subsequent consulting behaviour, medical treatment, adherence and health. Delay may seriously affect a patient's risk of disease progression and the development of complications.

The symptom iceberg

Over a 2-week period about 75% of the population will experience one or more symptoms of ill health. About one-third of these people will do nothing about their symptoms. About one-third will self-medicate or seek the advice of an alternative practitioner (see pp. 98–99), and about one-third will consult their general practitioner (Fig. 1).

Hannay (1979) has shown that the proportion of people with significant medical symptoms who do not consult a doctor is higher than the proportion of people with minor medical symptoms who do consult a doctor (26% and 11% respectively).

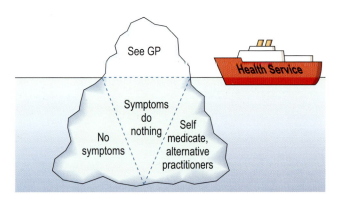

Fig. 1 **The symptom iceberg.**

 STOP THINK

- A GP in Scotland (Usherwood 1991) produced a booklet to help parents decide when to seek professional advice for children with symptoms. The overall effect of the booklet was a small reduction (28%) in daytime home visits for booklet symptoms, but a large increase (173%) in out-of-hours, night-time consultations.
- Why do you think the booklet had this effect on consultation behaviour?

Differences in symptom perception

Three features of symptoms are important for people's perceptions of their seriousness: the intensity or severity of the symptom, the familiarity of the symptom, and the duration and frequency of the symptom. For example, a severe headache may cause a person who has rarely had a headache to go to the doctor, whereas a person who has experienced migraine for some years is unlikely to consult. This person may consult, however, if the symptoms are unusual in some way or if the headache persists for longer than usual or recurs more frequently than usual.

Differential explanation

At the same time as they perceive their symptoms, people try to make sense of them, and to explain them within the context of their lives. They do this using their own lay knowledge and experience, and the knowledge and experience of their family and friends (pp. 98–99). Lydeard and Jones (1989) investigated the health concerns of a sample of consulters with symptoms of dyspepsia and a sample of non-consulters with similar symptoms, and shows that consulters were significantly more likely to be worried that their symptoms indicated a serious or fatal condition, particularly heart disease or cancer. People with a family history of stomach cancer were also more likely to consult, seeing themselves as 'more vulnerable'.

Differential evaluation

People weigh up for themselves what the relative costs and benefits will be of going (and of not going) to the doctor or other health practitioner. People often decide that other things in their lives are more important than dealing with symptoms of ill health; indeed, doctors themselves are classic examples of people who battle on at work because they perceive themselves as indispensable. Many patients 'temporalize': they wait, possibly take some medication that they already have with them, and see if the symptoms go away over time and only decide to consult if they do not.

People also weigh up what they think the doctor will think of them, and what the doctor or other health worker can actually do for them and their symptoms. Research with people with breathing difficulties has shown that people who perceive their symptoms to be serious may delay going to see their doctor if they believe that they will not be able to communicate the seriousness to the doctor.

It is also common for people to consult their doctor with symptoms that appear minor to the doctor but the decision to consult reflects anxiety that things might be serious, and they are consulting in order to confirm that they've reached the right explanation and to reassure themselves that there is nothing seriously wrong.

Mothers of children, for example, are very aware of the 'moral dilemma' they face every time they perceive their child not to be well: do they consult with what might be 'trivia' and risk being seen as 'bad' consulters, or do they delay and risk being labelled as 'bad' parents (see Case Study)?

Access

People experiencing symptoms are less likely to visit their doctor if they live farther away from the clinic/surgery. Studies in the UK of the use of accident and emergency (A&E) services have shown that the relative distance from the GP's surgery and the A&E department is a key factor in deciding which to consult: the closest being the most favoured.

Access to child-care arrangements or the provision of a sitting service for a dependent relative, the availability of a telephone to make an appointment, the availability of a

Case study

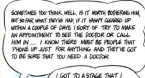
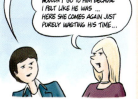

Fig. 3 **Mothers' consultation dilemmas.** (Adapted from: Cunningham-Burley and Maclean 1991)

A qualitative study of mothers' accounts of how they recognized and dealt with children's illness found that 'not wanting to bother the doctor' and 'not wasting his time' were dominant themes for mothers when they were deciding whether or not to consult.

suitable appointment slot, and the approachability and friendliness of the doctor and the practice staff are also important factors affecting accessibility.

In some countries, but less so in the UK where most medical care is free at the point of use, the financial cost of payment may act as a deterrent to consulting a doctor.

Influence of family and friends

According to some studies, up to 50% of symptoms are taken to a doctor on the advice of family or friends. It appears that family are more likely than friends to recommend a visit to the doctor, possibly because they have the responsibility for caring for the individual.

Research with pregnant women has found that social class V women with extensive and strong lay support and advice, sometimes referred to as people's lay referral network, are less likely to attend hospital ante-natal classes compared with women from social classes I and II with less lay support. It has been suggested that both the relative number of lay advisers and the degree of congruence in culture between the woman and the doctor will affect the woman's decision whether or not to consult.

People who move to a new area away from their friends and family have been found to make more visits to a doctor in their first year after moving. This raised consultation rate may reflect not only the absence of social support, but also the increased risk of ill health arising from the stress of moving house.

Triggers

Several studies have shown that it is not always the experience of symptoms that brings a person to see the doctor. A symptom or an anxiety may have been present for some time, but something else in the person's life 'triggers' the person to consult. A relative may become concerned about a continuing problem and suggest a visit to the doctor; a change at work or in one's personal life may make the symptom more noticeable or incapacitating than before, precipitating a consultation.

Delaying

A good example of the problems associated with patients who delay when they experience symptoms relates to the symptoms of having a heart attack. There is good evidence that delay in receiving medical care is associated with higher mortality, which might have been avoided had treatment (defibrillation and/or thrombolytic therapy) been instituted earlier.

Ruston et al (1998) found that people who did not delay seeking medical care had a better knowledge than 'delayers' of a wider range of symptoms of a heart attack, and were more likely to consider themselves 'at risk'. Delayers were also more likely to be taking medicines for other conditions, like dyspepsia, and would take these medicines and temporalize. Similarly, Horne et al (2000) identified a mismatch between symptoms expected of a heart attack and symptoms actually experienced, leading to delay.

In a study of people experiencing angina (chest pain on exertion), Richards et al (2002) found that, compared to residents living in an affluent area of Glasgow, residents from a deprived area reported greater vulnerability to heart disease but that this was not associated with higher reported use of a general practitioner. Instead, they interpreted their symptoms as 'normal' and did not present to their doctor for fear that they would be reprimanded by the GP for bothering them with trivia.

Deciding to consult

- The decision to consult a doctor is a complex interplay of physical, psychological and social factors.
- Many people go with relatively minor symptoms because they are anxious that something serious may be indicated.
- People may delay with serious symptoms because of anxiety, lack of knowledge, mismatch of knowledge, use of substitute medication and the relative greater importance of other things in their lives.
- There is often a mismatch between what doctors and patients perceive as appropriate reason for consulting.
- The perception of what the doctor can do for them and how they will treat them is a significant factor in a person's decision to consult.
- A change in a person's social setting or relationships may trigger a consultation even when there has been no change in the symptoms.

Seeing the doctor

Every day in the UK about 1 million people consult their general practitioner, and about 8% of them are referred to a hospital consultant for further specialist care. Patients with very different personalities and from very different backgrounds consult with very different problems and are seen by doctors with very different styles. The consultation between patient and doctor is at the core of all medical practice, be it with a general practitioner or hospital doctor, be it in the UK or elsewhere. Although an intensely personal and private meeting, usually conducted behind closed doors or curtains, there are rituals and social norms (expected ways of behaving) that provide structure and coherence to what happens in a particular culture.

Doctor–patient relationship

Four models of the doctor–patient relationship have been described.

Paternalistic

The 'paternalistic' relationship has, until recently, been the most commonly observed type of relationship, and is relatively disease focused. The doctor, a medical expert, makes a systematic enquiry, with the patient answering relatively specific and closed questions, carries out appropriate tests and reaches a diagnosis or a range of possible diagnoses. The doctor then decides on the appropriate treatment, which the patient is expected to follow without question. The process is relatively technical and specific to the symptoms/problem that the patient presents.

In the 1980s, studies of doctor–patient relationships demonstrated that patients were also 'experts' in what the symptoms/problem meant to them and their families (Tuckett et al 1985). This and other research suggested that patients sometimes held different ideas from their doctors about their illnesses, why they were ill or what they wanted to do about it.

Mutual

The 'mutual' relationship is now becoming more common, partly as a result of greater patient knowledge particularly about chronic disease, and partly because of a general cultural shift for individuals not to be passive followers of authority but autonomous agents in their own right. It is characterized by the doctor recognizing both this patient autonomy and the importance of the patient's own beliefs and knowledge of their health and illness, and the social context in which the illness is dealt with. This model involves the doctor working with a 'patient-centred' approach and is discussed in more detail below.

Consumerist

The 'consumerist' relationship is relatively uncommon in Britain but is becoming more common as a result of the extension of private health insurance, the introduction of patient charters, the increasing emphasis on extending patient choice and initiatives to provide quicker access to a doctor. It is characterized by patients 'shopping around' for their preferred care, and is accompanied (as exemplified in the USA) by relatively high levels of investigation, treatment and litigation.

Default

The fourth model, sometimes labelled 'default', is characterized by low levels of engagement between doctor and patient. It is most commonly observed in situations where the doctor can find nothing organically wrong to explain the patient's symptoms, and where the patient is labelled as 'somatizing'. There are very particular problems associated with the way patients and doctors respond to such situations, and there is a considerable risk that patients will become trapped in a cycle of over-investigation and treatment.

The 'patient-centred' approach

In its latest recommendations for undergraduate education in the UK, the General Medical Council (2002) has emphasized the importance for all students of learning the 'patient-centred' approach. Table 1 highlights five key features of the approach.

Stewart (2001) contrasts the 'patient-centred' approach with 'what it is not – technology centred, doctor centred, hospital centred, disease centred'. This is unfortunate as there are equally good reasons for hospital doctors to use the patient-centred approach, particularly as many in-patients and out-patients are attending/in hospital with acute episodes of illness often associated with, or complicated by, chronic illness. They have important information needs and their own perspectives on what is happening to them (p. 100).

The skilled doctor, whether in hospital or in the community, should be able to move easily between dealing quickly and effectively with acute, life-threatening symptoms using a disease-centred approach to taking a more patient-centred approach as soon as the threat to life has diminished. Furthermore, the acute, disease-centred approach does not have to be at the expense of treating the patient with dignity, respect and humanity. Rather than being seen as two separate and incompatible styles, it is better to think of them as two approaches working in parallel, so that the doctor is skilled in both approaches. The importance of being able to work with both approaches is well illustrated by Kinmonth et al (1998), who reported

---

Table 1 **Patient-centred care**

- Explores the patient's main reason for the visit, concerns and need for information
- Seeks an integrated understanding of the patient's world – that is, their whole person, emotional needs and life issues
- Finds common ground on what the problem is and mutually agrees on management
- Enhances prevention and health promotion
- Enhances the continuing relationship between the patient and the doctor

(Adapted from Stewart 2001)

Table 2 **Negotiation strategies**

Patients	Doctors
Disclose	Physical setting of room
Suggest	Language
Demand	—technical/non technical
Leading question	—open/closed questions
Non-verbal behaviour	—tone of voice
Hesitation/silence	Clarifying/functional uncertainty
Delaying tactics:	Listening/interrupting
'While I'm here...'	Picking up/ignoring cues
See a different doctor	Non-verbal behaviour
	Interest/uninterest
	Calm/haste
	Prescription

evidence of poorer disease management of people with type 2 diabetes by doctors who had received extra training in the patient-centred approach.

The research evidence for the practice of patient-centred care is complicated by different definitions of and methods of measuring patient-centred care. Similarly, definitions of and methods of measuring the outcome of care are not precise. Although not all studies have reported a positive association between the practice of patient-centred care and the outcome of that care (Mead and Bower 2000, Mead et al 2002), the weight of the evidence is that patients are more satisfied when they receive patient-centred care (Kinnersley et al 1999, Little et al 2001, Stewart 2001).

This judgement is confirmed by a recent review of 'longer' consultations (Freeman et al 2002). There is good evidence that patient-centred consultations generally take more time (Howie et al 1992), and the review reported that longer consultations were associated with:

- less prescribing (judged as desirable)
- more advice on lifestyle and health-promoting activities
- better recognition and handling of psychosocial problems
- better patient enablement (see Howie et al 1998)
- better clinical care of some chronic illnesses
- higher patient satisfaction.

The 'patient-centred' consultation still involves taking a systematic history of the patient's presenting and underlying problems, but it differs from the more traditional paternalistic relationship by integrating it with an enquiry into the patient's ideas, knowledge, beliefs, concerns and expectations (see pp 36–37, 146–147). In their study of doctor–patient relationships, Tuckett et al (1985) showed that consultations were most likely to break down, and patients were most likely to be dissatisfied and non-compliant (pp. 92), when doctors failed to elicit and respond empathetically to patients' beliefs and expectations. Of course, patients will sometimes hold unrealistic or inappropriate expectations. In such cases it is important that

STOP THINK

- Not all studies have found that patients prefer patient-centred care. Why might this be?
- Will the consumerist model become the dominant type of patient–doctor relationship, and if so, how will this affect the patient-centred approach?

the doctor and patient are clear what the patient's expectations and beliefs are, and that the doctor explains in a manner that does not make the patient feel stupid or defensive, why the belief or expectation is inappropriate. In some cases this will involve negotiation. Some of the strategies that patients and doctors use to control consultations are summarized in Table 2. Working-class people may sometimes express themselves rather directly, which doctors may interpret as a demand for a particular test or treatment. On occasion, no resolution may be found, and both patient and doctor are likely to feel dissatisfied with the consultation.

It is also important to remember that a single consultation between a patient and a doctor does not occur in isolation, particularly in general practice. A 5- or 10-minute consultation may be but one of a series of consultations during which patient and doctor may negotiate the diagnostic and treatment possibilities, and the implications for the patient's general well-being.

Lack of time may frequently constrain a doctor from being as person centred as he or she would like, and this puts pressure on the doctor and on the patient. Patients themselves are very conscious, not only of their responsibility not to consult with trivia (pp. 86–87), but also not to take up too much of the doctor's precious time. Patients often feel intimidated by doctors and are reluctant to ask questions or mention anxieties. Given that people frequently have anxieties that relatively minor symptoms may indicate something more serious, and given their reluctance to present with mental-health problems (see pp. 86–87), it should not be surprising that they often feel unable to mention their worries lest the doctor think that they are either wasting their time with trivia or 'stupid' (see Case study).

Case study

Time and guilt

All patients, except the two with consultations under 5 minutes (patients 88 and 101), complained of shortage of time. Although most patients said that they were not rushed and could have asked more, this was the major reason given for not asking questions.

'. . . you're thinking of the person behind you so you don't want to keep him waiting too long and I wasn't sick, so I'm forgetting the things I want to ask him . . .' (Patient 73)

The doctor's time was seen as short and valuable. Patients felt that they themselves actively limited the length of their consultation. Most patients felt guilty while consulting, for two reasons – wasting the doctor's time and taking more than their fair share:

'You always feel you want to cut corners if you can and get it over as quick as possible so he's not too late finishing because he works so many hours.' (Patient 51)

'The only reason I feel guilty is for taking up other people's time . . . I feel personally that, you know, let's hurry up because he's got other people waiting especially sometimes when you go in there and there's four or five people behind you . . .' (Patient 73)

(Cromarty 1996 BJGP 46: 525–528)

Seeing the doctor

- Doctors and patients have different knowledge, beliefs, wants and expectations, and consultations often involve negotiation.
- The process and outcome of care differs not just between patients but between doctors and especially in doctor style.
- Patient-centred doctors are more likely than disease-centred doctors to identify patients' psychosocial problems, and to deal with their anxieties.
- Patients are often reluctant to voice their ideas and anxieties in case they are thought of as inappropriate, stupid or time-wasting.

Placebo

A remedy without any direct action on a disease, given to keep the patient happy, or to persuade the prescriber that he is doing something positive and useful, or both.
Penguin Medical Encyclopaedia

The placebo effect (from the Latin 'I will please') is important to understand because it can have a great effect on the treatment of patients. Placebos are used and abused, but often little understood.

The emergence of placebo effects

Until recently there could be no neat distinction between drugs whose mode of action for a specific disorder was known and understood, and any other drug (see Fig. 1). With the development of scientific medicine, people then began to identify active ingredients and to become more suspicious of drugs whose action was not understood. This introduced the notion that there were drugs that would treat a particular condition by a particular route and other substances that might be placebos.

However, placebos have been shown to bring about clinical improvement in many branches of medicine: surgery, the treatment of cancer, dentistry, psychiatry, paediatrics and numerous others. They can produce the same phenomena observed with other drugs:

- habituation (a tendency to increase the dose over time)
- withdrawal symptoms
- dependency (an inability to stop taking them without psychiatric help)
- inverse relationship between severity of symptom and efficacy of placebo.

The nocebo phenomenon

It is also possible for a drug or procedure to produce adverse effects that are not the result of any known pharmacological mechanism. These are called 'nocebo effects' from the Latin 'I will harm'. In one study women who believed they were prone to heart disease were nearly four times as likely to die as women with similar risk factors who did not believe (Eaker et al 1992). While effects *can* be severe, reported nocebo symptoms are more usually generalized and diffuse, such

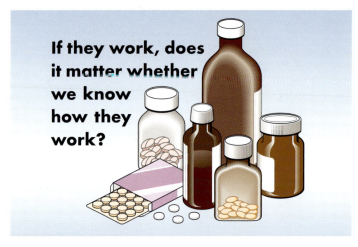

Fig. 1 **Drugs and mode of action.**

as drowsiness, nausea, fatigue and insomnia. In clinical trials these nocebo effects can be severe enough to lead to discontinuation and dropout.

Placebos and clinical trials

In order to demonstrate the efficacy of any new treatment now, clinical trials include a placebo for comparison so that such effects can be separated from the effects of the experimental compound. These are often 'double-blind' trials, i.e. neither the patient nor the member of staff who gives it knows which is the experimental drug and which is the placebo. This ensures that nothing can influence a patient's expectations about the drug and, therefore, the response.

Types of placebo

- Pure placebo: thought to contain no active ingredient, for example, a sugar pill.
- Impure placebo: contains an active ingredient, but one which is not known to have any effect on the condition being treated, e.g. a vitamin C tablet being given for headache.
- Placebo procedure: a procedure, for instance taking blood pressure, which is not known to produce any clinical change.

What makes someone susceptible to placebo effects?

There are no personal characteristics that will predict whether or not a patient will respond positively to a placebo. Circumstances and presentation are more influential. For

example, people's perception of pain depends on the situation: people injured in combat appear to tolerate pain better than those with similar injuries in hospital. In war, an injury means evacuation to safety and thus brings great relief; this is not the same in civilian life. With placebos, experiments have demonstrated a number of factors that produce a response, for instance:

- The physical appearance of the placebo; for example, green tranquillizers reduce anxiety more than yellow or red ones (Shapira et al 1970).
- The reputation of the setting, e.g. a university research unit will enhance treatment more than a backstreet clinic.
- The patient's perception of staff attitudes affects response – for example, where doctors are judged as more interested and enthusiastic, the results are more positive.

The nocebo phenomenon has been found to be more common in women than men, and while cultural and ethnic factors are thought to be important, there is little empirical evidence (Barsky et al 2002). Nocebo effects are more likely to be found in:

- people who expect to experience side effects
- patients who have been previously conditioned to experience side effects
- patients with certain psychological characteristics, such as anxiety, depression or neuroticism.

	First dose	Second dose		Levels of pain reported	
				First dose	Second dose
Group 1	Morphine	Morphine			
Group 2	Naloxone	Placebo			
Group 3a	Placebo	Placebo	Responders		
			Non-responders		
Group 3b	Placebo	Naloxone	Responders		
			Non-responders		

Fig. 2 **Levels of pain reported in double-blind trial, naloxone/placebo.** (Reproduced with permission from Levine et al 1978, pp. 654–657)

Case study

Levine and colleagues hypothesized that placebo effects that relieve pain are mediated by endorphin release. If that were the case, then naloxone (an opiate antagonist) would block them. They gave medication to patients after surgery in a double-blind trial (Fig. 2). The patients had all had wisdom teeth removed. Group 1 were given morphine, Group 2 had naloxone and Group 3 got a placebo. Of those initially given a placebo (Group 3), half were given another placebo 1 hour later (Group 3a), and half were given naloxone 1 hour later (Group 3b). Our interest lies in these two groups of patients. When they were initially given the placebo, 39% reported a significant decrease in pain, but if they were in Group 3b, those given naloxone, the pain increased again. For those who had not responded to the placebo, the naloxone made no difference. So it appeared that some patients obtained significant pain relief from a placebo, but this was reversed by an opiate antagonist. The experiments concluded that endorphin release must have occurred with the placebo.

How do they work?

There are various possibilities:

- Social influence – doctors are perceived as people in authority and, therefore, their direction and expectations are followed.
- Role expectation – the doctor's role is to organize treatment, and the patient's role is to get better, so he or she plays that role.
- Classical conditioning – for a patient, past experiences of taking drugs led to improvement, so the administration of a new drug is more likely to produce the same response (see pp 20–21).
- Operant conditioning – the doctor rewards the patient who shows any sign of improvement, thus increasing the probability that the patient will continue to report improvement (see pp 20–21).
- Cognitive influence – the patient has firm beliefs about medical treatment, such as 'modern medicine is based on scientific evidence, therefore this drug will be effective.' Of course, the opposite would also be true: if the patient believes modern medicine to be harmful, he or she may be less likely to respond and may, in fact, experience adverse effects.

What are doctors' attitudes to placebo effects?

Many doctors have strong feelings about the use of placebos in medicine: some are positive, but many are negative, perhaps because the placebo effect is similar to faith-healing, when many doctors prefer to see medicine as a science. While most health professionals are aware of the therapeutic aspect of placebo, fewer are aware of the nocebo phenomenon. Views about placebo effects can range widely:

- Placebo effects are a nuisance that interfere with the understanding and practice of medicine.
- Placebo effects are powerful, but to use placebos in practice is a betrayal of trust between doctor and patient.
- Placebo effects are powerful and should be usefully incorporated to enhance treatment.

STOP THINK

- Many people in prison are vulnerable and have in the past been dependent on drugs or alcohol. They feel the need to continue to take something 'to help with nerves'. Part of this dependence is psychological rather than chemical and they frequently come to the medical officer asking for medication.
- Should a medical officer prescribe a placebo in this case, 'to keep the patient happy, or to persuade the prescriber that he is doing something positive or useful, or both?'

Placebo

- Placebo effects have been demonstrated in many branches of medicine.
- Nocebo phenomena are usually generalized and diffuse adverse symptoms.
- Placebo effects ought to be controlled in experimental trials of medical procedures.
- There are no established personal characteristics that will predict a therapeutic response to placebo.
- Nocebo phenomena are more likely among people who expect to experience adverse effects or have been previously conditioned to experience adverse effects.
- Effects are influenced by context: culture, expectations and beliefs.
- There are ethical issues involved in the clinical use of placebos.

Patient adherence

What is adherence?

Adherence means following the advice of health-care professionals. This includes taking preventive action (e.g. reducing alcohol consumption), keeping medical appointments (e.g. screening or follow-up appointments), following self-care advice (e.g. caring for a wound after surgery) and taking medication as directed (e.g. in relation to dose and timing). Non-adherence is usually defined as a failure to follow advice, which will lead to a harmful effect on health or a decrease in medication effectiveness. Most medical interventions rely on patient adherence. For example, diagnosis and prescription can only affect patients' health if they pick up prescriptions and take medication as advised.

Measuring adherence

Patients' own reports, pill counts and analysis of blood or urine samples can be used to measure adherence. Patients appear to consistently overestimate their adherence when self-report measures are compared to objective measures (Ley 1997, Myers and Midence 1998). However, some simple, direct self-report measures can offer good estimates of adherence (Morisky et al 1986).

How good is patient adherence?

Rates of adherence vary across behaviours. However, it has been estimated that 40–45% of patients are non-adherent (Ley 1997). This implies that: (i) almost half of all prescribed medication has a reduced health impact; (ii) doctors may only be effective with 55–60% of their patients; (iii) patients are becoming ill unnecessarily due to non-adherence.

It has been suggested that 10–25% of hospital admissions are due to non-adherence. Even when patients' lives depend on taking medication as directed, as in the case of heart and liver transplants, between 5% and 33% of patients have been found to be non-adherent (Rovelli et al 1989).

Why do patients not follow advice?

Patients may be non-adherent for different reasons and in different ways (see Donovan and Blake 1992). Some patients may intend to take recommended medication but forget to do so or find it difficult. Others may disagree with the diagnosis or the medication regimen and decide not to take the medication, or deliberately to take more or less than was advised. Knowing why patients do not adhere is important to promoting adherence.

Key questions that influence patients' decisions to adhere, or not, are: Do I really need this treatment? Am I at risk of symptoms without doing what was advised? How effective/beneficial is the recommended action? What side effects will it have? Will adherence conflict with other things I want to do? If consultations with health-care professionals result in misunderstandings regarding illness or treatment this may also lead to non-adherence.

When do patients follow advice?

Reviews of adherence research have identified a number of factors influencing adherence (see Fig. 1). Adherence is most likely when patients understand what they are being asked to do and why. Patients must also remember what they are told if they to act on it later and, finally, satisfaction with the doctor and the consultation makes adherence more likely.

How can doctors increase adherence?

Patients are more likely to feel satisfied and to understand advice when doctors find out what they think is wrong and discuss this. The doctor should seek to reach an agreement with the patient about what is wrong and what should be done about it. The

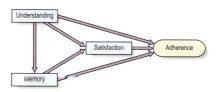

Fig. 1 **Key determinants of patient adherence.** (Adapted with permission from Ley 1997.)

importance of such co-operation has been underlined by the proposal that, instead of encouraging adherence, doctors should seek to establish 'concordance' in their consultations (Mullen 1997). If doctors can facilitate joint, negotiated decision-making, or 'concordance', about treatment then patients are more likely to intend to adhere. For example, if a drug and regimen are jointly agreed then the patient is likely to be more committed to taking the drug as recommended. This implies that the feasibility of any particular regimen needs to be assessed for each patient, that is, doctors should consider whether the patient will able to take the medication as advised.

If doctors are to ensure that the recommended treatment is clearly understood, and also consider the difficulties the patient may have in following an agreed plan, they must make time for discussion and negotiation in consultations. This is especially important because some patients may be reluctant to raise doubts or ask questions for fear of appearing stupid (pp 88–89). Below we consider particular steps doctors can take to enhance patients' satisfaction,

---

Box 1 Changing health beliefs to increase adherence

Jones et al (1987) showed how the health belief model (p 146) could be used to increase adherence amongst patients attending an accident and emergency unit with asthma symptoms. Patients' health beliefs were assessed and they received information relating to their suscept-ibility to asthma complications, the seriousness of such complications and the benefits of visiting their GP to obtain treatment and avoid complications. Ninety one per cent of this group made a follow-up appointment with their doctor compared to 43% in a control group who had not received the educational intervention. 75% kept these appointments compared to 10% in the control group.

Box 2 Helping patients remember in general practice

Ley et al (1976) assessed the amount of information that the patients of four doctors remembered. The researchers then developed a brief manual for the doctors, which explained how they could simplify information, use explicit categorization and repetition, and give specific rather than general advice. The amount of information patients remembered after their doctors had read the manual increased from an average of 56% to an average of 71%, suggesting that memory-enhancing communication increased the amount patients remembered.

Information remembered by patients (%)		
	Before	After
Doctor A	52	61
Doctor B	56	70
Doctor C	57	73
Doctor D	59	80

increase their understanding and maximize their memory for advice.

Promoting patient satisfaction

If a patient feels his/her doctor is not interested in his/her problem or has not understood it this will undermine confidence in the doctor's advice. For example, in a well-known study of paediatric consultations, Korsch et al (1968) found that mothers who were very satisfied with their doctor's warmth, concern and communication were three times more likely to adhere than dissatisfied mothers. Satisfaction depends upon the patient's perception of the doctor's sensitivity, concern, respect and competence. Reducing waiting time, taking time to greet the patient in a courteous manner and engaging in friendly introductory exchanges are all likely to increase satisfaction. Asking open-ended questions which cannot be answered 'yes' or 'no' and allowing the patient time to express his or her worries is also likely to make the patient feel satisfied with the consultation (pp 94–95).

Increasing patients' understanding

Using simple words to describe the body or treatments and encouraging patients to express their views is essential to ensuring that patients understand. Clear communication depends upon knowing what others already know and what they expect from us. The doctor's task may be a little like giving directions. Deciding upon the most effective directions involves establishing some common understanding of local geography. Similarly, the doctor may need to assess the patient's health knowledge, beliefs and expectations before deciding how to explain the problem

- A patient taking anti-hypertension medication returns for a routine check-up. You find that his blood pressure is high. What do you do – increase the dose, change the medication, refer the patient for further tests or talk to the patient about the medication and any problems which may be involved in taking it?

Case study

Janice was using a bronchodilator inhaler to control her asthma symptoms. She also had a preventive steroid inhaler but was reluctant to use it because she worried about the potential side effects of taking steroids. She needed more medication and wrote a short letter to her GP asking for her usual repeat prescription.

She was asked to make an appointment because she had already had five previous repeat prescriptions. Janice was disappointed because work was hectic and she had little time to spare. She arrived at the surgery on time but had to wait 30 minutes before being called. Her doctor took a few minutes to finish some notes while she waited in his room. When she explained that she needed a new prescription for her inhalers the doctor asked about her use of the bronchodilator inhaler. The doctor explained that she should be using the preventive steroid inhaler every day to control her symptoms and that she was relying too heavily on the bronchodilator. The doctor asked her if she understood. Janice did understand and said so. The doctor wrote the prescription and Janice, who was worried about missing her driving lesson in 15 minutes time, left without asking any questions.

Janice started taking the preventive steroid inhaler morning and night as advised. Then she watched a television programme about the side effects of steroids on body builders and, again, began to worry about potential long-term effects of using the steroid inhaler. Combined with her concerns about oral thrush, this was enough to discourage Janice. She stopped using the steroid inhaler and reverted to controlling her asthma by using the bronchodilator. Three months later Janice needed another prescription and got a repeat prescription without seeing a doctor.

and treatment. Assessing the *health beliefs* (pp 146–147) specified by the health belief model and clarifying any misunderstandings regarding, for example, symptom severity, treatment effectiveness or side effects may motivate the patient to follow an agreed treatment plan (see Box 1). Assessing how motivated the patient is and what others' may think of their illness or of the suggested treatment may also help identify problems that could lead to poor adherence.

Helping patients to remember

Telling someone what you are about to tell them makes it more likely they will remember because this assists with the process of encoding in memory (pp 26–27). This labelling of information is called 'explicit categorization'. For example, a doctor might say, 'I'm going to tell you what I think is wrong with you' or 'I'm going to remind you when you should take your tablets and how many you should take' before conveying these important pieces of information. Instructions may also be remembered more easily if the doctor stresses that they are important and repeats them.

Specific advice, for example, 'cut the number of cigarettes you smoke by half' or 'make an appointment for 2 weeks' time', is easier to remember than general suggestions such as 'cut down the amount you smoke' or 'come in again soon'.

Simple advice and regimens are easier to understand and remember. Where possible, doctors should negotiate regimens that suit the patient. For example, the progestogen-only pill may not be an appropriate contraceptive for a woman who thinks she is unlikely to remember to take it at the same time every day.

Encouraging patients to take notes in consultations and providing printed information can ensure that patients have accurate information. Using such techniques has been shown to improve the amount of information remembered by patients in general practice (see Box 2).

Patient adherence

- Up to 45% of patients are non-adherent.
- Adherence is more likely when patients understand advice, remember it and feel satisfied with the consultation.
- Doctors can increase satisfaction by being friendly and considerate.
- Adherence is more likely when doctors consider and discuss the patient's perspective, understanding and motivation.
- Doctors can increase understanding by simplifying information and by discussion of patients' health beliefs.
- Doctors can increase patients' recall by using explicit categorization, stressing and repeating instructions and giving specific advice.

Communication skills

Medical science has provided increasingly sophisticated diagnostic and treatment techniques. However, there is no point in being expert in those techniques if you cannot enable your patients to understand how they may be helped by them. The consultation is central to effective medical care and is characterized by two primary communicative tasks: relational development and informational exchange (Cegala et al 1996). If doctors are poor at accomplishing these tasks there is increased risk of:

- failing to identify the patient's main problem
- inaccurate diagnosis, inappropriate investigations (Stewart et al 1979)
- poor adherence with treatment (Ley and Llewelyn 1995)
- patient dissatisfaction and complaints (Richards 1990)
- patients choosing litigation if an error is made (Shapiro et al 1989).

It is therefore important for doctors to be aware of factors that affect the quality of their communication with patients and to seek to improve their skills as part of maintaining 'fitness to practice'.

Factors affecting doctor–patient communication

These can be considered under four broad headings.

1. Physical setting

The environment within which a doctor interviews a patient is important:

- **Seating**. It is helpful if a doctor sits at an angle of about 45° to the patient. A patient is likely to feel more uncomfortable if the doctor sits directly facing them, sits behind a desk, or stands when the patient is sitting or lying down.
- **Privacy**. Unless patients believe they won't be overheard they are unlikely to talk freely.
- **Noise and interruptions**. Intrusions that disturb the patient's (or doctor's) concentration can make a consultation less effective.

2. Non-verbal behaviour

Non-verbal communication (NVC) refers to behaviour, other than speech, which influences social interaction. NVC is not normally under conscious control and can at times contradict what is said. Among the most important aspects of NVC are:

- **Proximity**. Sitting a comfortable distance from a patient assists communication. Being too distant makes the doctor seem aloof, while being too close may feel overly threatening.
- **Posture**. Sitting upright but relaxed, with arms and legs uncrossed and leaning slightly toward the patient, conveys attentiveness. Leaning back or slouching may suggest lack of interest.
- **Eye contact**. This is the most powerful NVC for initiating, maintaining and ending communication. The doctor's gaze should be in the direction of the patient without staring. This allows the patient to make eye contact as wished. Avoiding eye contact for long periods inhibits communication.
- **Facial expression**. Facial expressions often give away how a

person is really feeling. Doctors can be alert to patients' expressions showing emotions such as fear, embarrassment or confusion, and can by their own facial expressions show interest, compassion and concern. However, if the doctor's expression reflects disgust, anger or disbelief, the relationship with the patient may be prejudiced.

- **Head nods**. Head nods convey understanding and encouragement to say more. However, vigorous nodding may be interpreted as impatience. Similarly, nodding when a patient expresses a strong opinion may inadvertently imply the doctor's agreement.
- **Touch**. Within medical relationships touch can be *facilitative* (e.g. in helping to establish a friendly relationship with the patient by shaking hands on meeting), *functional* (e.g. to carry out physical examinations) or *therapeutic* (e.g. touching a distressed patient on the hand, arm or shoulder to console). However, not all patients find the latter comforting so its appropriateness must be judged for each individual.
- **Paralinguistic features**. This refers to aspects of verbal messages that serve to modulate their meaning. Variations in vocal attributes such as tone, pitch and volume can determine whether the same words, e.g. 'You took all the tablets', are expressed as a statement of fact, surprise, or as a question.
- **Silence**. Silences may occur when a patient is taking time to decide how to answer a question, trying to recall a detail or is experiencing a difficult emotion. It is important not to 'fill' this silence immediately with another question but instead to allow the patient time to respond. If the patient begins to appear very uncomfortable with the silence, use of a reflection, e.g. 'You seem upset', can often lead to a clarification of thoughts or feelings.

Awareness of NVC can assist a doctor to form a good therapeutic relationship with a patient. Used skilfully, non-verbal behaviours offer powerful tools with which to encourage a patient to talk, and to demonstrate interest in, understanding of and empathy with the patient's predicament.

- Patients often complain that doctors do not ask about their feelings or emotional responses to illness. But some doctors argue that their job is just to treat disease, not deal with how people cope with it.
- What's your opinion on this view of medical practice?

3. Verbal communication

Effective exchange of information with a patient is vital if a doctor is to clarify presenting problems, explain diagnoses, and discuss treatment options sensitively. It is therefore important that language is used effectively to achieve these goals. Different aspects of verbal clinical communication can be identified.

Questioning

There are different types and functions of questions but two broad categories can be distinguished:

■ **Closed/narrow questions**. These are so called because they tend to limit the patient to one- or two-word answers. Closed questions are useful for obtaining or clarifying details. Examples include questions which invite:

 – an item of detail – When did the pain start?
 – choice of alternatives – Is it sharp or dull pain?
 – yes/no response – Is the pain still there?

■ **Open/broad questions**. These questions allow patients more discretion in replying and are good for eliciting beliefs, opinions or feelings. Open questions are also useful early on in an interview for encouraging a patient to describe fully their problems, for instance:

 – what's been troubling you?
 – what do you think is wrong with you?
 – how do you feel about the operation?

Blended skilfully, questions of these two types will allow you to explore, and confirm understanding of, a patient's difficulties. It is also important to avoid asking more than one question at once and to avoid leading questions.

Reflecting
Reflection is an important verbal skill for encouraging a patient to talk and for demonstrating active listening. Thus if a patient says, 'I can't believe it's cancer', a doctor might reflect back:

 – using the patient's words – You can't believe it.
 – an interpretation of those words – It's too much to take in.
 – or an impression of the patient's feelings – You feel shocked.

Summarizing
A summary draws together the significant aspects of what has been said. Doctors may summarize their understanding of the patient's symptoms or the key points of treatment. This provides an opportunity for clarifying misinterpretations on the part of the doctor or patient.

Explaining
The ability to deliver lucid, coherent explanations is critical to providing patients with an understanding of their illness, diagnosis, investigations or treatment. An explanation should be presented in a way that takes account of the patient's needs and is easily understood. When giving an explanation it helps to:

■ use a series of logical points
■ avoid or explain any jargon
■ repeat and emphasize key points
■ use examples and diagrams
■ give specific rather than vague advice
■ ask for feedback on understanding.

4. Psychosocial context
This refers to characteristics of doctors or patients which may affect how they relate to each other. Such attributes include personal values, attitudes and beliefs, which may reflect the influences of family, socio-economic, religious or ethnic background. These factors may have particular significance when issues with ethical or moral overtones arise, e.g. sexual matters, drug taking, AIDS. Organizational context is also very important, with short appointment times providing little opportunity for patient-centred consultations (see pp 88–89).

Case study

Consider the following different responses of a consultant to a patient.
How successful is relational development and information exchange in each example? Why are they different?

Peter was a 26-year-old physiology PhD student with a recent history of passing blood following mild exercise. At a busy out-patient clinic he had just undergone an IVP to X-ray his kidneys and was called to see the consultant, Mr Brown.

Mr Brown (looking at X-ray on screen): *Well, Peter, I can find nothing wrong with your kidneys. I think you have a touch of long-march haematuria, which sometimes happens to people who exercise a lot.*
Peter (in a hesitating voice): *Oh? I . . . I've read a bit about that condition and I don't think it fits with what happens to me.*

Response 1
Mr Brown (turning to stare at Peter with an expression of disbelief and annoyance): *Oh, you don't!* (pause) *Well young man, in that case you've just talked yourself into a cystoscopy! We'll send you an appointment for a few weeks' time.* (Walks off briskly.)
Peter (looking very anxious): *Oh dear. Thanks.*

Response 2
Mr Brown (turning with an expression of surprise but interest): *What makes you say that, Peter?*
Peter: *Well, the blood I pass is bright red and in this condition I believe it's usually a dark brown colour.*
Mr Brown: *I see! That's possibly significant.* (pause) *Well, we could do a cystoscopy to have a look in your bladder. That would mean giving you a general anaesthetic and passing a fine optic fibre up through your penis. How would you feel about us doing that?*
Peter (looking apprehensive): *Well . . . OK, if you think it will help find out what's wrong with me.*

Peter underwent cystoscopy and was found to have calculi that had been causing inflammation in the lining of his bladder.

Communication skills

■ Doctor–patient communication is central to effective medical practice and can affect quality of care
■ Effective information exchange and relational development are key tasks in medical interviewing.
■ Four factors which influence the effectiveness of doctor–patient communication are:
 – physical setting
 – non-verbal communication
 – verbal communication
 – psychosocial context.
■ Effective clinical communication requires the ability to use the relevant skills flexibly in response to the needs of different patients.

www.wansford.co.uk/skills/skills2.htm

Breaking bad news

What is bad news?

Bad news has been defined as 'any news that drastically and negatively alters the person's view of her or his future' (Buckman 1994). Bad news may be giving a terminal or life-changing prognosis, e.g. metastatic cancer or multiple sclerosis, but it could also be news of sudden loss, e.g. telling a young wife that her husband has died after a massive heart attack or parents that their teenage son has been killed in a motorbike accident. It may also be about something much less dramatic for patients, such as having to tell them that their medical notes have been lost after a long period of waiting at an out-patient clinic.

Why is it difficult?

There are several reasons why breaking bad news is an especially difficult task for doctors, irrespective of their age, speciality or professional experience. These may be personal (related to their own personality or past experience), social (to do with society's attitudes), professional (influenced by role or peer values), or legal/political (Buckman 1994). Some of these are listed in Table 1. In addition, it may be made more difficult if family members want to protect the person from bad news and distress (Kaye 1996). Under these circumstances, the doctor may be asked to collude with the relatives in order to maintain a conspiracy of silence. This situation often puts strain on a previously healthy relationship, and can lead to feelings of mistrust and isolation on the part of the patient. Nowadays, most doctors believe that people should be made aware of their diagnosis and prognosis if they wish, and will tell the person if asked directly. Studies also show that most patients want the truth about their diagnosis but the depth of information sought will vary according to individual needs (Meredith 2000, Yardley et al 2001).

Research has shown that doctors find the breaking of bad news so stressful that they adopt a variety of strategies to make the task easier for themselves (Taylor 1988). The use of these strategies in turn can affect the amount and type of information doctors give to patients, i.e. their policy of disclosure. The way a doctor breaks news of this kind can affect how patients later adjust to and cope with their illness. Numerous guidelines have now been developed that describe ways in which a doctor can manage this situation to make it easier for those receiving the news.

Table 1 **Difficulties involved in breaking bad news**	
Personal	Fear of own illness/death
	Fear of expressing own emotions, e.g. crying
	Recent bereavement
	Identification with own experience (for example victim may be same age)
	Embarrassment/distress/discomfort
Social	Removal of death from home to institution makes death unacceptable and taboo
	Sickness stigmatized
Professional	Lack of experience or training
	Fear of eliciting a difficult response, e.g. anger
	Fear of being blamed by person or superiors
	Failure to provide cure
	Fear of causing pain/emotional damage
	Fear of destroying hope
Political	Fear of litigation
Source: Buckman 1994	

Managing the consultation

1. Check the person's physical ability to take in news

Before attempting to give any information of this kind it is important to make sure that the patient or relative is physically and mentally able to understand (Faulkner et al 1994). In the case of a serious diagnosis, such as cancer, the patients may already be experiencing symptoms that are preventing them from thinking clearly, such as confusion or drowsiness. It is necessary, therefore, to treat any condition that will prevent the person from comprehending the news, before attempting to impart it.

2. Check own appearance and readiness

The way doctors present themselves during consultations can also help patients to accept the news more easily. Making sure that you appear comfortable, relaxed and not rushed will communicate to patients that you have the time to spend with them and feel at ease with the task. Appearing in a blood-stained coat and looking tense and harassed will only serve to heighten patients' stress.

3. Setting the scene

The context of where the news will be broken is as important as how it is broken. The most appropriate place will be a quiet side room on the ward to ensure the person's privacy and concentration. People will absorb the news better if they feel as relaxed and comfortable as possible. Most doctors find it helpful to be accompanied by another member of staff, e.g. a nurse, social worker or chaplain, as well as allowing the person to be joined by a relative or friend. The presence of other people can often help to clarify information that was given by the doctor after the interview, as well as providing emotional support when the news is broken.

The process of breaking bad news

The process of breaking bad news can be described as a series of stages to be worked through by the doctor and the recipient (Buckman 1994, Faulkner et al 1994, Kaye 1996, Twycross 1999).

Stage 1

It is essential before breaking the news to find out what the person already knows and understands about his illness. This will inform the doctor of the degree of insight and provide a baseline on which to build. Sometimes the person will indicate that he already suspects that something is seriously wrong. This may be especially true of people who have been experiencing difficult symptoms or have known a relative or friend who has had the same illness.

Stage 2

Before continuing, the doctor should find out what the person wants to know about his/her illness. This can be done by asking the person directly, and should leave the doctor in no doubt about how much information to give. For example, some people will require only to know about their treatment without wishing to speak about their diagnosis or prognosis.

Stage 3

If the person wants to know more, the news should be broken frankly and clearly. To begin with, some information should be given by the doctor to warn the person that the news is not good. For example, 'The results of the tests are more serious than we thought', but avoid euphemisms.

Stage 4

Leave silence and allow time for news to sink in.

Stage 5

Listen and respond to how the person reacts. You can keep giving information as long as the person is asking for it and understands what is being said.

Stage 6

Plan treatment or next course of action with the patient or relatives (for example, with bereaved relatives this may be viewing the body). It is also vital that the doctor arranges to see the patient at a follow-up interview in order to help clarify any misunderstandings or anxieties the person may have about the news.

No news is bad news

An important part of communicating news to patients is conveying the results of tests. It can be difficult to reassure patients who have been anticipating bad news that the news is good. Studies show that patients who are experiencing symptoms but have negative test results may remain anxious long after the consultation and continue to experience the same symptoms, often leading them to consult again. Reasons for this anxiety may be a misunderstanding of what the doctor has said or disbelief. Doubt may be also fuelled by conflicting evidence from an individual's personal circumstances – for example, knowing someone with the same symptoms who has died or who has had a false negative result. In these circumstances direct discussion of the patient's concerns is advocated rather than referring the patient on for further tests (McDonald et al 1996).

Sudden bad news

In cases of trauma, the task of breaking bad news may be even more difficult because of the suddenness and unexpectedness of the death, illness or accident. In addition, there will usually have been no time to establish a relationship with the person beforehand or warn him/her that the news is serious. Often the situation is complicated by the fact that the victim may be young, the next of kin may be difficult to establish or contact, and it may be less easy to control the context in a busy accident and emergency department or intensive care unit (McLauchlan 1990). In these situations the police may be a useful source of help in contacting and supporting relatives.

Reactions to bad news

The way a person reacts to bad news will vary widely. Its impact will depend on the difference between what the person hopes for and the medical reality (Buckman 1994). Reactions may be dictated by the person's past experiences, personality, coping strategies or the impact of the news on the individual. They may be unrelated to the type or stage of the disease. Reactions may vary from calm or resigned acceptance to acute distress, anxiety, anger, shock and denial.

Case study

John is a 34-year-old man who is engaged to be married next year. For the past 2 years he has periodically experienced pins and needles in his arms and legs. Although his fiancée and family urged him to go to the doctor he had shrugged the symptoms off. In the last few weeks, however, an episode of blurred vision and a temporary loss of power in his right leg precipitated his referral to a neurologist by his general practitioner. A series of tests confirmed a diagnosis of multiple sclerosis. Unfortunately, the neurologist was unable to give the news himself because a prior commitment to present a paper at a conference meant that he had to be absent from the ward for a few days. He therefore asked his house officer to break the bad news in his place. This worried the house officer because he had never had to do this before. To minimize his anxiety, he decided he would do it while taking blood from John as this would give them both something to concentrate on. On hearing the news, John was devastated. He began to cry and then became angry with the house officer and demanded to see the consultant. Not knowing how to respond to this reaction, the house officer fled to find the ward sister.

Breaking bad news

- Ensure the person is physically able to take in the news.
- Find a quiet room where the news can be broken in privacy and undisturbed.
- Allow the person to be accompanied by a friend/relative/staff member of their choice.
- Check what the person already knows, understands and requires to know further.
- Give warning to alert the person that the news is serious.
- Continue giving information if the person is understanding and responding positively to it.
- Monitor the person's reaction and respond.
- Plan next course of action with the person and always arrange follow-up.

Imagine you were the house officer in the situation given in the case study.

- How would you have broken the news to John?
- What factors might have caused John to react the way he did?
- If you were the ward sister, what would you do to help John now?

Self-care and the popular sector

People experiencing physical discomfort or emotional distress do not always turn to a doctor for advice and treatment. In all societies there is a range of ways in which people either help themselves or seek help from others. Kleinman (1985) has suggested that health-care systems are composed of different sectors or arenas – the popular sector, the folk sector and the professional sector – although they may partly overlap with each other (Fig. 1). In Western industrialized societies, the professional sector is predominantly biomedicine. However, doctors certainly do not see all the illness and disease that occurs in a community. Indeed, they only see what has been called the tip of the iceberg of both symptoms and disease (see pp. 86–87). This means that there is a considerable amount of unmet need in the community, where people may be experiencing health problems that would respond to medical treatment. However, it also means that many people are dealing with a range of both self-limiting and chronic illness themselves, by using self-care (popular) or complementary treatments (pp 142–143). We can begin to understand this by examining the popular sector in more detail.

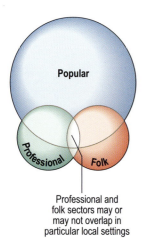

Fig. 1 Three sectors of health care.
(Redrawn from Kleinman 1985)

The popular sector

The popular sector is where ill health is first recognized and defined. It is also where much ill health is treated, and where various health-maintenance activities take place (for example, ensuring healthy diets, taking vitamin supplements). It includes all the therapeutic options that people use without consulting either medical or folk/complementary practitioners. Three components of the popular sector are important: the lay referral system, self-care and self-help.

The lay referral system

Most people discuss their symptoms with someone else, whether this is a member of their family or a friend. Indeed, some people in the community have an important place in these lay networks – those with experience of an illness, those with experience of raising children, and those who are or were health professionals. This system of lay referral may influence health and illness behaviour. For example, if the network or subculture is incongruent with doctors, in terms of beliefs and situation, there may be a low rate of uptake of medical services (Friedson 1975, McKinlay 1973). Alternatively, friends and family may encourage attendance at a doctor's surgery or hospital.

Self-care

How people deal with illness themselves will depend on their beliefs, attitudes, resources and access to formal health care. Self-care, and specifically self-medication, is a large and important part of the popular sector of health care. Self-care can include both over-the-counter medicines and home remedies. In research conducted in Scotland involving three generations within a family, the older generation were found to be the most likely to use home remedies, and the younger generation over-the-counter remedies (for themselves and their children) (Blaxter and Paterson 1982). Other research involving mothers with young children (Cunningham-Burley and Irvine 1987) found that self-care was the most common response to children's symptoms. In this study, mothers were asked to complete health diaries and participate in an in-depth interview: 42 women completed health diaries, and the results showed that the mothers closely monitored their children, and often noticed changes which may indicate illness. Something was noticed on 49% of all recorded days. On 65% of these days the mothers took some kind of action in dealing with their children's symptoms, yet they made contact with a health-care professional on only 11% of these days.

The mothers thought that you could 'catch an illness early', thus obviating the need to go to the doctor for a prescribed medication. They also knew from their own experience that many illnesses were self-limiting – they would thus try something first, and only go to a doctor if symptoms did not clear up. They also did not want to bother their doctors when they could attempt to treat the child themselves. The main ways in which mothers dealt with the symptoms that their young children were experiencing were through home nursing and home remedies (some of these activities may have been previously recommended by doctors), and by providing over-the-counter remedies, particularly analgesics and cough medicines. Using the pharmacist was an important part of the lay referral system and self-care activities amongst this group. The extracts from interviews, shown in Figure 2, illustrate this.

There has been a rise in the range of over-the-counter medicines available to consumers due to drug deregulation. Some drugs formerly only available on prescription from a doctor are now

"...the chemist told me to take Actifed and I found out it really did her some good, so I just get the Actifed now and if she has got a cold I just give her that."

"...it was the chemist who told me to get them. I mean they are quite expensive but I don't bother. I'd rather that than go to the doctor. I mean I think I would go to the doctor if they were really ill or anything."

"...well, they had lots of things like throat infections, colds, constant colds, and I would sort of rub them with Vick and give them paracetamol. If it lasted a couple of days, I would take them to the doctor."

Fig. 2 The chemist and self-care: mothers' views. (Source: Cunningham-Burley and Irvine 1987)

available from a pharmacist. This has led some to suggest that there is now greater consumer choice in relation to medicine taking, and greater autonomy in self-care. However, others suggest that the efficacy of some traditional formulations, such as expectorants, is not well proven (Bates 2001).

An extended role for the community pharmacist is being emphasized by the profession and by governments. The community pharmacist operates on the boundary between the popular and professional sector. The pharmacist may give specific health advice, but consumers may also use the pharmacy (or indeed supermarket) to purchase a specific product that they have used before for a similar symptom (Williamson et al 1992). Research suggests that people like the convenience of the pharmacist, and may use the pharmacist as an alternative to the doctor or as a stepping stone to the doctor; in both cases some form of self-care occurs (Cunningham-Burley and Maclean 1987, Hassell et al 1998). However, some customers have experienced a lack of privacy (Hassell et al 2000), and other research suggests that, although pharmacists are held in high regard, there is not a high expectation of their diagnostic and therapeutic role. Pharmacists, however, do offer something different from doctors: the purchase of over-the-counter medicines, along with advice about these and the minor symptoms for which they are intended, seem to form an important part of self-care.

Self-help

A third component of the popular sector is self-help (see also pp. 138–139). Self-help groups in relation to health have grown in recent years, often providing an alternative to formal medical care. They are important both for the individual members of the group, but also at a more collective level, where they may lobby for a change in attitudes or in the provision of health care. Some groups emphasize the former and are 'inner-focused', and some the latter and are 'outer-focused' (Katz and Bender 1976). There are different reasons why self-help groups have developed to be an important part of the popular sector of health care. Firstly, existing services sometimes fail to meet the needs of people with a particular condition; secondly, self-help groups

provide a panacea to the isolation many feel when experiencing a chronic illness. Self-help groups have several characteristics that give mutual support and help. Members have a common experience of the problem, and there is no distinction made between helper and helped. Reciprocity is an important part of self-help, and the sharing of problems. Groups may provide important information to members, and may help people overcome stigma or feelings of being different.

Practical application

Recognition of the vast amount of health care which takes place in the popular sector is important both for doctors working in the community and for those planning health-care services. When self-care represents appropriate treatment, doctors should respect this expertise when someone does eventually consult them. Reassurance that the initial response to symptoms is appropriate is one way of doing this; and education about other options helps to develop a patient's own resources for care. It is also important for doctors to recognize the value of self-help, to be aware of groups in the area, and to alert patients to them. This may be particularly important for people living with a chronic illness, although other problems and conditions are also relevant. Working with other professional and lay groups should be an important component of a doctor's approach, thus bridging the divide between the different sectors of health care.

■ People may well be experts about their own illnesses, and they certainly may well have self-treated before contacting a general practitioner about symptoms. Why is it important for a general practitioner to ask a patient 'What have you done so far?'

Case study

Kelleher (1994) investigated self-help groups for people with diabetes. These are a recent development in the UK, and reflect grass-root activities and recognition of need. They are affiliated to the British Diabetic Association, which is a large national organization, but are small locally run groups. They meet to discuss problems around managing diabetes. This provides an important forum for people to express their worries, to learn from others about how they manage, and to admit to temptation. Members begin to feel less guilty about how they manage their condition as part of their everyday lives, and become more confident.

Self-care and the popular sector

■ Most illness does not come to the attention of doctors but is dealt with by people themselves through self-care within the popular sector of health care.

■ The community pharmacist is an important figure in self-care strategies.

■ Self-help is a growing area of health care, based on mutual aid and support.

The experience of hospitals

More and more people visit hospital at some point in their lives (see Fig. 1) but hospitals are changing from places where one goes to die, to places for acute conditions and specialist care. In the past there was a greater risk of dying in hospital, so it is not surprising that for many older people hospitals are places with negative associations. Modern hospitals may appear quite different, and offer cafés and shops to serve patients, visitors and staff.

Nearly all first births in the UK take place in maternity hospitals. This means that about 90% of women will experience a stay in hospital, and nearly everyone will have known a relative who has stayed in hospital. Elderly people are more likely to be admitted than younger people, although efforts are made to care for them in the community (see pp 14–15, 154–155). However, less time is spent as inpatients and there are more day cases and earlier discharge into the community. Hospitals also play a part in maintaining health, and many people go to hospitals for check-ups or rehabilitation programmes.

The experience of being a patient

When someone is admitted to hospital, even if only for a day or overnight stay, then they enter the role of a *hospital patient*. Goffman (1968a) suggested that the person becomes invisible, leaving only the illness visible. Doctors and nurses may talk about patients as if they were not present (see Fig. 2). Being a patient also carries certain expectations. They must move parts of their body on command, respond to probes in parts of their anatomy with declarations of pain and answer questions about the name of the current Prime Minister.

Patients may also resent their loss of freedom. They may wear night clothes throughout the day, and be dependent on others for basic functions. They may have little or no choice about the timing of meals or visits. Lights will go off at a set time and they may be forbidden to get out of bed, or not allowed to stay in bed. They lose their familiar social rôles at work and at home.

Not all patients are perceived in the same way by medical and nursing staff. The patients who obey instructions, make no demands, do not ask questions, and never complain may be labelled as 'good patients'. 'Good patients' are appreciated by staff and may be easier to manage, but their health may actually suffer. Taylor (1986) points out that 'good patients' may not ask for information and may not report important clinical symptoms. The hospital environment may actually encourage patients to become helpless. The more that

patients feel they cannot control the environment around them the more they will feel helpless.

The patients who ask questions, demand attention and complain may be labelled as 'bad patients'. 'Bad patients' who are not seriously ill may be perceived as difficult patients. However, they may be angry and demanding because they are anxious. These patients may assert their sense of control and independence by breaking the rules. Being a 'bad patient' could be good for health. If more questions are asked, more information will be given, and if symptoms are reported, they may help the diagnosis and treatment.

Control

The feeling of losing control is unpleasant. Taylor (1986) divides control into behaviour control, cognitive control, decision control and information control.

- **Behaviour control** involves being able to influence procedures in some way. Allowing a patient to control the progress of a painful procedure such as an enema can reduce anxiety. If anxiety before an unpleasant event can be reduced it will be more tolerable.
- **Cognitive control** is used in cognitive therapy and is very effective. The idea is to think about something neutral or irrelevant (distraction technique) or to concentrate on the positive aspects of the procedure. In childbirth the pain of contractions can be borne by learning to apply distraction techniques such as recalling a tune, or a poem.
- **Decision control** – If a patient can choose when to have an unpleasant procedure, e.g. an injection, then they will experience less discomfort.
- **Information control** – It is often assumed that the more information the patient receives the better, but this is not so for everyone. Information may be reassuring because it may reduce fear of the unknown and enable people to adopt coping strategies.

Stressful aspects of hospitals

Medical students may quickly get used to hospitals, but patients and relatives may find them stressful.

Privacy

In a single-bedded ward patients have more control over their own activities, but a multiple-bedded ward can be a friendly place.

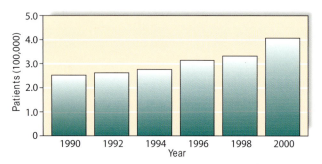

Fig. 1 **Hospital outpatient visits in Scotland 1990–2000.**
(Source: National Statistics: Annual Abstract of Statistics 2000 edition no.138)

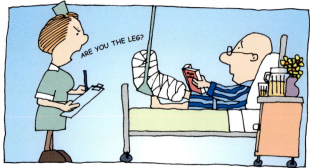

Fig. 2 **The person may become invisible on admission, and be identified only by the condition.**

The ward environment

Patients and visitors may find noise, smells and elaborate instruments stressful.

The professional role

In a joint report (Royal College of Physicians and Royal College of Psychiatrists 1995) it was emphasized that medical patients also need psychological care. Health professionals may find it difficult to discuss psychological problems with patients in hospital and may avoid this by offering false reassurance or by switching the discussion to a safer topic. Nurses, junior doctors and medical students have different social identities and rôles. Each social rôle has rôle-related rights such as being allowed to inflict pain, to administer drugs, or to ask intimate questions. Each rôle also has obligations to be respectful, to be caring and to preserve confidentiality.

- In what ways may a hospital's teaching and research interests conflict with the interests of patients? What could be done to reduce this conflict?

Stressful medical and surgical procedures

Many people undergo minor, but potentially stressful, medical procedures in hospitals as inpatients. A diagnostic procedure such as a laparoscopy may be the cause of anxiety because of the fear of what might be found. Some procedures can be very painful, e.g. pelvic floor repairs, and in most surgical procedures an anaesthetic is given. However, although this alleviates the pain it also means that there is a loss of control.

Some studies of preparation for stressful procedures in adults have shown benefits (Mathews and Ridgeway 1984). Information given about the procedure beforehand can reduce anxiety. In a study of cervical screening, anxiety was reduced by giving information, reassurance and the opportunity to ask questions (Foxwell and Alder 1993). Many women find the procedure of taking a cervical smear distressing and do not fully understand the meaning of a negative result. One group of 30 patients (the study group) was given routine care plus an extra 10 minutes of

- Talk to someone who has been a patient recently or has visited someone. How do their experiences relate to the above?
- Do you think there are gender differences in patient behaviour? What are they?
- Contrast your experience of hospitals with a recent television drama.

information, reassurance, and an opportunity to ask questions. The control group was given brief information and a leaflet. The two groups were no different in anxiety scores before the smear was taken, but when they received the results 3–4 weeks later, anxiety levels were significantly reduced in the study group, but not in the control group.

Research into anxiety

Janis (1958) suggested that people differ in their approach to surgery. Some people worry a great deal, feel very vulnerable and have difficulties sleeping. A second group show moderate levels of anxiety. They are somewhat anxious, worried about specific procedures, but ask for information. The third group are unconcerned about the operation. They sleep well and deny that they feel worried.

Although these early studies claimed a *curvilinear* relationship between fear level and outcome, this has not been confirmed by other studies. There is more likely to be a *linear* relationship between anxiety and recovery. The greater the level of fear before surgery, the poorer was the recovery. Those who are anxious beforehand have more pain, more medical complications and slower recovery (see pp. 102–103).

The experience of hospitals

- Hospitals are changing as more medical care takes place in the community.
- The experience of being a patient may be stressful, and not all patients react in the same way.
- Stressful aspects of hospitals include lack of privacy, the ward environment, identification of professionals, worry about surgery, worry about the outcome, and anxiety about the family at home.
- Many medical and surgical procedures are stressful, but the stress can be alleviated by preparation.

Case study

Mrs McNab, aged 75 years, had never been into hospital before. Her two children had been born at home, delivered by the local midwife. She was frightened by the ambulance ride from her remote croft into the city, although the paramedical staff were kind and gentle. On arrival she was undressed and given a hospital nightgown. The hospital bed was in a large ward full of strangers. Mrs McNab had never before slept in a bed outside her own home. The operation to remove her appendix was explained to her and she signed a consent form, although she had not brought her reading glasses with her. Following the successful operation she experienced great pain but did not ask for pain relief because she thought this would damage her brain. She missed her family acutely and was frequently found weeping.

- What could be done to alleviate her distress?
- How might her distress affect her recovery?

Psychological preparation for surgery

Psychological preparation for surgery has been developed to reduce patients' anxiety and to improve recovery in the post-operative period.

Anxiety

Anxiety is an unpleasant emotion associated with threatening situations or thinking about threat (see pp. 110–111). People differ in their propensity to experience anxiety; those with anxious personalities generally tend to have higher levels of anxiety, but are also more likely to experience heightened anxiety when exposed to a threatening situation such as exams, surgery or speaking in public. Increased anxiety is associated with changes in cognition, behaviour and physiology.

Anxiety is likely to make it more difficult for the patient to understand information given or to cooperate fully with instructions. In addition, physiological processes associated with anxiety may interfere with recovery.

Anxiety in surgical patients

Patients are anxious before surgery for a number of reasons: they have an illness requiring surgery, they have to undergo the surgical procedure, and there may be uncertainty about the outcome and the likely speed of recovery. In addition, patients worry about being away from home and how the family is coping, as well as continuing to worry about their usual preoccupations, such as money, relationships, etc.

Using the standard measures of anxiety, which have been developed to deal with the problems of subjective reporting, patients are found to have high levels of anxiety both before and after surgery. For example, Figure 1 shows daily anxiety levels from 4 days before to 14 days after major gynaecological surgery. Compared with normal levels of anxiety as measured 5 weeks after surgery, patients show high levels both before and after surgery.

Anxiety before surgery has been found to relate to many post-operative outcomes, including:

- distress
- pain
- use of analgesics
- physiological functioning

- return to normal activities
- length of hospital stay.

Therefore methods of reducing anxiety are likely to improve patient outcomes.

Methods of psychological preparation

A variety of methods of preparing people for surgery have been developed and typically they are administered on the day before surgery, although some have been used in outpatient visits prior to admission. Some methods have been used with groups of patients, and others incorporate the use of booklets, audio and video tapes.

Methods used include:

- information giving: procedural and sensation information
- behavioural instruction
- cognitive coping
- relaxation/hypnosis
- emotion-focused or psychotherapeutic discussion
- modelling.

Information giving – procedural and sensation
Procedural information

Patients are informed about the procedures they will undergo, when they will happen, and where they will be. For example, they would be told about waking in the recovery room and the possibility of having a drip or catheter.

Sensation information

As well as procedural information, patients are informed about the sensations they are likely to experience. For example, they might be told that pre-medication will not necessarily make them feel drowsy or that following major abdominal operations they may experience pain due to wind.

Behavioural instruction

Patients are instructed and may be encouraged to rehearse things they can do post-operatively to reduce pain and facilitate recovery. For example, they may be taught how to cough without pulling on the wound incision or how to turn over in bed without causing unnecessary pain.

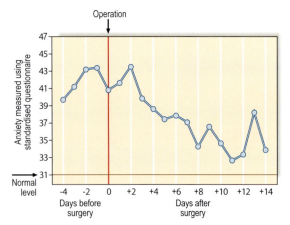

Fig. 1 **Anxiety levels before and after surgery.** (Reproduced with permission from Johnston 1980 Anxiety in Surgical Patients. Psychological Medicine 10: 145–152)

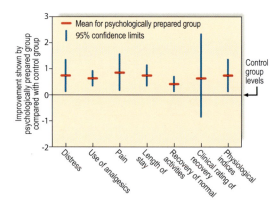

Fig. 2 **Benefits of psychological preparation for surgery.** This is a summary of 40 clinical trials. (Diagram based on data from Johnston and Vogele 1993)

Cognitive coping

Based on the assumption that patients' thoughts about what is happening may serve to either raise or reduce their anxiety, interventions have been designed to encourage more adaptive cognitions. For example patients may be trained to reinterpret events in a more positive manner – e.g. a patient thinking that a doctor passing the end of her bed is a sign that her condition is giving rise to concern may, after training, propose that this is a sign that she is making progress. Or she may be trained to use cognitive-coping techniques that they have found useful in other situations – e.g. if she says that distraction has been useful in previous anxiety-provoking situations, she may be advised on how to use such a technique before and after surgery (see pp 132–133).

Relaxation/hypnosis

A variety of general relaxation procedures and hypnotic techniques have been used, which patients can practise in bed before surgery, sometimes using taped instructions.

Emotion–focused/ psychotherapeutic discussion

Patients are invited to discuss their worries, either on their own, with a therapist or in groups. There are no very clearly specified instructions for this type of intervention.

Modelling

This method, which is most commonly used with children, involves showing the patient a film of a similar-aged patient going through various stages of the surgical procedures. The method communicates a considerable amount of procedural information and may demonstrate use of any of the other methods.

Results of psychological preparation

The first properly controlled trial (Egbert et al 1964) randomly allocated 97 patients to special preparation or normal care. The specially prepared group had less pain, used fewer analgesics post-operatively and their hospital stay was on average 2.7 days shorter than for patients in the control group.

Since then, there have been more than 40 controlled trials involving comparison of groups randomly allocated to psychological versus normal care. The results of these studies have been aggregated using statistical techniques (meta-analysis). Clear benefits for patients have been demonstrated. Figure 2 shows the mean difference between the psychologically prepared and control groups, expressed in units of standard deviations, and the 95% confidence intervals, for each outcome.

The group receiving psychological preparation shows statistically significant benefits where the mean difference is greater than zero and where the confidence interval does not pass through zero. Thus there is evidence of benefit on measures of distress, pain, use of analgesics, physiological indices, such as heart rate and blood pressure, and behavioural indices, including resumption of normal activities, and length of hospital stay. Clinical ratings of recovery do not show a reliable difference. One might expect to find improved patient satisfaction, but too few studies have examined this variable to draw conclusions.

- While the benefits of psychological methods of preparing patients for surgery have been known for at least 20 years, they have not been widely implemented. Why might this be?

The limitations in implementing these techniques may be due to the lack of appropriately trained staff. The development of booklet or taped instructions may facilitate the use of these techniques, but needs to be more fully evaluated.

Psychological preparation for surgery

- Patients are anxious before and after surgery.
- High pre-operative anxiety is predictive of poor post-operative outcomes.
- A variety of methods has been developed for preparing patients for surgery (e.g. information giving, behavioural instruction, cognitive coping, relaxation, emotion-focused discussion and modelling).
- These methods have been shown to improve post-operative outcomes in well-controlled clinical trials.

Case study

The following case describes a man whose anxiety interfered with his ability to have surgery.

Mr Aspell was admitted to a surgical ward, for abdominal surgery on the day after admission. He was anxious about the procedure, but particularly in anticipation of undergoing anaesthesia. After receiving his premedication on the morning of surgery, he could not contain his anxiety and discharged himself. Since there was nothing further the hospital could do, he returned to his GP, who was now faced with a patient who required surgery but could not tolerate the procedures.

The GP referred Mr Aspell to a psychologist, who used psychological preparation procedures involving relaxation training and cognitive techniques. Mr Aspell was trained to use relaxation as a distraction technique, especially when experiencing worrying thoughts. He was taught to recognize negative thoughts such as 'What if I die during surgery?' or 'What if I am still aware of what is going on even if the doctors think I am unconscious?', and to deal with them by thinking of counteracting thoughts, such as 'I've never heard of that happening to anyone I know – why should it happen to me?' or 'These doctors are experts – I am in safe hands'.

Mr Aspell was able to return to the surgeon and to proceed with treatment without further interruption.

Heart disease

Coronary heart disease (CHD) describes a number of conditions including angina pectoris and myocardial infarction (MI). Angina pectoris refers to a sensation of tightness or chest pain because of brief obstruction or constriction of an artery and MI refers to death of heart muscle (myocardium) as a result of blockage of the arteries that prevents oxygen reaching the myocardium.

The main medical interventions are: pharmacological (medications to reduce blood pressure, prevent clotting, etc.); re-vascularization: percutaneous transluminal coronary angioplasty (PTCA), coronary artery bypass grafts (CABG); coronary care; cardiac rehabilitation; risk-factor reduction (primary and secondary).

Prevention

CHD is the most common cause of premature mortality and a frequent cause of morbidity in Western societies. Major well-established risk factors are smoking, hypertension and high serum cholesterol. Additional lifestyle risk factors include lack of exercise, obesity (pp. 82–83), hostility and stress. The Type A behaviour pattern (hard-driving, time urgent, hostile) was identified in the 1960s as typical of the coronary-prone individual, but recent research has indicated that high hostility alone is the factor most associated with greater risk of CHD (see also pp. 124–125). The best evidence that stress causes heart disease comes from animal rather than human studies (Fig. 1). In surveys, patients and healthy populations believe 'stress' to be the most common cause of MI (i.e. heart attack) (pp. 84–85; 124).

CHD is related to socio-economic disadvantage (p. 42). This may in part be due to patterns of smoking, diet and work experience, as working-class men smoke more, have a poorer diet and are more likely to have jobs where they have little control and high demands compared with middle-class men. While some have argued that socio-economic disadvantage is an important risk factor and that reductions in CHD require greater socio-economic equality, others have suggested that individual risk may be reduced by changes in behaviour and lifestyle (pp. 68–69).

Thus, changes in behaviour and lifestyle offer opportunities for prevention (both primary and secondary), and countries such as the USA, where there have been major changes in lifestyle, have shown significant reductions in CHD. Nevertheless, as it is so common, many of the people who actually suffer from CHD are those at average or low risk. This is known as the prevention paradox.

Response to symptoms and MI

Individuals may misinterpret symptoms. A large number of patients referred to cardiology departments present with non-cardiac chest pain probably due to anxiety about physical symptoms. Equally, many patients experiencing an MI do not recognize the symptoms as those of an MI and therefore delay seeking help (pp. 86–87; 88). Average delay between first symptoms and arrival at hospital is 3–4 hours in the UK (Birkhead 1992). Given the importance of early thrombolysis, such delays may critically determine the patients' treatment and survival (see Case study 1). A rapid response ensures more effective treatment and therefore better outcomes. MI is a sudden life-threatening event and many patients experience high levels of anxiety and depression following MI. Close family members may be even more distressed than the patient in the early period, while the patient is in hospital. These high levels of distress are unrelated to the severity of the MI and may persist for months or years.

In addition to its immediate debilitating effects, depression is associated with higher mortality rates. In a study of 222 MI patients, depressed patients were over three times as likely as non-depressed patients to die within 18 months. This remained true even when other factors, such as severity of MI, were controlled for (Fig. 2). In addition, patients who were socially isolated were also more likely to die in this period.

Cardiac rehabilitation

Cardiac rehabilitation programmes have been shown to:

- reduce psychological distress for patients and their families
- improve cardiovascular fitness

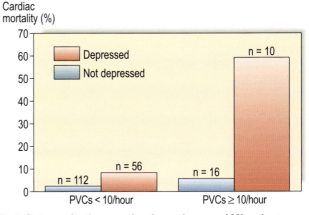

Fig. 1 **Effects of social stressors on coronary artery in monkeys.** The diagrams show cross-sections of coronary artery of monkeys subjected to different living conditions. Greatest occlusion of the coronary artery was found in (c), dominant monkeys subjected to the stress of having the group they lived with broken up regularly. Less occlusion was found in those living in stable groups (a and b) or in subordinate monkeys in unstable social groupings (d). (Drawing based on photograph in Manuck et al 1983)

Fig. 2 **Outcome for depressed and non-depressed MI patients.** Depressed patients were more likely to die than those who were not depressed. This was true for both those with a low rate of preventricular contractions (PVCs) and those with a high rate. (Source: Frasure-Smith et al 1995)

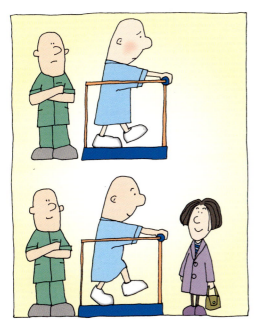

Fig. 3 **Following MI, patients whose rehabilitation exercises were observed by their spouses did better than those only seen by the rehabilitation team.**
- reduce mortality
- increase rate of return to paid employment
- reduce health-service costs.

Benefits from such programmes persist for years. Programmes may involve education, exercise, dietary and vocational counselling, and psychological components such as stress management. The addition of psychological components to exercise- and education-based programmes results in greater patient benefit.

In a randomized controlled study, 862 cardiac patients were allocated to an educational programme or to this programme plus an additional psychological programme in which patients met weekly in small groups and were trained to make the following changes: (a) cognitive, e.g. 'I must always arrive first at work' may be reconstrued as 'As long as I arrive by 9 a.m., I can complete a good day's work' (b) behavioural, e.g. learning to walk at a more relaxed steady pace (c) emotional, e.g. learning to relax in response to early signs of anxiety or anger. After 4.5 years, the latter group had experienced significantly fewer non-fatal cardiac events and fewer deaths – 12.9% versus 21.2% (Friedman et al 1986).

Rehabilitation may be enhanced by involving spouses or lay carers in routine medical procedures. For example, allowing spouses to observe routine treadmill testing of cardiovascular fitness (Fig. 3) increases both patient and spouse confidence in the patient's ability to engage in energetic activities, with resulting greater activity levels at home in the period following the test.

Response to stressful medical procedures

Medical procedures may be stressful due to the discomfort or pain experienced as well as the uncertainty about the outcomes. Psychological preparation can reduce the stressfulness of the procedures and improve the outcomes (p. 102); for example, compared with patients receiving normal care before CABG, patients receiving cognitive and behavioural preparation were less distressed and recovered more quickly. In addition, they were less likely to suffer from acute post-operative hypertension, a life-threatening condition (Anderson 1987).

Case study

Delay to treatment for symptoms of a myocardial infarction

On the way home from their wedding anniversary meal, Mrs MacDonald feels pressure in her chest. She thinks it unlikely to be anything more serious than indigestion at her age (51). She does not like to mention it as it would spoil the evening. Going upstairs to bed the pain intensifies and she comes out in a cold sweat, so she lies down to see if she feels better. Her husband worries that it is a heart attack, but Mrs MacDonald says 'I don't think so – women don't have heart attacks. It's more likely to be the menopause!' After some hours of increasing symptoms, she calls her GP. By the time the ambulance takes her to hospital, she is too late for the full benefit of thrombolytic drugs.

STOP THINK

- Psychological factors are involved in many aspects of CHD. How might a psychologist contribute to the work of a cardiology department?

Heart disease

- CHD may be prevented by changes in behaviour and lifestyles.
- Socio-economic disadvantage is associated with a high incidence of CHD.
- Patients may fail to recognize the symptoms of MI, with resulting delays in seeking medical treatment.
- Anxiety and depression are common responses to MI of both patients and their spouses.
- Depression following MI is an independent predictor of mortality.
- Cardiac rehabilitation, including psychological components, enhances patient outcomes and survival.
- Psychological preparation for medical procedures reduces their stressfulness and improves post-operative recovery.

Social aspects of HIV/AIDS

HIV (human immunodeficiency virus) appeared at a time when it was widely believed that science had brought infectious diseases under control, and it seemed that all of a sudden a new incurable disease presented itself. Until recently it was only possible to treat some of the secondary effects of HIV and AIDS (acquired immune deficiency syndrome – the disease stage of most infected people) and since the infection is currently not curable the main remedy still lies in prevention. Since the virus can be transmitted in different ways (Table 1), prevention requires targeting different types of behaviour.

Although HIV is widespread (over 40 million cases were reported worldwide by December 2001) it is clear that the infection is not equally spread amongst members of society or between societies. Even within the UK (Fig. 1) we see great differences in the proportion of people infected through sexual intercourse between men and intravenous drug use (IDU). The figure for women as a percentage of the total number of people diagnosed with AIDS differs considerably between Scotland and the UK as a whole (Fig. 1). The proportion of women among the people diagnosed with AIDS in Scotland (20.6%) is 50% higher than the UK (13.8%). Thus certain groups of people have a far higher infection rate than others.

The disease has distinct social aspects. At a social level it involves several taboos, such as sex, drugs, and death and dying; consequently it is heavily stigmatized. Secondly, at a personal level, the acceptance of being diagnosed as HIV positive can be very difficult. People can feel isolated, shocked, frightened, panicked, guilty, profess denial and become depressed, but some also display a sense of coming to terms with themselves, and even acceptance. Such emotions are understandable, as awareness of one's own mortality will be increased.

- Why is society's reaction to people with HIV generally negative?

Double stigma

HIV has what is called a 'double stigma' attached. Stigma refers to the identification and recognition of a bad or negative characteristic in a person or group of persons and the treatment of them with less respect or worth than they deserve due to this characteristic (pp 60–61). The double stigma refers to 'terminal illness' and 'sexually transmitted diseases'. The former stigma is also applicable to cancer and other terminal diseases. The latter refers to stigma attached to 'deviant', 'unnatural', or socially undesirable activities, such as men having sex with men, injecting drug use, or prostitution. Alonzo and Reynolds (1995) explain that stigma is the 'identification of some sort of moral contamination that causes others to reject the person bearing it'. Thus people living with

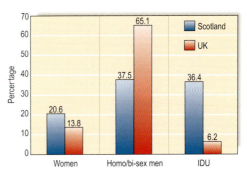

Fig. 1 **Percentage women, homo/bisexual men and intravenous drug users among cumulative number of AIDS cases in Scotland (March 2002) and UK (December 2001).** (Source: SCIEH Weekly Report 2002).

HIV are regarded as 'dangerous, dirty, foolish and worthless' in comparison to descriptions of cancer or stroke patients.

Experiencing stigma (stigmatization) may lead to low self-esteem in the infected person, reduced willingness to seek medical and social help, and increased difficulty in sharing worries with friends, relatives and neighbours. At a societal level, widespread fear of HIV/AIDS still exists, despite the fact that it has been scientifically demonstrated that AIDS is not communicable by day-to-day social contact. This fear and stigmatization can easily be translated into discrimination and victimization of people with HIV. HIV/AIDS is branded a plague, which implies that people living with HIV are threatening and dangerous rather than threatened, because they carry the potential to contaminate the healthy through transmission of a contagious disease. This led to some dentists and doctors refusing treatment in the past even when safe procedures were available.

Society also often makes a distinction between 'innocent' and 'guilty' victims. It is believed that the people with HIV bring it on themselves through their own doing, and they are blamed for their disease, and as a result are branded as 'guilty' victims. In contrast, 'innocent' victims are infected through mistakes by the medical profession or infected blood. Babies of HIV-infected mothers are included as innocent, while their mothers may be seen as guilty.

The use of the phrase 'risk group' reinforces the idea that HIV can only happen to certain people. The idea of stressing risk behaviour is far more meaningful both in terms of reducing the stigma attached to being HIV positive and in terms of preventing the spread of the infection. It is not what people are that gives them a higher risk, but what people do.

HIV and the media

The media are a major source of information for people, as well as influential in forming or at least confirming people's opinions (pp. 50–51). Many people in industrialized countries will not personally know anyone who is infected with HIV; consequently, the perception of the disease is likely to be mediated or even formed by mass media. This includes 'facts' in, for example, newspapers and television news programmes, and 'fiction' in soap operas and cinema films.

In an interview with The Independent newspaper (3 November 1993, p. 23) Suzanna Dawson, who in a soap opera played the wife of a character who had AIDS, said:

Table 1 **Routes of transmission of HIV**
■ Unprotected penetrative sex (vaginal, oral or anal)
■ Unsterilized needle/syringe which has been used by someone infected with HIV
■ Mother to child during pregnancy, labour and breastfeeding
■ Infected blood or tissue transfer
■ Receiving semen from an infected man for artificial insemination.

. . . I've had some terrible experiences of the kind of prejudice HIV-positive people face . . . I've been slapped and spat at in the street, booed off the field in a charity match . . . it makes you feel so alone, so scared . . . I've picked up the phone at 2 a.m. to hear some guy screaming: 'You're a dirty bitch, spreading disease throughout the world.'

Ms Dawson suffered this level of abuse even though she was merely the actress playing that rôle.

Psychological issues

One key set of psychological issues centres around the question: 'Who do you tell?' Being diagnosed HIV positive may involve having to adapt one's behaviour and outlook on life. Telling a partner or family could mean having to admit to injecting drugs, or having sex with another man, or being sexually unfaithful. Telling employers might mean losing a job, not necessarily because the employer wants to get rid of you, but because your colleagues do not want to work with you any longer. Bringing up the issue of using safer sex methods can also be problematic. It is a difficult enough issue for most, especially at the time of first sexual intercourse. However, people with HIV might find suggesting the use of condoms with prospective sexual partners difficult, because of the fear of being rejected, emotionally or physically (see pp. 84–85).

Health promotion and HIV

HIV health-promotion activities have often focused on the sexual transmission of the virus. Since (a) people with HIV are generally not recognizable until the end stages of the disease, and (b) the virus has a long incubation time, the health-promotion message had to be aimed at all men and women who are sexually active, not just the high-risk groups.

Figure 2 shows one of the posters/postcards with a safer sex message targeting the general population. The message is clearly aimed at men, unlike previous health-promotion activities for condoms, when condoms were 'only' contraceptives, and often seen as a woman's responsibility (see pp. 84–85).

Despite all the health-promotion messages over the past decade and a half, talking about condom use and sexual desires still proves to be difficult for many people.

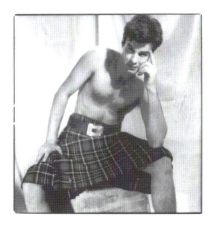

Fig. 2 **One HIV health promotion in Scotland.** The slogan read, 'What should a real Scotsman wear under his kilt?' Answer: 'A condom!' (Courtesy of Scottish AIDS Monitor and Lothian Health)

HIV/AIDS in developing countries

The majority of people with HIV live in developing countries. Many of these developing countries have poor economies and, consequently, underfunded public health systems. In Africa HIV is transmitted mainly by heterosexual contact; in Europe and the USA homosexual contact is still the leading factor, although heterosexual transmission is increasing. Many areas of Africa do not have the means to screen blood consistently, which means that HIV is still being transmitted through blood transfusions, and very few medicines or social services are available for people with AIDS. It is worth remembering that for some African nations hit hardest by AIDS, the entire national health budget is equal only to that of one large hospital in the USA.

Consequently many developing countries cannot afford to offer the kind of treatment that has made long-term survival of HIV patients common in industrialized countries.

Social aspects of HIV /AIDS

- Prevention is the main, the only approach to stop the spread of HIV/AIDS.
- People living with HIV/AIDS often suffer from a double stigma.
- Mass media have played an important role in influencing public perception of the disease.
- We should move away from thinking in terms of risk groups to risk behaviour. It is not important who you are, but what you do.
- The majority of people with HIV live in the developing world, where much less funding is available for prevention and care.

www.unaids.org/hivaidsinfo/index.html

Case study

Andrew (age 20 years) is a third-year medical student. He took an HIV test with his new partner when they started a sexual relationship. He felt it was a waste of time, a fashion, and really went along to please his partner. Although he was counselled at the time, he was very shocked to be told that he tested HIV positive. His thoughts jumped back and forth between his partner and what would happen to the relationship, his study and career. He wondered: 'Who gave me the virus?' and 'Which private habits do I have to disclose, and to whom? Will I die young and horribly?'

STOP THINK
- What other issues might this medical student face after his recent diagnosis?

Cancer

Despite differences in the progress of different cancers and the increasing effectiveness of medical treatments, cancer continues to be the most widely feared group of diseases. It creates greater anxiety than coronary heart disease, which has approximately double the fatality rate. Psychological and social factors are involved in the aetiology and response to the disease and its treatment.

Aetiology

In a review of the preventable causes of cancer, behavioural factors were implicated in the majority of cancers (Doll and Peto 1981): smoking (involved in 30% of cancers); diet (35%); reproductive and sexual behaviour (7%); alcohol use (3%).

Other psychological factors, such as stress, may also be important. Animal studies have shown that tumour growth is faster and resulting death is earlier in mice subjected to uncontrollable stress (electric shocks), compared with animals receiving a similar amount of controllable shock. It has been proposed that Type C personality (characterized by lack of emotional expressiveness and resigned acceptance of negative events) increases the risk of cancer, but there is little scientific support for this proposal. There is some evidence that depressed individuals are more prone to cancer.

Communication about cancer

Cancer is associated with many social and clinical taboos. In popular language and in medical settings euphemisms such as 'growth', 'tumour', 'lump', 'shadow' are used to avoid the word 'cancer' (see pp. 96–97). These communications may arise from the fears and misconceptions surrounding cancer, but they, in turn, also give rise to such fears. Thus patients with benign disease sometimes suspect that they have malignant disease but that their doctor is withholding the information.

Doctors may refrain from using the word 'cancer' because they believe patients prefer not to be given a potentially terminal diagnosis. However, research studies show that members of the general public are much more likely to say that they want to be informed of a terminal

---

Case study

Providing test results in an oncology clinic

Miss Browne returns to the oncologist for test results following biopsy for a breast lump. The consultation goes as follows:

Doctor: *The tests on your breast lump are negative . . .*
Miss Browne: *So there's nothing you can do . . .*
Doctor: *Oh yes. Don't worry, we don't leave things like this. We'll be proceeding with local excision of the necessary tissue. It's all quite routine, and under general anaesthetic.*
Miss Browne: *That means I'll have to have the operation after all. What's the point?*
Doctor: *That's how these lumps are always managed. Everything will be fine. Try not to get upset. We'll fix a date for doing this as soon as possible. What about Wednesday next, coming in on Tuesday evening. OK?*

- What did the doctor understand by the word 'negative'?
- What did Miss Browne understand?
- What are Miss Browne's thoughts as she comes into hospital for surgery?

---

diagnosis than doctors estimated they would be. Members of the general public are also more likely to say that they would want to be told personally, rather than have other people (such as a relative) told first (pp. 96–97). Nevertheless, people may not take opportunities to detect cancer when these are offered, for example, through health screening. Screening for the detection of pre-cancerous cells or for the early diagnosis of treatable cancers has often resulted in poor uptake rates (pp. 64–65).

Reticence about communicating about cancer may also be associated with unduly pessimistic views of the impact of the disease. Doctors' ratings of the quality of life of cancer patients are significantly worse than the patients' own ratings. Communications about cancer are fraught with problems due to these negative attitudes of patients, their families, health professionals (including doctors and nurses), other hospital personnel and the wider lay community (pp. 94–95 and pp. 96–97).

Response to diagnosis

Even when the term 'cancer' is used in giving the diagnosis, patients may subsequently report that they have never received such a diagnosis.

In order to ensure that patients can recall the full description of their condition and the potentially reassuring communication about treatment and prognosis, some clinicians have provided patients with an audio-taped recording of the diagnostic consultation. Initial results suggest that these tapes may help patients to communicate information about their condition and its treatment to their family, and patients have responded favourably to receiving the tapes.

Patients have varied ways of coping with a cancer diagnosis. Kubler-Ross has proposed a sequence of staging of the response to a poor prognosis ranging from shock and denial, through anger, depression, and, finally, to acceptance. While there is considerable doubt about the actual sequence of stages, this range of response is commonly observed in patients with cancer (pp. 16–17). Researchers have investigated whether some coping methods may result in better adjustment or prognosis. In general, coping strategies that focus on emotional aspects of the response are associated with poorer emotional adjustment. By contrast, patients whose strategies focus on thinking about the issue in a different way, e.g. by acceptance of the condition, or on seeking solutions to problems, show better subsequent adjustment. Coping strategies may also influence prognosis: patients showing 'denial' or 'fighting spirit' were found to survive for longer than patients whose coping responses were stoic acceptance or 'helplessness/hopelessness' (Greer et al 1979 – see Fig. 1).

Psychological interventions

Various patient support groups and psychological interventions have been designed. Professional-led groups, provided in clinical settings, have aimed to: provide emotional support; allow expression of emotion; enhance self-esteem by being able to support others; increase the range of coping strategies; enable patients to learn from successful coping attempts by others.

A number of controlled clinical trials show that these groups improve emotional adjustment, reduce pain and may increase survival. For example, Spiegel et al (1989) randomly allocated 86 patients with metastatic or advanced breast cancer to either a control group, which received normal care, or an experimental group, who additionally participated in a weekly small group led by professional staff that ran over 1 year (see Fig. 2). The experimental group showed the following benefits:

- decreased emotional distress
- decreased pain
- increased survival time (mean survival time for experimental group = 36.6 months, for control group = 18.9 months).

Response to treatment

Where two medical treatments are thought to have a similar prognosis, patients may be offered a choice of treatment. While doctors originally expected patients to prefer the less mutilating cancer surgery, e.g. lumpectomy rather than mastectomy, this has not been borne out in studies. For instance, in patients with advanced prostate cancer, orchidectomy (surgical removal of testicle) or bi-monthly hormonal injection (synthetic luteinizing hormone) with minimum side effects have similar survival rates. Yet, when given the choice of treatment, a large proportion, 23 out of 50 men, opted for the mutilating surgery rather than the minimally invasive injections (Chadwick et al 1991) (pp. 100–101).

Just as patients' choice of treatment may be unexpected, their response during treatment may also be somewhat surprising. In a study of patients receiving chemotherapy, levels of distress were associated with some side effects of

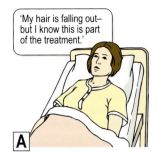
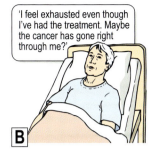

Fig. 3 **Which patient is likely to be more depressed – A or B?**

treatment but not others. Distress was associated with tiredness and lack of energy rather than with hair loss or nausea. The authors argue that patients had been informed that the treatment would result in hair loss and nausea, and were therefore less concerned by those side effects. By contrast, they had not been told to expect general tiredness and therefore attributed this symptom to advances in the disease rather than to the chemotherapy (Nerenz et al 1982 – see Fig. 3).

Many patients experience anticipatory nausea and vomiting as the course of treatment progresses. For the initial treatments, nausea is experienced during and after the treatment. With later treatments, the nausea can occur before treatment, on arrival at the hospital or even on the journey to hospital. This effect has been explained in terms of classical conditioning (pp. 20–21) – the patient learns to associate the visit to hospital with the administration of chemotherapy and therefore responds as if to chemotherapy, with nausea and vomiting. Considerable success has been achieved in training patients in relaxation techniques, to practise in anticipation of and during chemotherapy, thus obviating the need for antiemetic drugs.

STOP THINK

- To what extent is fear of cancer, in patients and in the general public, increased by:

– taboos on using the word 'cancer'
– poor communications with cancer patients
– mass-media images of cancer.

Cancer

- Cancer is the most widely feared of all diseases.
- Behavioural factors are important in the aetiology of cancer and, therefore, offer opportunities for prevention.
- Communication about cancer may be limited by social taboos, concern to avoid upsetting patients, and undue pessimism about the impact of the disease.
- Patients' coping strategies can affect subsequent adjustment and survival.
- Psychological interventions can reduce emotional distress and may prolong survival.
- Patients' choices of, and response to, treatment may be unexpected from a medical point of view, but may be psychologically meaningful.

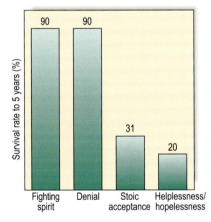

Fig. 1 **Initial psychological responses to breast cancer by 5-year outcome.** (Adapted with permission from Greer et al 1979)

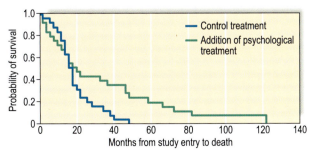

Fig. 2 **Patients with metastatic breast cancer receiving psychological treatment showed longer survival.** (Reproduced with permission from Spiegel et al 1989)

Anxiety

Anxiety is part and parcel of daily life. It is adaptive: it provides the motivation to study for exams and it prompts the rush of adrenaline that gives a certain sparkle to a public performance, whether this is sport or presenting a seminar paper. Most of us have experienced episodes of unpleasant anxiety. Usually these are time limited and resolve themselves. But even when they do not warrant treatment, their physiological effects can still interfere with health by making other conditions worse (e.g. asthma or eczema), or by confusing the clinical picture (e.g. in diagnosis and management of heart disease).

Anxiety in health-care situations

Many aspects of health care are anxiety provoking in themselves. Waiting to see a doctor makes most patients anxious because they often feel ill and, therefore, vulnerable. They are dependent on the doctor for help, do not know what to expect and may find it difficult to say exactly what they want to say. Coming into hospital produces the same effect, but has the added stress of being taken into a strange institution and having loss of control imposed upon them (pp. 100–101). It is easy to underestimate the degree of anxiety that patients feel when faced with a doctor. They may react in maladaptive ways: by not giving the right information, or by being defensive, hostile or tearful. They are frequently too anxious to listen or remember what is said to them. They may show clinical signs of anxiety that may be mistakenly attributed to some other illness. Every effort should be made to reduce anxiety in order to get the most out of a clinical encounter (pp. 94–95).

What is anxiety?

Anxiety refers to an emotional state that can usefully be divided into three components:
1. Thoughts – these often act as the trigger for creating the state of anxiety, e.g. 'What if my foot slips off this ledge and I fall down the rockface?', 'What if I can't answer key questions at the interview?' or 'What if we split up and I'm left on my own?'
2. Physical symptoms – these are numerous; most commonly they include an increased heart rate, increased blood pressure, feelings of tension in the muscles, sweating, nausea or indigestion, trembling, blushing, tightness or dryness in the throat, and dizziness.
3. Behaviour – this is what you do in order to reduce anxiety, for example, refusing to go on up the rockface, or avoiding interviews, or doing deep breathing in order to ease the physical symptoms of anxiety in an interview. Behaviour that reduces anxiety without damaging health or welfare is adaptive, but many of the ways in which we respond to anxiety are maladaptive, e.g. avoiding social occasions, or using alcohol for relief (pp. 124–125).

How is anxiety maintained?

The three components listed above can interact to maintain anxiety and can also make it worse. The case study illustrates how anxiety can escalate.

Whatever the initial cause of Andrew's symptoms, he had interpreted the sensations as potentially threatening (the risk that he would faint in the shop and how embarrassing this would be). These anxious thoughts set off further symptoms (through the release of adrenaline and noradrenaline). Escaping reduced symptoms and avoidance prevented them.

Types of anxiety problem

High anxiety that interferes with everyday functioning may be categorized as follows (Davison and Neale 2001):

Phobias

A phobia is a fear that is out of proportion to the potential threat posed by a particular object or situation. Being afraid of a pit bull terrier dog would not be classed as a phobia, but being afraid of a moth would. There is a significant risk to your safety in the first, but not the second.

Common specific phobias are to blood and injections, enclosed places such as lifts, animals and aspects of the natural environment, such as heights and water. Phobias to blood and injections are characterized by a decrease in heart rate, often causing fainting, whereas other phobias are associated with an increased heart rate. Social phobias may develop from the common social anxieties experienced in adolescence. They can be debilitating, leading to acute embarrassment in the company of others and avoidance of social situations.

Generalized anxiety

Generalized anxiety refers to the experience of all-pervasive anxiety, not apparently linked to any specific situation, event or object. The person experiences a high state of arousal for much of the time and a general sense of dread. They are likely to experience uncontrollable worry, a variety of somatic complaints, tension and restlessness.

Panic attacks

Panic attacks are sudden waves of acute anxiety that seem to come out of the blue. People may be overwhelmed by feelings of loss of control, going mad or even dying. Panic attacks that occur in public places and involve feelings of being trapped are called agoraphobia. They may be associated with fears of shopping, crowds or travelling.

Case study

Andrew was recovering from 'flu' when he went into a supermarket on a Saturday afternoon to stock up on food. He was dressed in warm clothing to combat the winter weather outside. Inside the shop it was hot and crowded, and he had to wait in a long queue for the checkout. While waiting he began to feel very hot himself, slightly faint and nauseous. He broke out in a sweat and thought that he might actually pass out in the shop. He put down the basket and went straight to the entrance for fresh air. He began to feel better, but decided just to go home.

The next time he went to the supermarket, he thought about his last visit, and wondered if it might happen again. He thought that people might notice if he looked flustered or nervous, and this would be embarrassing. Thinking and imagining the scene was accompanied by a quickening heart rate, and then sweating and a feeling of dizziness and nausea. He thought again that he might faint and that this would be terrible. He made straight for the door and on getting outside, began to feel better again.

STOP THINK ■ Think of the last time that you sat a difficult exam. When did your anxiety peak? Was it a week before, the day before, the morning of the exam, waiting outside to go in, sitting down at the desk, looking at the paper, or answering the questions? It differs from person to person, but commonly the anxiety peaks at some point before the exam, rather than during it. This is a common feature of anxiety: anticipation of an event is often worse than the actual event. Anxiety-provoking thoughts initiate and maintain the anxiety while waiting, but are replaced by the thinking necessary to actually tackle the feared situation itself. It may help to remind yourself of that when you are next anxious.

Obsessive-compulsive disorder (OCD)

People with OCD suffer from obsessional ruminations, which are intrusive and recurrent, and often distressing thoughts or images, e.g. about contamination or harming others. They may also experience compulsions to perform certain repetitive behaviours, such as checking and re-checking, and lengthy cleaning rituals.

Post-traumatic and acute stress

This is an extreme response to an extreme stressor, such as assault, environmental disaster or war. Its symptoms form three categories: frequently re-experiencing and being distressed by the traumatic event (e.g. nightmares), avoiding or forgetting or feeling numb towards the trauma, and being highly aroused (e.g. sleep and concentration problems, feeling jumpy).

Treatment

Methods of treatment depend on the nature of the anxiety, its impact on everyday functioning and the individual's preference.

Drugs

These work by reducing the physiological symptoms of anxiety. The most commonly used group of drugs are the benzodiazepines, but these can cause dependence. Beta-blockers, which control heart rate, are sometimes used to reduce symptoms for a one-off occasion, e.g. a musician giving an important performance. For generalized anxiety and OCD, anti-depressants may be used.

Psychological therapies

Behavioural approaches are effective treatments for anxiety problems. For a simple phobia, graded exposure to the feared object is combined with learning to use relaxation techniques (called systematic desensitization; see pp. 20–21). In this way, the patient learns that the feared object is tolerable (see Fig. 1). Exposure-based treatments are also effective in reducing agoraphobia. For PTSD, exposure is to the traumatic images, and therapy seeks to help people gain control over the images and their emotional responses to them. As a general principle, cognitive-behaviour techniques aim to identify the situations and thoughts that cause and maintain anxiety problems, and then break the cycle of anxious thoughts, physical symptoms and maladaptive behaviour (see pp. 134–135).

Relaxation and cognitive therapy may also be used for panic attacks and generalized anxiety. Learning social skills may help social phobics to feel confident and to behave appropriately in social situations. Modelling, or observational learning (see pp. 20–21), is another effective technique, in which someone demonstrates a non-anxious response to situations feared by the anxious person.

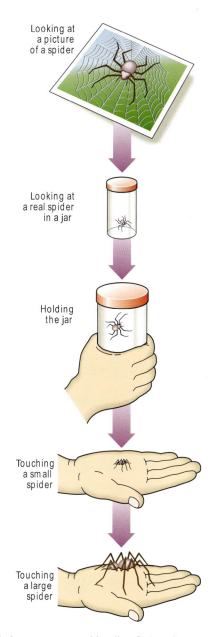

Looking at a picture of a spider

Looking at a real spider in a jar

Holding the jar

Touching a small spider

Touching a large spider

Fig. 1 **Graded exposure to a spider.** (from Puri 1996)

Anxiety

- Anxiety is common and usually time limited.
- Persistent anxious thoughts, physical symptoms and maladaptive behaviour can interfere with healthy functioning.
- Anticipation of anxiety and avoidance of feared situations can maintain and increase anxiety in a feedback system.
- Behavioural and cognitive therapies are used either with or without drug treatments, which may run the risk of dependency.
- The prevalence and effects of anxiety among patients are underestimated.

Depression

Depression is a common and serious disorder. At any one moment in time, about 1 in 20 individuals suffers from a significant depressive disorder, and it is estimated that 17% of the population will suffer from a major depressive disorder at one point in their life (Hammen 1997). Depression can be a disabling condition, and patients may be unable to function effectively for several months. It is becoming increasingly recognized that children and adolescents can suffer from depression, and that this is often not diagnosed or treated. Depression is currently rated the fourth leading cause of disability throughout the world, and it is predicted to rise to the second leading cause by the year 2010.

What is depression?

The major features of depression are outlined in Box 1. Typically patients have a negative view, not just themselves, but also of the world and their future (the *negative cognitive triad*). It can be a chronic or recurring condition. Suicidal thoughts and attempts are the most worrying and disturbing features of depression. It has been estimated that between 11 and 17% of individuals with a diagnosis of major depression eventually die by their own hands.

Types of depression

At one time it was common to distinguish between two sub-types of depression: *endogenous* (coming from within the individual) and *reactive* (where an external event precipitated the illness). However, the current view is that no such neat distinction can be made. While diagnostic schemes such as the international classification of diseases (ICD) and the diagnostic and statistical manual (DSM) present disorders as discrete categories, there is clearly a continuum of depression severity. Mild depression is largely treated in general practice, but some patients with severe depression may have psychotic features such as delusions, and may require hospitalization for medical and nursing care, and to protect the patient from the risk of suicide.

Gender

Consistently, studies throughout the world report approximately a 2:1 rate of depression for women compared to men (Hammen 1997). However, this may reflect, to some extent, a greater readiness on the part of women to admit distress and to seek help from health professionals. Men, it is argued, present their distress in a disguised manner, e.g. presenting with physical complaints such as pain. On the other hand, similar data on sex differences in rates of depression have also been derived from community surveys. It has also been suggested that men may be more prone to 'self-medicate' in response to depression, e.g. by alcohol abuse.

Social factors

Over and above the heightened risk in females, working-class women with children have considerably higher rates of diagnosed depression and admission rates to psychiatric hospitals compared with middle-class women, whether or not they have children.

Brown and Harris (1978) proposed that working-class women are more at risk for two reasons. Firstly, they are more likely to experience one or more **vulnerability factors** (Table 1) leading to low self-esteem. They are also more likely to experience a **provoking agent**: a severe life event or major difficulty, particularly in relation to housing, partner's job, finance or marriage (Table 2). A major life event is unlikely to be the sole cause of depression, but will combine with vulnerability factors, such as the loss of a mother in childhood, the lack of a confiding relationship and the stress of isolation at home with small children, to precipitate a depressive episode.

The experience of loss can precipitate a depressive episode. It is easy to see how this could happen in bereavement, but it can also occur due to the loss of a partner through divorce, the loss of friends through moving to a new area, or the loss of a role through unemployment or children leaving home.

Box 1 Diagnostic criteria for a major depressive episode as defined by the American Psychiatric Association Diagnostic and Statistical Manual, 4th Revision (DSM-IV).

A

Five or more of the following over the same 2-week period, representing a change from previous functioning and featuring either 1 or 2.

1. Depressed mood
2. Loss of interest or pleasure in activities
3. Significant weight loss or gain
4. Insomnia or hypersomnia
5. Psychomotor agitation or retardation
6. Fatigue or loss of energy
7. Feelings of worthlessness or guilt
8. Diminished ability to think or concentrate
9. Recurrent thoughts of death

B

The symptoms do not meet criteria for a mixed affective episode.

C

Symptoms cause clinically significant impairment in social or occupational functioning

D

Symptoms not due to direct effects of drug or general medical condition

E

Symptoms not better accounted for by bereavement

Table 1 Specific 'vulnerability' factors for women

- Lack of intimate or confiding relationship
- Loss of mother before age 11 years
- 3+ children aged < 15 years old at home
- Unemployment

Table 2 Examples of severe life events and difficulties

Events

Long-term (>1 week) marked threat focused on woman, or woman and partner

- Deaths
- Illness/accidents to subject
- Relationship changes
- Crises, e.g. burglaries
- Illness/accidents to others
- Job change
- Residence change.

Difficulties

Problems that have gone on for at least 4 weeks.

Social support

An important environmental factor that markedly affects risk for depression is the availability of good-quality support from friends and family. This seems to offer protection in helping individuals deal with stressors that may otherwise precipitate a depressive episode. The lack of an intimate or confiding relationship, one of the vulnerability factors in Table 1, is a good example of lack of social support increasing the risk for depression.

Genetic factors

Some types of depression tend to run in families. McGuffin et al (1996) reported concordance for life-time major depression of 46% for monozygotic twins compared with 20% for dizygotic twins, with both rates being higher than life-time depression in the general population. Evidence such as this suggests a strong genetic contribution to the development of major depression. However, genetics cannot be the whole story, if it were, the concordance rate would be 100% for monozygotic twins. From the McGuffin et al (1996) study, it is clear that the majority of the variance (i.e. over 50%) must be explained by environmental factors.

Treatment

A particular problem with depression is that many patients are reluctant to seek treatment. They may be concerned about the 'stigma' of being labelled as having suffered from a psychiatric disorder. Some patients do not recognize themselves as being ill, but rather believe that they are lazy, wicked or simply undeserving of treatment. Of those that do seek treatment (often after persuasion by family), many will be treated by their general practitioners, using antidepressant medication, such as selective serotonin re-uptake inhibitors (SSRIs), and counselling. It usually takes some weeks before patients will note any benefit, and they may need to be encouraged to persist with treatment. Many antidepressants have side effects, particularly in the early stages of treatment, and this often leads to discontinuation of treatment.

Cognitive-behaviour therapy (CBT) (see pp. 134–135) and inter-personal psychotherapy (IPT) have also been shown to be effective psychological treatments for depression. CBT is useful for patients without psychotic symptoms who are able to engage in the learning process involved. By enabling patients to see the link between thinking, mood and behaviour, they can be helped to develop the ability to evaluate evidence regarding their beliefs objectively, with associated benefits to the way they feel and behave. CBT is clearly more expensive than drug treatment in the short term, but there is accumulating evidence that CBT reduces the risk of future depressive episodes (Scott 2001). For many patients, a combination of antidepressants and psychotherapy is most helpful. This may be because the drug treatment provides a boost to increase activity and aid concentration, enabling the patient to take an active part in a psychological intervention, which in turn may reduce the risk of future relapse.

STOP THINK ■ If you developed the features of a depressive episode as described in Box 1, how would you feel about going to see your GP? Would you have any concerns about attending? If you did require treatment, what type of treatment would you prefer?

Electro-convulsive therapy (ECT) is a controversial treatment for severe depression. ECT has been shown to be effective in controlled clinical trials. It is not usually given as the first method of treatment, but can be helpful for people who have not responded to any other approach. Patients often complain of memory loss following ECT, but the evidence for this is inconclusive, as depression itself is often associated with both subjective and objective cognitive impairment.

There is no perfect treatment for depression and many have high dropout rates. This is likely to be due to a number of reasons: depressed patients lack energy and concentration and will find the effort of attending clinics difficult. They are also likely to have a pessimistic view of the treatment (one of the symptoms is a sense of hopelessness). No therapy offers an instant cure, so patients receive little positive reinforcement for attending initial treatment sessions.

Depression in the general medical setting

Many patients who suffer from general medical conditions also suffer from depression. For example, in a recent study of 300 consecutive new attenders at a neurology outpatient clinic, 27% met diagnostic criteria for major depressive disorder (Carson et al 2000). Unfortunately, many such patients do not get their depression diagnosed or treated, yet even in terminal disease states, such as metastatic cancer, treating an underlying depressive illness can markedly improve the patient's quality of life.

Case study

Susan, a 34-year-old bank clerk, has been married for 12 years and has three children all under the age of 10 years. In the past 3 years, both her parents died and she was promoted at work to a more demanding position, with a difficult superior. The family moved to a new home 6 months ago. Two of the children had problems settling in at their new school. For 6 weeks, Susan was wakening at 4 a.m. in the morning and was unable to get back to sleep. She worried constantly that they made the wrong decision moving home and she also regretted taking up her promoted post. She became increasingly convinced that she was failing both in her job, and as a wife and mother. She lost her appetite and 12lbs in weight in 1 month. She was constantly exhausted and irritable. She felt joyless and saw the future as bleak. She was convinced that her husband and children would be better off without her. Her husband became increasingly concerned about her, and this made her feel even more guilty for giving cause for concern. Eventually, her husband persuaded her to go to the GP, who diagnosed a major depressive episode. She was treated with a combination of antidepressant (paroxetine) and cognitive-behaviour therapy. Susan then reduced her working hours and joined a gym so that she could get some exercise and time away from work and the family, and this also enabled her to meet new people. Over a 2-month period she gradually improved and felt back to her 'old self'. The GP recommended that she stay on her medication for a further 6 months.

Depression

- Depression is a common and serious illness, which can prove fatal.
- Symptoms lie on a continuum from mild to severe.
- Vulnerability factors and stressful life events increase the risk of depression.
- Effective treatments include antidepressant medication, cognitive-behaviour therapy and interpersonal psychotherapy.
- Primary prevention includes alleviating material and emotional deprivation.

Inflammatory bowel disease

Inflammatory bowel disease (IBD) illustrates how social and psychological processes impact on the response to and the experience of illness, and some of the issues which these processes generate for medical care. Ulcerative colitis (one type of IBD) will be used to demonstrate some of these features.

Clinical features

Ulcerative colitis is a disease of the lining layer of the large gut. It can occur at any age. Its principal symptoms are chronic unpredictable diarrhoea accompanied by heavy anal bleeding, weight and appetite loss and abdominal pain. Its causes are unknown at present. There is no medical cure. The mainstays of treatment are rectal and systemic 5-aminosalicylic acid derivatives and corticosteroids, with azathioprine in steroid-dependent or resistant cases (Ghosh et al 2000).

The complications of colitis can be severe. There may be perforation of the bowel, and the effects on the overall health of the patient can be very marked. Where the disease is present for more than 10 years there is a very greatly enhanced risk of the development of bowel cancer. At present, the best treatment option available in the face of unremitting symptoms and/or the development of cancer is the surgical removal of the bowel. This involves either creating an internal pouch to collect the waste matter of digestion with normal anal evacuation, or simply redirecting the faeces through the abdominal wall via a stoma. The operations are major and have a profound effect on one of the body's major systems.

Onset

When the first symptoms – usually diarrhoea – appear, the most typical response by the sufferer is to minimize them. Diarrhoea is quite common, so the sufferer often makes the not unreasonable assumption that the symptoms will remit of their own accord. This may continue until such time as blood appears in the motion. This is usually taken as a critical and frightening symptom by the patient. Whereas diarrhoea is common, anal bleeding is not. Contact with the medical profession is frequently made some time after the appearance of blood.

I was working. I had two children . . . I began to feel, y'know, unwell. Went to my GP. Didn't examine me at all, and told me I was suffering from piles, haemorrhoids, and gave me some medication. The piles wouldn't go away, and I was back there. And by this time it was terribly painful. And I started to get really worried because I was losing blood. So I made another appointment with another doctor in the practice, and she took me into the examination room, examined me straight away, and within a week I was up at St George's Hospital.

38-year-old teacher (Kelly 1992)

The important social–psychological concept involved here is help-seeking (see pp. 86–87). Diarrhoea comes well within the range of the normal experience of most people, who will wait and see whether it passes in a day or two ('temporizing behaviour'), but for most people the appearance of blood will trigger the person to consult the doctor. From a medical point of view a patient consulting for the first time with rectal bleeding would also be seen as having a significant symptom requiring investigation, but it would possibly not engender the same degree of anxiety as experienced by the patient, and as far as colitis is concerned bleeding does not necessarily indicate an exacerbation of the illness. Thus the patient's estimation of the seriousness of the symptom may not necessarily correspond to the doctor's. However, in order to manage the patient's symptoms and anxieties successfully the doctor must be aware not only of the physical symptoms but also how they are being interpreted by the patient. The fact that the patient believes a symptom to be grave is what is important in understanding why the patient has consulted.

Diagnosis and treatment

Confirming the diagnosis will involve inspecting the patient's colon with a colonoscope or a sigmoidoscope. Alternatively, a barium enema will provide radiologic confirmation. From the patient's perspective these procedures are undignified, uncomfortable, frequently painful, and often highly stressful, as this patient described:

So I got the appointment for the X-ray Department, went in, without a care in the world. I came out absolutely devastated . . . it was terrifying . . . And you go into this place, which had this revolving table and everything and this room, and they pump all this stuff into you. It was ghastly.

33-year-old female school teacher (Kelly 1992)

Most X-ray departments have little or no time to prepare people for these procedures, and the fear and anxiety that may be generated are considerable because the patient is uncertain as to what is happening. The stressfulness of these kinds of experiences has been shown to be significantly reduced if patients have been well prepared in advance (see pp. 100–103). Furthermore, recognizing the indignity of the procedures can also be reassuring for the patient.

Having made the diagnosis, the physician faces a dilemma. If the disease can be brought under control, all well and good. However, what the physician also has to convey is that this may only be a temporary respite and that the patient may face a long period of chronic illness of varying severity. This raises some very important ethical and legal issues about how much information a patient needs to know. If doctors do provide a full account of the potential seriousness of the illness, the patient can be terrified and lose hope. If the doctor keeps the information from the patient and the illness takes a grave turn, and surgery has to be recommended, the patient may feel angry and may feel they have legal grounds on which to sue their doctor.

It is usually the case that the patient enters treatment for this disease in the expectation of a cure. Even if the physician has not explained all the likely complications and difficulties, eventually the patient will come to realize that they are not going to recover fully. This is further complicated by the fact that if the patient is trying to live as normal a life as possible, they face a tension between the demands of fulfilling usual social responsibilities and accepting the limitations imposed upon them by the illness.

Although this is not easy, people do manage to cope with their illness in spite of the difficulties it presents. Doctors can help here, by encouraging the patient to live as normal a life as they can, but also by helping them to recognize the limitations the illness can produce.

- To what extent might there be a conflict between the medical and psychological management of colitis? Is the refusal of some patients with colitis to have surgery adaptive or maladaptive?

Living with the illness

Many aspects of life are likely to be affected by the illness. The chronic, unpredictable diarrhoea means that things like travel, shopping, walking, eating, socializing are interrupted as the sufferer has to go off and find a toilet. The nature of the symptoms are such that the patient usually has very little warning (perhaps less than 30 seconds) of the need to evacuate. Sufferers become highly skilled in breaking off from social interaction, arranging journeys and trips so that toilets are always with easy reach, and carrying a change of clothes for the occasions when they self-soil.

I didn't enjoy shopping or anything. I was always wanting to be near a toilet; I, well, always felt nauseated with it. I didn't have the energy to go shopping like everybody else . . . we couldn't plan anything . . .

46-year-old housewife

It is sometimes remarked that patients suffering from colitis exhibit odd behaviour: obsessive attention to detail, concerns about personal cleanliness. However, the general consensus is that this behaviour is an adaptive product of the struggle with the illness, rather than a cause of it, which allows them to survive and function in the world, in spite of their illness.

Surgery

For some patients with colitis, the prospect of surgery has to be confronted. There are two important behavioural issues. First, the patient has to deal with the prospect of major body-altering surgery, which, with some operations, will leave them with a stoma. Second, the patient now faces a new psychological threat. While the medical decision may be relatively straightforward, it is not automatically viewed in that way by the patient. Some will refuse surgery, believing that the threats arising from the illness are preferable to the threats arising from the surgery. Helping the patient adapt to

surgery is, therefore, a key problem in this procedure. Preparations for surgery should not involve trying to make the patient 'accept' their illness or the fact that they need an operation. Helping the patient prepare for surgery should be about allowing them to acknowledge the psychological pain and distress, and the associated feelings of loss that this surgery engenders. It should aim to help them work through their feelings of hurt. This is a difficult and traumatic procedure from the patient's perspective and one which requires considerable social and psychological skills on the part of the people caring for that patient (see pp. 102–103).

Case study

Gillian is 52. She was first diagnosed as having colitis when she was 46. She is married with two teenage children. Her doctor has just told her she needs to have a total colectomy and ileostomy. She is completely distraught at the prospect. She thinks of herself, and always has, as an attractive woman. She is horrified at the prospect of wearing a bag. Yet, she is very ill. She has not had a proper night's sleep for nearly 3 years. She has to get up in the night three or four times to go to the toilet. During the day it is even worse. She usually cannot go for longer than an hour before she has to open her bowels. Her work as a secretary is becoming increasingly difficult. Her boss is very understanding but the fact that she constantly has to leave the office has made things very awkward. Her appetite is poor, and when she does eat she sticks to a diet of minced breast of chicken and white bread. She and her husband used to go out a lot, but they stay at home all the time now. Her doctor has told her that the operation will make her better. Gillian, however, is resolute in her refusal to have the operation.

Inflammatory bowel disease

- The process of making decisions about seeking help are governed by social and psychological factors as well as the degree of medical seriousness of the condition.
- Symptoms which are regarded as critical by the patient will not necessarily be the same ones as those identified as medically serious.
- In a disease like colitis social and psychological symptoms may be evident, but they are usually a consequence rather than a cause of the illness.
- The treatments for colitis, as with many illnesses, are frequently viewed as more psychologically threatening by the patient than the illness itself. These threats condition patient behaviour as much as the threats from the disease and its symptoms.
- The surgery performed to cure colitis is often associated with very powerful feelings of distress and loss.

Website: http://www.nacc.org.uk

Physical disability

Physical disabilities are limitations in the ability to perform activities and can be the result of such diverse conditions as cerebral palsy, rheumatoid arthritis, stroke, multiple sclerosis or accidental injury. As shown in Figure 1, the commonest disabilities in Western industrialized countries are in locomotion, hearing and personal care. The prevalence of disability increases with age, so that approximately half of those over 75 years have locomotion limitations.

Activity limitations can result in social disadvantage. Disability present from birth, e.g. in cerebral palsy or cystic fibrosis, may disadvantage the individual throughout their lifetime and affect school, employment, marital, parenting and other social opportunities. By contrast, an injury as a young adult, a myocardial infarction in middle age or a stroke after retirement will have very different impacts both on the individual and on his/her family.

Assessing disability

In research or clinical practice, levels of disability are assessed to ascertain the severity of the condition or to evaluate improvement or deterioration. Clinical assessments may be used to make decisions about medical care, referral to rehabilitation services (especially physiotherapists, occupational therapists, speech and language therapists), provision of aids or adaptations to the home, or recommendations for absence from work, pensions or welfare benefits.

Disability is typically assessed by measures of activities of daily living (ADL), which assess the person's ability to perform everyday self-care or mobility activities. These measures assess activities that virtually everyone would wish to perform and, therefore, do not include activities that may be important for particular individuals. For example, the Barthel Index (Johnston et al 1995) includes:

- personal toilet (wash face, comb hair, shave and clean teeth)
- feeding
- using toilet
- walking on level surface
- transfer from chair to bed
- dressing
- using stairs
- bathing.

There are two main methods of assessment: *self-report* and *observation*. The first requires the individual to describe difficulties experienced, and in the second they perform defined activities while a trained observer notes successes and failures. Using self-report allows the clinician to assess a wide range of activities, occurring in home and private situations, covering all times of day and night, and over days, weeks or months. Observational methods are restricted to what can be assessed in the limited setting of the hospital or in the limited period available for a home visit; patients who can use the toilet independently in the hospital setting may not be able to do so at home if there is less space to manoeuvre or no support to lean on, and they may be even more disabled if they need to go to the toilet during the night if this involves additional flights of stairs. These methods may be supplemented by electronic monitors, which can be used to record activity levels throughout the day, in the individual's normal environment, without risk of the bias that may be involved in self-report.

Models of disability

Three different models or perspectives on disability have developed. These are not necessarily in conflict, but each contributes to a broader understanding and possibly to achieving better medical, social and psychological outcomes for patients.

Medical model

In a medical context, activity limitations can be seen as a direct consequence of an underlying disease or disorder that causes impairment with resulting disability. Adopting this model, disability can only be reduced by treating the medical condition. A good example of this kind of model was the World Health Organization (WHO) model, which conceptualized disability as a consequence of impairment, and social limitations or 'handicap' as a result of impairment and disability. This model has been criticized both for the stereotyping and stigmatizing language used (see pp. 60–61), and for lack of recognition of social and psychological factors. It has recently been modified and updated (see Fig. 2) as the ICF (international classification of functions) model, which recognizes three components of health conditions (impairment, activity limitations and participation restrictions). In this model, disability is largely represented as activity limitations and the process of disablement includes both activity limitations and participation restrictions. All of the components are affected by personal and environmental factors.

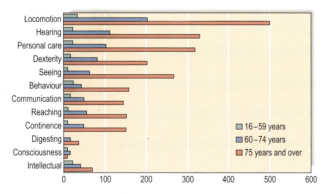

Fig. 1 **Prevalence of disabilities by age** (rate per thousand population). (Adapted from Martin et al 1988)

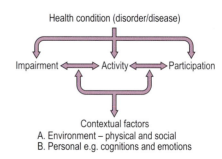

Fig. 2 **International classification of functions.** (Source: adapted from WHO 2001)

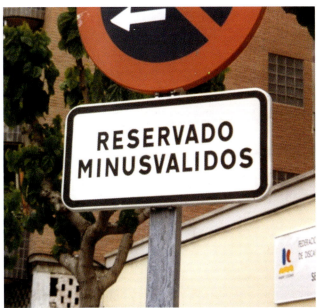

Fig. 3 **Social values.** Would a disabled person feel valued by a society that offered this 'special' car-parking space ('Reservado minusvalidos' means 'reserved for the disabled')? Or would they feel that they were 'minus validity'? English uses similarly stigmatizing vocabulary, e.g. 'invalid' (with two pronunciations) or 'handicap' (derived from the 'cap in hand' of the person begging).

Social model

A social model of disability emphasizes that activity limitations and participation restrictions result from social and environmental constraints. So the individual is limited not by their medical condition per se, but by the behaviour of other people towards them and by environmental barriers, such as the inaccessibility of buildings or poor sound systems, that make it impossible for the individual to participate fully. A person may be less disabled when activity is supported than in a protective social environment; there is evidence that compassionate attention to activity limitations can increase levels of disability. In Figure 3 we see an attempt to overcome problems of access for individuals with locomotion impairments, but the language used reflects the stigmatizing attitudes that can make participation difficult (pp. 60–61).

Psychological model

A psychological model of disability emphasizes that activities performed (or not performed) by someone with a 'health condition' are influenced by the same psychological processes that affect the performance of these behaviours by non-disabled people. So the individual will be motivated to engage in the activity because it results in things they like, because they believe that other people who are important to them would like them to do it and because they believe they can (see Case Study 2). Thus, two people with identical medical conditions, living in identical social and environmental situations, may have very different activity limitations because of their cognitions, emotions or coping strategies (see Stop and Think box and pp. 108–109).

Depressed or anxious people are likely to be more limited. People may differ in their beliefs about their condition or about the activity; someone who believes that they can overcome their disability, who finds the activity more rewarding or sees family and friends to be more supportive will be more likely to engage in the activity than someone with different beliefs (pp. 146–147).

There is ample evidence that such psychological factors predict disability outcomes. For example, stroke patients with a stronger belief that they can influence their recovery are found to do more than patients with less belief in personal control, and this difference persists for at least 3 years following stroke. Treatments that enhance perceived control beliefs have resulted in reduced activity limitations.

- Mr Harrison was disabled as the result of a spinal-cord injury incurred by falling from a lorry. From being an able-bodied lorry driver, he was now confined to a wheel-chair. However, he felt his quality of life had improved as he was now studying for a degree rather than being a manual worker. The clinical team believed that Mr Harrison could learn to walk again but seemed unmotivated. What factors are likely to be influencing Mr Harrison's degree of disability? What would be the appropriate clinical approach?

Case study 1

Mrs Patel was interviewed when she had symptoms of motor neurone disease, which meant that she could not contain her saliva and she had difficulty in speaking and eating. She had been born with only one eye and had started to become blind in this eye as a result of diabetes, a condition that had resulted in her losing a leg. Despite this accumulation of disabilities, Mrs Patel did not appear down-hearted and scored in the normal range of a test assessing mood disorder. She had good social support and coped by concentrating on the positive aspects of her lifestyle. Her mental representations and coping style appeared to protect Mrs Patel from becoming depressed.

Case study 2

Following a road traffic accident, Miss Lopez did not resume eating and drinking when she was physically capable. She only regained normal ingestive activity following a behavioural programme which socially reinforced taking sips of water and enabled her to have the confidence that she could do it.

Physical disability

- Disability is assessed by ADL measures, using both self-report and observational methods.
- Disability and its impact can be explained in terms of disease and social and psychological factors
- Disability is influenced by impairment due to disease or disorder, the physical environment, the social environment, emotions, cognitions and coping strategies.

Learning disability

The implications of a learning disability for the health of individuals who are affected and their families can be far reaching, and they may need considerable clinical care, and psychological and socio-economic support.

Approaches and prevalence

It is important to recall the WHO definition of disablement, which distinguishes between impairment, disability and handicap. This medical definition of disability and handicap should be contrasted with the view of some groups of disabled people that 'disability' is created by society through various physical, social and psychological barriers (Fig. 1): the 'social model' of disability (see pp. 116–117). This approach informs both the 'self advocacy' movement (for example: People First Scotland 1997), which is founded on the assumption of the competence and humanity of people with learning disabilities (Chappell et al 2001), and the recent UK government White Paper *Valuing People* (DoH 2001), which identifies four key principles: legal and civil rights, independence, choice and inclusion. These principles are also embodied in the Disability Discrimination Act.

The White Paper defines learning disability as: 'a significantly reduced ability to understand new or complex information, to learn new skills (impaired intelligence), with a reduced ability to cope independently (impaired social functioning), which started before adulthood with a lasting effect on development' (DoH 2001).

Estimates of the numbers and prevalence of people with learning disabilities suggest that about 25 people per 1000 have mild to moderate learning disabilities, and a further three per 1000 are severely disabled (DoH 2001).

Advances in neonatal care and in screening for learning disabilities (particularly Down's syndrome) before birth have enabled parents to choose whether or not to proceed with the pregnancy. Both of these have reduced the incidence (number of new cases per year) of children with learning disabilities. However, medical advances have also enabled children with learning disabilities to survive into adulthood and middle age when previously they would have died. So, although the overall prevalence has not changed over recent years, the age distribution of people with learning disabilities is showing a shift towards a larger proportion of older people, and they are likely to make relatively heavy use of community and hospital services.

Causes

In the case of people with mild learning disabilities, the cause is generally multifactorial and the precise mechanisms are unclear. It is generally found that environmental

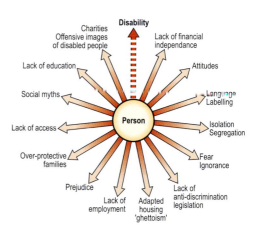

Fig. 1 **It is the 'barriers' present in society that truly disable people.**

problems like poor housing, poor nutrition, excessive smoking, alcohol and drug abuse can retard foetal and infant development, as can premature birth, difficult delivery, low birth weight and infections. It is, therefore, not surprising that mild learning disabilities are more commonly found in working-class families (nine times higher). There is less of a class association with severe learning disability, where the causal agents are more specific.

Related disabilities and problems

It is relatively common for children with severe learning disabilities to experience other disabilities, and for disabled children and adults to experience higher than average episodes of ill health. For many people, difficulty in communicating causes frustration and anger, which contributes to behaviour problems. Table 1 illustrates the problems that parents faced over one year. Of particular importance are their feelings that they have to provide continuous supervision to prevent something negative happening to their child. This can lead to social isolation, to deterioration in the principal carer's own mental and physical health, and to strains on family relationships.

The experience of having a child with a learning difficulty

It often takes some time for a baby to be identified as having a learning disability, and it is often the mother who begins to realize that something is wrong. She is likely to be very anxious (see pp. 110–111) and to have many, often confused, concerns that she may find difficult to express. It is very

STOP THINK

- Look out for posters and advertisements – how do they portray people with a disability?
- Is the social model of disability simply an extension of the concept of social handicap (see pp 116–117) or is it fundamentally different?
- In what ways do you think that medicine and research contribute to disability?

Table 1 **Problems faced by parents of child with learning disability in previous year**	
Incontinence	19%
Giving continuous care	18%
Lack of freedom, social isolation	14%
Strains in the family	14%
Worry about injury, illness, surgery	12%
Night care	12%
Lifting, carrying	10%
Mental/physical illness, fatigue	8%
Bathing, washing, personal hygiene	8%
(Source: Holland and Youngs 1990)	

important that doctors take these concerns seriously and do not dismiss them as the product of an over-anxious mother's worries.

Parents are very likely to experience strong feelings of loss, in many cases similar to the loss associated with bereavement (see pp. 16–17). They will need time and support to grieve for the child they had been looking forward to, and to adjust to the implications of having a child with learning disabilities.

As the child grows older, particularly when it is time for school, the extent and implications of cognitive impairment become clearer, and parents have difficult decisions to make about schooling. The decision will be strongly influenced by how vulnerable they feel their child to be, his/her social abilities, emotional adjustment and physical abilities, and their own feelings of protectiveness. Both the family GP and the paediatric specialist can be helpful in listening to parents, and in helping to identify and mobilize appropriate support and services.

Integration and community care

Over the last 30 years, the policy of community care has seen the closure of many long-stay hospitals and the discharge of people with learning disabilities into society (pp. 154 155).

The principles behind this policy are summarized in Table 2.

A review of community-care developments for people with learning disabilities in Britain, reported that community care that was well structured and resourced resulted in improvements in material standards of living, more satisfaction with life, and people became more competent and made more constructive use of their time. However, some people continued to show serious challenging behaviour and some experienced isolation, little integration into the local community, and experienced restrictions and problems similar to those experienced in institutional care (Emerson and Hatton 1994).

It is with a view to addressing some of these deficiencies, and concerns that some people with learning disabilities are being 'lost' in the community without adequate care and support, that the UK White Paper, 'Valuing People' (DoH 2001), recommended. These are that all people with learning disabilities will: have access to a health facilitator by June 2003; be registered with a GP by June 2004; and have a 'Health Action Plan', which is part of the individual's 'person-centred plan', in place by June 2005. We will have to wait to see whether these proposals will be adequately resourced and whether they will meet the aspirations of people with learning disabilities themselves.

Case study

Jill's first child, Sarah, was not an easy birth, but there was nothing in her pregnancy or delivery to suggest that anything might be wrong with Sarah. It was only some months later, when Jill felt that Sarah was not developing as she had expected, that she decided to check with her doctor. Although he reassured her that there was nothing to worry about, she felt that she was being dismissed as an over-anxious, first-time mother. Her husband, too, tried to reassure her that Sarah 'would soon catch up'. Some weeks later, and still concerned, Jill took Sarah to see another doctor in the practice, who suggested that Sarah should see a paediatric neurologist. Although this confirmed her fears, Jill at least felt that her concerns were being taken seriously. At the hospital, the specialist reassured Jill that Sarah would not be severely disabled, a reassurance that she now strongly resents as it turned out to be false.

Jill says that coming to terms with Sarah's disability has been like losing the healthy child she was expecting. Aged 5 years, Sarah started to have fits but drugs help to control them. Sarah cannot speak but uses a basic sign language. She finds sudden noise frightening and can throw tantrums. Sarah has no sense of danger so Jill feels that she requires constant supervision, from the special school, her parents, or the family that takes Sarah every other weekend to 'share the care'.

Over the years, Jill feels she has had to 'fight all the way' to get the services that Sarah and her family need. Her GP has been a key person, not in terms of expert knowledge, but as a support and an ally in getting things done.

Table 2 **Principles of service delivery to people with a learning disability**

- Enable people, where possible, to live ordinary lives by using means that are common, accepted and valued in their local community and culture
- Enhance the status of disabled people
- Acknowledge and respect disabled people as individual human beings with their own needs, preferences, abilities and social networks
- Work with disabled people, letting them retain, where possible, the initiative, choice and direction of their own lives
- No segregation from the rest of the community in housing, work, education or recreation
- Special, easily accessible services to meet needs inadequately served by ordinary means
- High professional standards in management, staffing and co-ordination of services.

Learning disability

- Although the prevalence of people with learning disabilities is relatively low, the impact on the family of having a child with learning disabilities is considerable.
- Doctors can be a great support to a family if they listen carefully and work with the family to obtain the services the family needs.
- Speech impairments often contribute to a person's feelings of frustration and can precipitate difficult behaviour.
- Parents often worry about what may happen to a child with learning disabilities and feel that they have to provide continuous surveillance.
- Community care for people with learning disabilities needs to be well structured and appropriately resourced.

Post-traumatic stress disorder

Post-traumatic stress disorder (PTSD) is a condition where exposure to an intense and frightening emotional experience leads to lasting changes in behaviour, affect and cognition. Typically after a life-threatening incident (e.g. a violent assault, rape or wartime experience), the individual re-experiences the event(s), e.g. via intrusive and distressing thoughts, images, 'flashbacks' or nightmares. The individual may exhibit phobic avoidance and/or physiological reactivity (e.g. increased heart rate) to reminders of the trauma. Increased arousal in terms of sleep disturbance, irritability, and exaggerated startle response are common. In addition, the individual may exhibit a restricted range of affect, sense of a foreshortened future, and may lose interest in previously rewarding hobbies or activities. As stated above, PTSD is characterized by intrusive distressing memories of the traumatic event. Paradoxically, it is also often associated with marked impairments in learning and memory for new material (anterograde memory), (pp. 26–27). Patients often complain that they remember what they do not want to, yet cannot remember what they now wish to. Heightened arousal at the time of encoding may result in modulation (strengthening) of the emotional memory trace, possibly via noradrenaline release in the amygdala. Subsequent anterograde memory impairment may be due to the deleterious effects of prolonged elevated levels of stress hormones (e.g. long-term hypercortisolaemia) on hippocampal functioning. Some MRI studies have shown that chronic PTSD is associated with reduction in volume of the hippocampus, a brain area critically involved in new learning and memory.

A psychological model

Brewin (2001) has recently outlined a dual representation theory of PTSD. He proposes that two memory systems are implicated in the disorder, verbally accessible memory (VAM) and situationally accessible memory (SAM). VAM memories can be retrieved either automatically or using deliberate, strategic processes, so that they can be edited and interact with the rest of the person's autobiographical memory. VAM memories are readily available for verbal communication with others and involve cognitive appraisals. SAM memories are difficult to communicate to others and are difficult to control. SAM memories are not encoded for context, e.g. time, and when they are retrieved they are re-experienced in the present. The emotions that accompany SAM memories consist mainly of fear, helplessness, horror and shame. Brewin proposes that VAM memories are hippocampally dependent, whereas SAM memories are non-hippocampally dependent, and involve the amygdala. In PTSD, a considerable amount of trauma information resides solely in the SAM system, and these SAM memories are particularly vulnerable to reactivation by trauma cues, e.g. flashbacks in response to sight or smells of trauma reminders (Brewin 2001) (see Fig. 1).

How common is PTSD?

The US National Comorbidity Survey (Kessler et al 1995) consisted of structured diagnostic interviews with 5877 community residents aged between 15 and 54 years. The estimated lifetime prevalence for PTSD was 7.8%. The most common precipitating traumas were combat for men, and rape and sexual molestation for women. When one assesses traumatized people, significantly elevated lifetime rates of PTSD have been reported, e.g. 32% for rape victims and 30% for Vietnam veterans. It is important to note, however, that: (a) most people do *not* develop a disorder after experiencing a stressful life event, and (b) many disorders other than PTSD often develop following adversity, in particular, phobias, depression, acute stress reaction and adjustment disorders. To take road-traffic accidents (RTAs) as an example, in one study of patients who were significantly injured in an RTA, at follow-up 10% had developed PTSD, but 25% had developed clinically significant phobias relating to driving. It is also clear that some individuals are more likely than others to develop PTSD following exposure to trauma. Predictive variables that have been identified include trauma severity, perceived threat, and prior emotional disorder, particularly depression.

Debriefing and PTSD

When disaster strikes there is an understandable need to act quickly to support survivors. With increasing recognition that PTSD can be a debilitating outcome in many individuals who experience trauma, rapid psychological interventions, i.e. 'debriefing', became popular during the 1990s. However, a recent systematic review of controlled trials in this area failed to find any evidence that debriefing reduced general psychological morbidity, depression or anxiety. In one trial at 1-year follow-up, there was a significantly *increased* risk of PTSD in those who had received debriefing (Wessely et al 1999).

Treatment

Cognitive-behavioural therapy (CBT) (see pp. 134–135) has been shown to be effective in the treatment of PTSD. Symptoms may be maintained via avoidance of reminders or thoughts about the event. CBT for PTSD generally involves two main elements, which may be used together or separately: (a) detailed and repeated exposure to traumatic

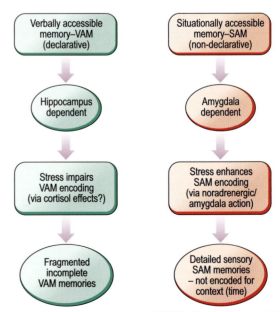

Fig. 1 **A dual representation model of PTSD.** (Source: Brewin 2000)

information, and (b) the modification of maladaptive beliefs about events, behaviours or symptoms. Exposure-based therapies have consistently been shown to be effective. These involve the common feature of having patients confront their fears, via either systematic desensitization (imaginal exposure to feared stimuli while in a relaxed state, in a graded, hierarchical fashion) or 'real-life' exposure. Eye-movement desensitization and reprocessing (EMDR) is a relatively new technique that consists of imaginal exposure while the therapist waves a finger across the patient's visual field with the patient tracking the finger. EMDR is a controversial treatment as some authors have made remarkable claims for its efficacy (Herbert et al 2000). Further well-controlled treatment trials are needed, and if EMDR is effective, this may be due in part to the exposure component. Pharmacological treatment is also effective in the treatment of PTSD. Antidepressant medication, particularly the selective serotonin re-uptake inhibitors (SSRIs) appear to be helpful, and in many cases the traumatized individual may fulfil diagnostic criteria for both PTSD and major depression.

PTSD in the medical setting

It is only relatively recently that attention has been drawn to the possibility that a significant number of individuals may be traumatized by their experience of medical events and procedures. In an important article, Shalev et al (1993) pointed out that modern medicine and surgery often use invasive procedures for which the patient has little or no preparation. For example, many individuals who previously would have died are now alive due to medical and surgical advances (e.g. electronic defibrillation following cardiac arrest). While such patients are now discharged as medical 'success stories', some survivors develop PTSD and become markedly disabled. Very often these cases are not identified in the general hospital setting, and appropriate interventions are not offered. Such individuals may subsequently avoid further contact with the medical profession, or show poor adherence with treatment regimes.

■ In a recent debate in the BMJ, Summerfield (2001) proposed that PTSD is a 'social invention' and that 'it was rare to find a psychiatric diagnosis that anyone liked to have, but PTSD is one'. He also stated that 'once it becomes advantageous to frame distress as a psychiatric condition, people will choose to present themselves as medicalized victims rather than as feisty survivors'. In reply, Shalev (2001) argued that the diagnostic criteria for PTSD are not built in stone, 'But neither are depression, psychosis or delirium'. He concluded that 'Doctors . . . have nothing to gain from claims that the pervasive and interminable personal disaster that is post traumatic stress disorder is not a disorder'. What do you think?

Case study

Mrs C., a 30-year-old woman, underwent a tonsillectomy. While in hospital her husband brought the baby to visit her. Mrs C. went to the baby and started to take off his hood. Suddenly, blood spurted out of her mouth all over the floor. Panic ensued and she was rushed in a state of hypovolemic shock to the operating room, where a bleeding artery was ligated. She remembers overhearing a doctor tell her husband that 'she had one foot in the grave'. For months following this event, Mrs C. lived in a constant state of anxiety. She feared that the pharyngeal scar would open and she would bleed to death. Intrusive thoughts and memories of the event kept her awake at night and disturbed her during the day. She was terrified to make a careless move in case it triggered a further episode of bleeding. She withdrew contact from her baby because of a fear that while hugging him blood would again spurt out of her mouth. Treatment involved controlled exposure, involving visiting the surgeon who had operated on her throat, and receiving accurate information regarding future risk, etc. Gradually she returned to her previous level of functioning. (Source: Shalev et al 1993).

Post-traumatic stress disorder (PTSD)

■ PTSD is an increasingly recognized, though controversial disorder.
■ PTSD is commonly reported following extreme trauma.
■ There is increasing evidence that some medical events (e.g. myocardial infarction) or treatments (e.g. defibrillation) can lead to post-traumatic symptoms.
■ Patients with PTSD following medical events are often not identified.
■ Sufferers may avoid further medical care and show poor adherence with treatment.
■ Improved recognition should lead to appropriate treatment and improved ability to make use of medical care.

Diabetes mellitus

The number of people worldwide with the chronic condition diabetes mellitus has increased dramatically over the past 10 years and is expected to go on rising. As a diagnostic category, diabetes includes numerous disorders, but the two most common are known as type 1 and type 2 diabetes. At least 1.4 million people in the UK have diabetes and there are probably another million people who have not been diagnosed. Approximately 85% of those diagnosed have type 2 diabetes. Both types of diabetes share the symptom of raised blood-glucose levels. Abnormally elevated blood-glucose levels have adverse consequences in both the short and long term.

Type 1 diabetes

Type 1 diabetes is typically diagnosed in childhood or adolescence. As a result of a combination of genetic and environmental factors, an autoimmune process progressively destroys the cells in the pancreas that produce the hormone insulin. Insulin is necessary to facilitate the uptake of glucose from the blood by body tissue. In the absence of insulin, blood-glucose levels continue to rise leading to the characteristic symptoms of Type 1 diabetes: frequent urination, thirst, fatigue, and weight loss. If untreated, there is a risk of ketoacidosis leading eventually to coma, which can be fatal. Type 1 diabetes is treated by replacing the insulin no longer produced by the body with exogenous insulin delivered by injection or pump. The complex treatment regimen requires the patient to use the results of blood-glucose monitoring to balance food consumption, insulin administration, and energy expenditure. Imbalance can lead to hyperglycaemia (abnormally high blood-glucose levels) or hypoglycaemia (abnormally low blood-glucose levels), both of which have negative health consequences.

Type 2 diabetes

Type 2 diabetes is predominantly a disease of the middle-aged and elderly, although, with increasing levels of juvenile obesity, it is now beginning to be seen among children and adolescents. Blood-glucose levels are abnormally high because of both impaired insulin production and insensitivity to insulin. The symptoms are similar to type 1, but often are less pronounced, so that Type 2 diabetes can go undiagnosed for years. Type 2 diabetes has a stronger genetic component than type 1. The lifetime risk of developing Type 2 is increased 40% by the presence of a first-degree relative with the disease. Overeating and a sedentary lifestyle are also risk factors for developing Type 2 diabetes. The treatment of Type 2 diabetes involves modifications to diet and exercise, and tablets for reducing blood-glucose levels. If these measures are not effective then insulin will be necessary.

Prevention of diabetes

A recent study conducted in Finland has demonstrated that Type 2 diabetes can be prevented by changes in lifestyle (Tuomilehto et al 2001). Participants were middle-aged, overweight and had impaired glucose tolerance (a diabetes risk factor). All received individualized counselling aimed at reducing fat consumption and increasing physical activity.

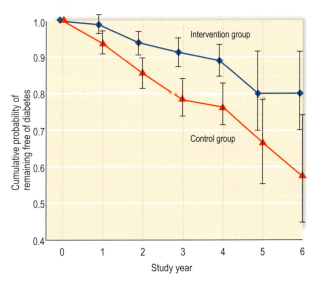

Fig. 1 **Results of a trial to prevent type 2 diabetes by improving lifestyle.** The proportion of subjects who developed diabetes was significantly higher in the control group than the intervention group from the second year of the study onwards. (Adapted with permission from Tuomilehto et al 2001)

The risk of developing diabetes in the intervention group was reduced by 58% over the period of the trial in comparison to the usual care control group (see Fig. 1).

Complications of diabetes

Abnormal blood-glucose levels increase the risk of diabetic complications resulting from damage to the small and large blood vessels. As a result, diabetes is a leading cause of blindness, kidney failure, amputation and coronary artery disease. Recent trials have demonstrated that some of these complications can be prevented or delayed by improvements in blood-glucose levels (DCCT 1993, UKPDS 1998), which underscores the importance of good self-management of diabetes.

Self-management of diabetes

For both types of diabetes, the person with the disease plays the central role in controlling the illness (Holman and Lorig 2000). The treatment regimen includes medical elements (blood-glucose monitoring and medication – tablets, insulin or both), and lifestyle elements (diet and exercise). People with diabetes find the lifestyle elements more difficult and more damaging to their quality of life than the medical elements (see Case study). Diabetes self-management presents different challenges depending on a person's age (Snoek and Skinner 2000).

Ways to support diabetes self-management

Patients benefit from support from health-care professionals to improve their self-management (Clement 1995). Such support needs to be ongoing and part of the routine care provided to diabetes patients. In a randomized controlled study, 206 diabetes patients were randomized to receive either a brief dietary intervention or usual care (see 'Tailored intervention' box). After 1 year, patients in the intervention group had improved significantly on measures of low-fat eating habits and on cholesterol levels. The cost of the intervention ($137 or £87 per patient in 1997 prices) was relatively modest (Glasgow et al 1997). Patients benefit from working in partnership with their health-care professionals, setting mutually agreed goals that are specific and tailored to the patients' particular circumstances (see Fig. 2). With optimal medical care and good self-management, people with diabetes can enjoy a healthy life for many years.

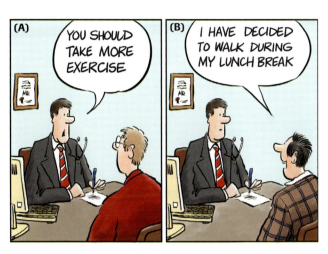

Fig. 2 **Which patient is more likely to increase their exercise levels – A or B?**

Tailored intervention for people with diabetes to reduce fat consumption

A tailored intervention that was brief, convenient and patient centred, and changed eating habits and lowered cholesterol was developed (Glasgow et al 1997). Successful achievement of one behaviour change will lead to increased confidence and further success.

■ **Brief**
Basic information about eating habits and barriers to healthy eating was obtained via a touchscreen computer. This information was used to guide the 20-minute session with the interventionist.

■ **Convenient**
The intervention occurred at the same time and place as their regular doctor's appointment.

■ **Patient centred**
Together, the patient and interventionist agreed upon a specific goal to reduce fat consumption (e.g. 'I will snack on raw vegetables instead of potato crisps when watching television'), anticipated barriers to achieving this goal, and agreed on ways to overcome these barriers.

■ Diabetes is more common among ethnic minorities in the UK. In what ways could health care for diabetes be made more culturally sensitive?

Case study

Part 1: self-management for a teenager with type 1 diabetes

Tracey is 16 and enjoys going clubbing. When Tracey stays out late dancing and drinking she misses her evening snack, and the alcohol and exercise lowers her blood-glucose levels. Her blood-glucose levels drop while she is asleep and she is often hypoglycaemic by the time she gets up. Her very low blood glucose makes her bad-tempered and uncooperative. Tracey has been rushed to hospital unconscious on several occasions. How can her health-care team help Tracey to take better care of herself?

Part 2: how can we help Tracey?

■ Encourage Tracey to attend sessions specifically for groups of teenagers with diabetes where they can discuss how to overcome the lifestyle challenges posed by their self-management.
■ Tracey's doctor may be able to suggest an adjustment to her insulin injections on evenings when she is going out.
■ The dietician may be able to recommend certain foods Tracey should eat before going out, and snack foods or soft drinks that she could have while clubbing.
■ Tracey or her mother could leave a favourite snack conveniently by her bed for when she returns home late.
■ Parents should not relinquish responsibility for their teenage children's diabetes too soon.

Diabetes mellitus

■ Diabetes is an increasingly common chronic illness, in part because of the ageing of populations in developed countries and the rise in obesity.
■ Type 2 diabetes can be prevented by changing diet and exercise patterns.
■ The onset of complications of both Type 1 and Type 2 diabetes can be prevented or delayed by improved blood-glucose control.
■ Day-to-day management of diabetes is primarily the responsibility of patients, who need empowering and supporting in their self-management of this disease.
■ Interventions to enhance patient self-management are most effective when they are patient centred and tailored to individual needs.
■ Diabetes occurs in all age groups from the very young to the very old, and different approaches to providing appropriate health care and support are needed for different age groups.

Stress and health

What is stress?

We are continually faced with demands from our social and physical environments. Stress is generated when we think we may not be able to meet perceived demands and expect negative consequences to follow. In other words, stress arises out of the relationship between our perceptions or 'appraisals' of environmental demands and of our own abilities and resources (pp. 132–133). Thus, the same event or situation may be stressful to one person but not to another. For example, some students may be very stressed by a forthcoming examination while others are not. Our experience of stress does not always correspond to others' assessment of the demands we face. Gifted students who have always done well in examinations may still feel stressed before an examination. Stress involves negative emotional responses and affects physiological functioning.

Factors influencing the experience of stress

When we are familiar with an event and when we feel confident in our abilities to handle it we are less likely to feel stressed. For example, a doctor who has previous experience of preparing a patient for surgery (pp. 102–103) or has been well trained in breaking bad news (pp. 96–97) is likely to feel less stressed than one approaching such tasks for the first time or one who has low confidence in their ability to control these situations (pp. 156–157). Feeling stressed may also undermine performance because we may be distracted by our own worries and seek to avoid the task rather than managing it well. This is why rehearsal and training are crucial to competent performance at work (pp. 56–57): when we feel confident in our abilities and resources we perceive demands as challenges rather than stressors.

We are less likely to feel stressed when we know the demanding situation will be short term, for example, a particularly busy day at work. When there seems no end in sight then we may doubt our coping capacity and feel overwhelmed by rising stress levels (pp. 158–159). Ensuring people have all the competencies they need to do their jobs effectively is important to avoiding stress at work. Stress at work is determined not only by job demands, but also by how much decision-making power people have, that is, how much control they have over work schedules and setting priorities (Karasek 1979). Greater control results in less stress. When people are unclear about their role at work or when there are contradictory demands on time this will increase work-related stress. For example, doctors and nurses may experience stress when they are unclear about management priorities or when they feel they have to compromise patient care because of administrative demands. Jobs that lack variety, do not involve the development of new skills and do not allow opportunities for social interaction are also more likely to create stress. Continued stress at work can undermine perceived control and motivation (see pp. 146–147) and lead to burn out.

Stress can also be caused by role conflict when the demands of one role (e.g. a work role) prevent one from fulfilling the obligations of other roles (such as friendships or parental roles). Similarly, losing a role that we value as part of our identity (e.g. being made redundant) can create stress. If alternative roles are not developed such loss may lead to depression.

Measuring stress

There are numerous self-report measures of stress. Holmes and Rahe (1967) developed the first 'life events' scale. This approach involves asking people to list events in their recent past that might be expected to be stressful and adding up the burden. For example, death of a close family member warrants a high score (100) as does losing one's job (47), while trouble with one's boss attracts a lower score (23). This scale also acknowledges that change in general, even what are commonly regarded as positive changes, can increase stress. Twelve points are added just after Christmas and 13 for a recent vacation. Psychologists have also measured the occurrence of more minor stressors, or daily hassles, such as taking examinations or getting a low grade in a test or examination. The main limitation of such measures is that they do not measure the different appraisals of these events made by different people. This is problematic because different people perceive the same event to be more or less demanding and undesirable. We can, instead, ask people directly to report how stressed they feel and how able they feel to cope with everyday demands.

Stress affects the sympathetic nervous system (SNS). Consequently, we can use measures of SNS activity as indicators of arousal and stress response. These include respiration rate, blood pressure, heart rate, skin conductance (which changes when we sweat) as well as concentrations of corticosteroids (e.g. cortisol) and catecholamines (e.g. adrenalin and noradrenalin) in the blood.

Stress and the cardiovascular system (see pp. 104–105)

Continued stress responses damage the cardiovascular system over time. For example, in studies of male baboons, lower-status animals, which are more likely to be attacked, were found to have higher average cortisol levels, and a lower ratio of high-density to low-density lipoproteins. These factors are thought to contribute to atherosclerosis, that is, accumulations of deposits on artery walls. Unsurprisingly, then, lower-status animals were also found to have greater narrowing of the coronary arteries and aorta, and higher blood pressure (Sapolsky 1993).

Personality factors make some people more likely to experience stress than others. Type A personality refers to people who are very ambitious in relation to the amount they try to get done in a given time, and are more likely to be competitive and hostile towards others. This may result in strong, frequent stress responses, which results in considerable wear and tear on the cardiovascular system. Such stress responses may precipitate a myocardial infarction earlier than would be the case for a Type B person (who is low on competitiveness, time urgency and hostility) with the same level of atherosclerosis. Hostility appears to be a particularly dangerous personality trait with those scoring highly on hostility measures being more likely to suffer a coronary heart disease (Miller et al 1996). High hostility is indicated by agreement with statements such as 'It's safer to trust nobody', 'No-one cares much what happens to me' and 'People often disappoint me'.

Stress and immune functioning

Research suggests that stress is associated with weaker immune responses and slower wound healing (Kiecolt-Glaser et al 1995). For example, medical students report higher stress during examinations and also show reduced immune response. This includes lower T-helper (CD4) counts, less-rapid proliferation of these cells in laboratory tests as well as reduced natural killer cell activity (Kiecolt-Glaser et al 1994). Similar evidence of compromised immune functioning has been observed amongst carers of people with Alzheimer's disease and amongst those who have been recently separated, divorced or bereaved. These results suggest that ongoing stress may leave us more susceptible to infection, slow wound healing and inhibit tumour surveillance.

There is also evidence suggesting that associations between stress and immune function are the result of communication between the nervous and immune systems. People who show strong SNS responses to stress also show the greatest immune responses. By contrast, only small immune effects are observed amongst those who have little SNS response to a stressor (Cohen and Herbert 1996). The field of research exploring relationships between the nervous and immune systems is known as psychoneuroimmunology.

Stress and risk behaviours

As well as affecting the cardiovascular and immune systems, stress may also increase the likelihood of illness indirectly by means of our behaviour. People who feel stressed may be less likely to take preventive health measures, including adherence to doctors' advice (pp. 92–93). They may also take risks with their health through smoking, drinking too much, poor diet, drug misuse and sleep loss. They may also take risks that increase the likelihood of involvement in accidents.

STOP THINK

- Examinations have been shown to increase students' stress. Which thoughts and perceptions increase this stress? What do students do as a result of stress that may affect their health? How could you help a friend who says they feel very stressed about a forthcoming examination?

Helping people deal with stress

Research has identified a number of factors that may alleviate the experience of stress. Social support may help. This includes emotional support, for example, providing intimacy that allows people to talk about their problems and fears (pp. 130–131), as well as providing information and actual resources (i.e. tangible social support), including money and time. Encouraging people to change their appraisals may also help. This could involve focusing on how they have managed to deal with similar demands in the past or by helping them to see that the stressor is less important than they think. People may also benefit from relaxation training so that they can reduce physiological stress responses. Exercising so that one keeps fit can also reduce the experience of stress and its impact on health. Some companies encourage such activities in stress-management courses designed to reduce the general level of stress amongst their employees.

Case study

Rethinking the problem

Jo is a young married woman who has a job she likes that is near her home. She is involved in a car accident that leaves her disabled with walking difficulties. This prevents her continuing with her job. Initially, Jo is very distressed and cannot see how her life will be worthwhile or happy again. She becomes depressed and anxious. Then, through counselling and the help of friends, she begins to rethink her life. She realizes she is better off than many other people, despite her problems. She comes to believe that, although she liked her job, it was limiting her potential. She enrols on a psychology degree course at her local university and embarks on a new career.

Stress and health

- Stress arises when we think that we may not be able to deal with perceived demands.
- Stress involves negative emotional responses and affects physiological functioning.
- Feeling familiar with an event, confident in our abilities and knowing the event will be short term reduce stress.
- Role strain and role conflict also cause stress.
- Continued stress responses damage the cardiovascular system over time.
- High hostility is associated with coronary heart disease.
- Stress is associated with weaker immune responses and slower wound healing.
- People suffering from stress may also damage their health through their behaviour.

Asthma and chronic obstructive pulmonary disease

Asthma, which is experienced by almost one in ten of the UK population, can occur from infancy to old age and is genetically based. Chronic obstructive pulmonary disease (COPD) is experienced by 8% of UK men and 3% of women and is an adult illness, in most cases the consequence of lung damage caused by cigarette smoking (less than 10% is due to occupational illness). Symptoms in asthma and COPD have many similarities, such as breathlessness, ranging from mild to severe, and a pattern of exacerbations that can be triggered by infections (for both asthma and COPD) or allergens in the case of asthma.

Medical interventions for asthma

For moderate asthma the most important intervention is anti-inflammatory medication. This is usually an inhaled corticosteroid. Used daily, and continuously, inhaled steroids reduce lung inflammation and thus prevent symptoms in asthma. Higher- dose oral steroids are used in short courses to manage exacerbations or, in severe asthma, may be taken daily for regular control.

Bronchodilating medication is the other main medical intervention. It relaxes airways and relieves symptoms, but does not reduce airway inflammation, the underlying mechanism that drives asthma. Patients use this medication when they feel mildly breathless or before exercise. It is usually given through a pocket-sized inhaler. In mild asthma, with only occasional breathlessness, this may be the only medication used.

Medical interventions for COPD

This consists of bronchodilating medication to relieve symptoms, taken daily through a pocket-sized inhaler or an electrically powered nebulizer, and antibiotics for COPD exacerbations resulting from chest infections.

Oral or inhaled corticosteroids are appropriate for some patients with COPD.

Quality of life in asthma and COPD

From the patient's viewpoint, the main difference between asthma and COPD is that for most people with asthma, lung obstruction is reversible. This means that breathlessness in asthma is relieved by regular use of inhaled or oral steroids, which control and diminish lung inflammation, and occasional use of bronchodilators to relax airways constriction. With appropriate medication almost all people with asthma can lead a non-restricted life.

COPD has more significant effects on quality of life, because lung damage is non-reversible. A diagnostic criterion of COPD is lung function (FEV_1) that is less than 60% of normal of comparable age. Constant moderate-to-severe breathlessness, cough, and phlegm production, with periods of acute symptoms triggered by infection are characteristic of COPD. About 15% of all hospital admissions are due to COPD. COPD is a disease of adulthood and old age.

In about 70% of patients with COPD, daily activities are limited by breathlessness, sleep is frequently disturbed and patients have severe attacks of breathlessness, which can lead to hospital admissions. In COPD, pulmonary rehabilitation can help patients cope with constant breathlessness, and manage everyday activities.

In about 90% of patients with asthma, activities need not be limited, and exacerbations can be reduced to a very low level.

Adherence in asthma

In mild to moderate asthma, lung inflammation can be controlled by daily use of inhaled corticosteroid, but most patients (60% or more) do not take their inhaled steroid as frequently as prescribed. This is for a variety of reasons. Patients may believe that they only need their medication at certain times of the year ('pragmatic' adherence) (Osman 1998). Patients may stop medication in order to test if symptoms reappear ('testing') (Osman 1998). Some patients also express 'steroid phobia', but dislike of taking any medication regularly may be as great an influence on non-adherence as specific dislike of steroids (Osman et al 1993). Patients who are depressed are more likely to be non-adherent (Bosley et al 1995). It has been shown that a 'fact-based' approach to persuading patients does not increase adherence (Hilton et al 1996), but a 'patient-centred' approach based on agreement on self-management is effective in improving outcomes (Osman et al 2002).

Self-management plans in asthma

In Patient adherence (see pp. 92–93), it was pointed out that adherence is most likely when patients understand what they are being asked to do, and why. Clear communication between patient and doctor and agreement on self-treatment increases the likelihood of adherence. Self-management plans (Fig. 1) are brief instructions on how to use asthma medication, and when to vary medication, such as increasing inhaled steroid when

YOUR ASTHMA DISCHARGE PLAN
These are the asthma medicines you should be taking when you leave hospital
Your GP may change this plan after seeing you

With hindsight, when did your asthma start to get worse and what do you think you could have done to prevent this admission to hospital?

Plans for controlling and preventing future attacks
Prevention inhaler use/oral steroid use/GP contact/trigger avoidance (circle)

YOUR ASTHMA MEDICINES

Your Relief Inhaler is
This inhaler quickly helps mild breathlessness
It does not prevent bad attacks

When you are well you should not need to use your relief inhaler more than 1 or 2 times a day

Your Long Acting Relief Medicine is
This inhaler should be taken every day
It does not prevent bad attacks

You should take ___ puffs ____ times every day

Your Prevention Inhaler is
This is an inhaled steroid. If you take it every day, it helps you have little or no breathlessness.
It also prevents sudden attacks

You should take ___ puffs ____ times every day

Oral steroid course
It is important to continue taking your inhaled steroid while you are taking any steroid tablets.
See your GP if you are not back to normal after finishing your steroid tablets

You should take every day after breakfast
____ tablets (mgs) for ____ days
____ tablets (mgs) for ____ days
____ tablets (mgs) for ____ days
then

Asthma warning symptoms
When you return to your usual level of prevention inhaler you know your asthma is worsening
• if you feel more breathless than usual and need to use your relief inhaler every two hours or more often
• if you wake at night feeling breathless
• AND IF YOUR PEAK FLOW DROPS BELOW

Remember 'What you can do'
• Act early. Don't wait until you are too breathless to do normal activities
• Double your usual inhaled steroid, or start tablet steroids when your peak flow drops
• Do not hesitate to contact your GP for guidance
• See your Yellow Book Plan for details

A GOOD PEAK FLOW FOR
YOU IS

SEE YOU DOCTOR IMMEDIATELY IF YOUR
PEAK FLOW DROPS BELOW

Fig. 1 **Hospital discharge self-management plan.**

symptoms increase, which have been discussed and agreed between the health professional and the patient. Use of self-management plans has been shown to improve outcomes for asthma and COPD patients, to reduce symptoms and to increase quality of life. A simple 'credit card' self-management plan can be used in general practice. Figure 1 shows a self-management plan used before hospital discharge of patients admitted with acute asthma. Patients who were given this plan were significantly less likely to be readmitted.

Smoking cessation in COPD

Smoking cessation is the main method of controlling further deterioration and early death in COPD (Fig. 2). (In asthma smoking cessation is important in limiting symptoms and controlling exacerbations and smoking cessation by parents is important in reducing the risk of asthma in children.)

Family and health-professional advice are the most important influences in encouraging attempts to stop. Brief doctor advice increases the likelihood that a smoker will stop by about 2–3%, advice plus nicotine-replacement therapy leads to increased cessation of about 10% (Fig. 3).

Pulmonary rehabilitation in COPD

COPD rehabilitation programmes include physical exercises aimed at building up patients' exercise tolerance, and techniques of managing breathlessness and education in techniques of efficient breathing. They are usually run by physiotherapists for small groups of patients, taking place one or two times a week for 6–8 weeks. Studies have shown that rehabilitation programmes of this kind can improve patient quality of life and respiratory muscle strength even when objective indicators of exercise tolerance and lung function do not change.

Psychological issues in asthma and COPD

Asthma deaths are uncommon, psychiatric morbidity is high among the small group of people (less than 1%) with a history of severe life-threatening asthma attacks. A summary of adverse factors associated with near-fatal asthma attacks is shown below:

Factors associated with near-fatal asthma attacks

(Campbell et al 1995, Innes et al 1998, Yellowlees and Ruffin 1989)

- depression
- denial
- psychiatric caseness
- alcohol or drug abuse
- severe domestic stress
- social isolation, living alone
- unemployment
- being female.

Intensive individual management programmes, with one-to-one contact, and fast access for patients to doctor or nurse support have been the most successful approach to reducing life-threatening attacks among this small high-risk group. Molfino et al (1992) followed 12 patients who had had near-fatal asthma attacks, and who had been recommended for closely supervised follow-up. Seven of the 12 agreed, and all survived. Five refused; of these, two died within 6 months of hospital discharge.

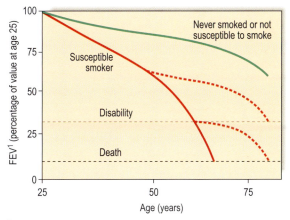

FEV^1 decline

^{1} Fletcher C and Peto R. BMJ 1977;1:1645-1648

Fig. 2 **Smoking and lung-function decline: Peto graph.**

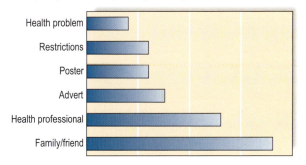

What prompted an attempt to stop smoking?

Fig. 3 **Influence on smoking cessation attempts.**

Case study

Adolescents and asthma (Slack and Brooks 1995)
In a focus group study 28 teenagers (13–17 years) with asthma talked about their experience with asthma and health care. The teenagers were concerned about adverse effects and the cost of medications and wanted more information about asthma and its treatment. They considered themselves compliant with therapy, but felt that they had had conflicting advice and inappropriate rules from adults about medication use. Members of the group wanted complete responsibility for medication, felt they did not disobey adults, and did not believe peers had a negative influence on them.

In 1997 the National Asthma Campaign carried out a national study of UK teenagers attitudes to asthma. This showed that worries about asthma attacks, and about use of inhalers were greatest among younger teenagers, and lessened as teenagers grew older.

Asthma and chronic obstructive pulmonary disease

- Regular inhaled steroids reduce risk of exacerbations in asthma, but many patients stop taking preventive medication when they have no symptoms.
- In asthma and COPD, agreement on treatment goals between patient and health professional improves patient outcomes. It is best achieved through developing a self-management plan with the patient.
- Smoking cessation is the most important intervention for aiding patients with COPD.

Death and dying

The medicalization of dying

Dying and death, like birth, are a normal part of everyday life. Over the past few decades, Western society has largely removed death and dying to the confines of institutions such as hospitals and hospices. Care of the dying and the dead is still, for the most part, the remit of professionals such as doctors, nurses and undertakers. As a result, death has become marginalized and stigmatized and, some would argue, increasingly medicalized (Clark and Seymour 1999). More recently, media images of death, dying and mourning, such as the Princess of Wales' funeral in the UK and the events surrounding 9/11 in the USA, have gradually re-introduced this topic to the public arena. Public outpourings of grief on national television seem more normal now.

Place of death

Paradoxically, though we know that most people would like to die at home, in their own beds, surrounded by family and friends, the majority of people will not (Townsend 1990). UK data on place of death showed that 66% of all deaths occurred in hospital in the year 2000 (Ellershaw and Ward 2003). A combination of factors, such as poorly controlled symptoms, lack of family support, the burden on carers, badly coordinated services and changes in people's preferences as their disease progresses, can result in people being admitted to a hospital or a hospice before they die. Thorpe (1993) suggests that improvements in care could enable more people to die at home (see Box 1).

Attitudes to death and dying

Many doctors find caring for those who are dying a stressful, but important part of their workload (Ahmedzai 1992). This may be because doctors feel guilty or frustrated at their failure to achieve a medical cure or because they have difficulty in knowing how to communicate with the dying and their relatives. In addition to these professional concerns, most doctors will face the common human fears when contemplating the inevitability and uncontrollability of death. The more anxious health professionals are about death then the more negative their attitudes and behaviour may be towards the terminally ill.

Stages of dying

Theoretical descriptive models have helped us to understand individual psychological responses to death. In her interviews with terminally ill cancer patients, Kubler-Ross (1970) described the dying process as a series of stages

Table 1	
Good death	**Bad death**
Lack of patient distress	**Negative effects on family**
■ Family acceptance	■ Unfinished business
■ Dying in presence of close people	■ Relatives' distress
■ At peace	■ Not dying with close people around
■ Continuing previous interests	■ Terrible physical symptoms.
■ No physical pain	
■ No anxiety	
■ Dying in place of choice.	
Patient control during dying process	**Patient non-acceptance**
■ Following appropriate cultural rules	■ Non-preparation of relatives
■ Dying in place of choice	■ Non-acceptance of illness
■ Cultural perceptions of good death	■ Fighting death to the end
■ Patient control	■ Badly managed death.
■ Dying in presence of close people.	
Role of staff	**Patient fears**
■ Comfortable process	■ Psychological distress
■ Peaceful death	■ Not dying in a place of choice
■ No anxiety	■ Terrible physical symptoms
■ No pain.	■ Fighting death to the end
	■ Not dying with close people around.
	Age of dying person
	■ Age

that the person passes through before finally coming to terms with his/her imminent death. These stages include shock, denial, anger, bargaining, depression and ultimately acceptance. Similar staged theories have been used to describe the bereavement process (pp. 16–17). However, not everyone passes through these stages in sequence and individuals may fluctuate between acceptance and denial as they try to maintain hope about their prognosis (Johnston and Abraham 2000). Carers and health professionals, therefore, need to be prepared for fluctuations in patients' moods so that they do not misinterpret them.

Caring for people from different faiths

The way we care for people as they die and prepare the body after the death should be guided by the person's cultural and religious beliefs. Unfortunately, such beliefs and associated rituals are often compromised by the organizational and bureaucratic barriers imposed by modern healthcare or by a lack of understanding on the part of health professionals. Yet, respecting these beliefs and ensuring prescribed rituals are adhered to can help patients to achieve a peaceful and dignified death, and facilitate the bereavement process for carers (Firth 2001).

Viewing the body after the death

Junior medical staff may often be involved in dealing with the relatives after the death. This may involve breaking the news of the death to the relatives and accompanying them to view the body, either on the ward or in the hospital chapel or mortuary where the body has been taken (pp. 96–97). Although this may be an uncomfortable duty, it is an important part of the grieving process and allows the relative to begin to absorb the loss and to say a final goodbye. It will be especially difficult, however, if the death has been sudden or unexpected.

Box 1 **Factors that would allow dying people to remain at home**

- ■ Adequate nursing care
- ■ Good symptom control
- ■ Confident and committed general practitioners
- ■ Financial assistance
- ■ Access to specialist palliative care
- ■ Effective co-ordination of resources
- ■ Terminal-care education.

The good death

Achieving a good death for patients is an important goal for health professionals who work with the dying (Ellershaw and Ward 2003). Studies of the dying process have led to a debate about the characteristics of a 'good death'. Table 1 describes the perceptions of one group of palliative-care professionals about factors that constitute a 'good' and 'bad death' (Low and Payne 1996). Good deaths occur when patients accept death and have control over the circumstances of their death, while bad deaths occur when patients are unprepared and the dying process is managed badly.

The importance of achieving a good death has led to the publication of guidelines and recommendations to help health professionals improve the standard of care for dying patients. A recent report by an English charity, Age Concern, identified 12 principles that facilitate a good death in elderly patients (Age Concern 1999) (see Box 2). The need to educate doctors to recognize care of the dying as an important component of their practice and to incorporate this subject in the core medical curriculum has also been highlighted (Ellershaw and Ward 2003). Such is the public interest that several publications have also been produced to guide lay people in achieving their own 'good death'.

Social death

The stigmas surrounding death and difficulties in knowing how to talk to those who are dying can mean that terminally ill people experience a type of 'social death' before their bodies physically fail. This may occur because family, friends and health professionals find it difficult to talk to people who are dying and therefore withdraw from them, or because the dying themselves begin a process of disengaging from people in an attempt to prepare themselves for their death (Johnston and Abraham 2000). This process may be initiated or exacerbated by physical symptoms that prevent patients from leading a normal life. Its result, however, may be that patients become lonely and isolated. Hospital staff may unwittingly compound this isolation by moving dying patients to side wards or hiding them behind bed screens. Maintaining good communication with terminally ill patients is essential to reassure them that they are still supported and valued as people, and have a purpose in life.

Box 2 Principles of a good death

- To know when death is coming, and to understand what can be expected.
- To be able to retain control of what happens.
- To be afforded dignity and privacy.
- To have control over pain relief and other symptom control.
- To have choice and control over where death occurs (at home or elsewhere).
- To have access to information and expertise of whatever kind is necessary.
- To have access to any spiritual or emotional support desired.
- To have access to hospice care in any location, not only in hospital.
- To have control over who else is present and shares the end.
- To be able to issue advance directives that ensure wishes are respected.
- To have time to say goodbye, and control over other aspects of timing.
- To be able to leave when it is time to go, and not to have life prolonged pointlessly.

Case study

You are a house officer on a busy medical ward to which an elderly Muslim man has been admitted. Investigations have shown that the patient's condition is terminal and that his prognosis is short. The consultant has informed the patient's wife that her husband's poorly controlled symptoms mean that allowing him to die at home would not be advisable. The patient has a large family, who are very distressed by the news. They want to visit every day and insist on bringing special food that they want the nurses to prepare. Their behaviour is causing disruption to the other patients, but there are no single rooms available. On the night of his death the nurses ask you to tell the family to go home and come back in the morning. You are uncomfortable about this, but do as you are asked. A few hours later the patient dies. On hearing of his death, Mr Ahmed's family are very angry and say that because they were not present at the death to perform special rituals his soul will never be at peace. You feel guilty and upset and wish you had done more to ensure that the wishes of the family had been respected (cf. Firth 2001).

- What steps could you have taken to ensure that Mr Ahmed had a 'good death'?
- How might you have found out more about the rituals that the family wanted to perform?
- How might this experience affect Mrs Ahmed's bereavement process?

Death and dying

- Our attitudes to death may affect the way we care for dying patients.
- Most patients want to die at home but most still die in hospital.
- Cultural differences will affect people's behaviour before and after the death.
- 'Good deaths' can be achieved if people are in control of the way they die.

Counselling

Counselling and medicine

Counselling is about supporting people to make constructive changes in their lives. Patients may benefit from counselling when they need to consider a complex problem, make an important decision, adjust to a change in their lives or contemplate changing their behaviour. For example, counselling is used to help people decide whether or not they want to take certain diagnostic tests (e.g. the HIV antibody test), have particular treatments (e.g. radical mastectomy or lumpectomy for some breast cancers) or undergo medical procedures (e.g. the termination of an unplanned pregnancy). It is also used to support patients in adjusting to new life situations (e.g. leading a healthy life after a myocardial infarction) or changing their behaviour (e.g. reducing Type A behaviour, see pp. 124–125). Recent advances in genetic testing mean that counsellors are employed to:
1) help prospective parents estimate the risks of their children inheriting certain diseases and make decisions based on this understanding, or 2) help patients assess their risks of developing illnesses and make life decisions based on this knowledge.

Counsellors may be professional or voluntary and counselling may take place in one session (e.g. deciding whether to have an HIV antibody test) or over a series of meetings (e.g. helping someone to give up smoking). Some doctors are trained counsellors, but many refer patients to others with counselling skills. Unskilled attempts at counselling can be harmful.

What is counselling?

Counselling aims to help people to achieve goals they have chosen. This is likely to involve developing a better understanding of themselves.

Counselling is often non-directive in the sense that it aims to support people in making decisions that take account of their particular circumstances and in setting goals that they can realistically achieve. For example, the aim of HIV-antibody pre-test counselling is not to advise patients on whether to take the test, but to help them understand the risk that has led them to consider testing, to clarify the consequences of being tested and to help them make a decision that they will feel content with.

Counselling may become directive when it is clear that a particular course of action is very likely to have negative implications. As well as clarifying the consequences of various options, the counsellor may wish to advise on one course of action rather than another. For example, directive counselling would be appropriate when supporting post-myocardial infarction patients in identifying life changes that could make a second heart attack less likely.

Whether directive or non-directive, counselling involves more than advising, information giving or teaching. It may also involve exploring: how a person can accept new information and relate it to their beliefs, hopes and desires, how they can develop plans based on this information, how they can gather the resources they need to translate those plans into action and how they can maintain new ways of behaving.

The counselling relationship

The counselling relationship is devoted to meeting the needs of the client. If a counselling relationship becomes distorted by the counsellor's needs it may become unhelpful to the client, unprofessional or unethical.

Carl Rogers, an influential figure in the development of counselling practice, defined three essential characteristics of an effective counselling relationship i.e. empathy, genuineness and unconditional positive regard.

Empathy

This refers to the ability to understand clients' experiences and feelings in the same way as they do. It involves adopting the client's own meanings and values when considering his/her experiences and communicating this so that he or she knows the counsellor has an accurate understanding. An effective way of achieving this is to *reflect back* what the client has said, summarizing what you think they *feel* and what they have *experienced*. For example, 'you feel anxious because the biopsy results aren't in yet'.

Genuineness

It is important to be genuine because the client must be assured that the counsellor is honest in his/her concern. This involves abandoning professional roles that may protect the counsellor from becoming personally involved with the client's emotions. Sharing personal experience may help a client realize that their problem is not unique and that other people have managed to overcome similar difficulties. Counsellors must, however, be careful to share their experience in a helpful manner. Seeking sympathy or counselling from the client will disrupt the counsellor–client relationship. Counsellors should also be able to acknowledge client complaints and share their concern that counselling is not working where they continue to feel that they are not helping. This may initiate a new approach or lead to a more productive referral elsewhere.

Unconditional positive regard

This refers to an unselfish concern for the client that does not depend upon their behaving in a manner approved of by the counsellor. It involves avoiding pre-judgements that may follow from the counsellor's own stereotypes. Unconditional regard provides a non-threatening context in which the client can disclose things that the client believes are disapproved of by others. Positive regard for others is conveyed through *non-verbal communication* (see pp. 94–95), as well as what we say.

Client responsibility

Counsellors can help people clarify their options and support them in making decisions but they cannot take those decisions or act on clients' behalf. Counselling seeks to clarify

Table 1 **What could a counsellor offer a bereaved relative?**
■ enable the client to admit his/her loss
■ help him/her to express the range of feelings this gives rise to
■ encourage him/her to explore the prospect of life without the deceased
■ help him/her anticipate and understand his/her feelings over time
■ question destructive coping strategies (such as social withdrawal)
■ offer support while encouraging the establishment of alternative social supports.
(See Worden 1991 for details)

what clients want to do, what they are choosing to do and how they view the consequences. Counsellors may, therefore, explore (and sometimes question) what is involved when clients say they want to do something for themselves but *cannot*, or when they say they *have* to fulfil social obligations that they view as destructive. In some cases such perceived barriers may conceal a fear of change.

What the client achieves

Drawing upon Egan's (1990) model of helping, we can identify five tasks which may be accomplished within a counselling relationship. These are described in terms of what clients achieve through the counsellor's help:

1. communicating a clear picture of their situation and feelings
2. constructing new ways of looking at their situation
3. defining goals and planning actions that could improve this situation
4. developing the motivation and abilities needed to implement change
5. becoming independent of the counselling relationship.

Not all of these tasks will be achieved (or given equal time) in any particular counselling relationship and a single counselling session may focus on one or all of these tasks. Table 1 shows how these can be translated into specific gains in the case of bereavement counselling.

The counsellor's task

By attending closely to the client's verbal and non-verbal communication, asking open questions, guiding the client towards clarification of their concerns, and reflecting what is being said, the counsellor can assure the client that he or she is understood. This may be a considerable comfort even in itself. It also deepens trust and encourages self-disclosure.

The counsellor may identify ways in which the client's understanding of his/her world creates barriers to problem solving and may question these understandings and explore new approaches or plans. Such intervention must be based on a trusting relationship and should be aimed initially at the problems causing the client most distress. Helping clients identify their needs and priorities is a key part of facilitating change and development. Counsellors may practise role-play interaction-sequences, which will help the client overcome social barriers or consider the use of rewards for different degrees of success.

Is counselling effective?

Counselling is not effective for all problems and one of the counsellor's skills is to know when a client should be referred for further psychological or psychiatric assessment. However, counselling has been shown to be effective with many patient groups. There have been many quantitative assessments of the impact of counselling and psychotherapy (e.g. Shapiro and Shapiro 1983). Effectiveness has been measured in terms of reduced psychological distress, fewer symptoms or behaviour change.

There is convincing evidence that counselling can be of benefit to smokers who want to give up, post-myocardial infarction patients and those who have recently suffered a bereavement. Parkes (1980), for example, reviewed evidence on bereavement counselling and concluded that it could

reduce the risks of psychiatric and psychosomatic disorders. Bereavement counselling has been evaluated by comparing those who have received counselling with matched controls who have received no counselling. Counselled groups have been shown to report fewer symptoms, have fewer consultations with doctors and receive fewer drug prescriptions.

- Read the statement below and summarize what the person has said using different words and showing that you fully understand their feelings, the options they are considering and what they are asking you.

I love my mother but she drives me mad. I don't know if she can go on alone. There's no one else to look after her. I don't know if I could stand having her live with me. I know I should look after her. Do you think she'll be all right on her own?

Case study

Counselling in terminal care

John had been told he had terminal cancer. He reacted by becoming perpetually cheerful and denying that he needed any help. This protected him from talking about his illness but also prevented anyone from offering him help or making plans about his care. His consultant persuaded him to talk to a psychiatric nurse who was a trained counsellor. By gently talking to him about his feelings about death the counsellor gradually allowed him to express more negative emotions. Over a series of sessions John began to express fear, self-pity, anger and sadness over his loss. During these sessions he recognized his feelings and accepted them as appropriate. He also began to talk about what was important to him now and clarified that relationships with his family were vital to his quality of life. This motivated him to talk openly to his wife and adult children about his cancer. He was also able to identify a number of decisions that he needed to make. He discussed treatment options and decided to limit radiation therapy and chemotherapy even though they might prolong his life. The quality of the time he had left became more important to him than its length. He also decided to spend a week visiting his brother and his family. The counsellor discussed his care preferences in the later stages of his illness and he identified a strong preference to die at home. Towards the end of his life John experienced periods of fulfilment and maintained that his nurse counsellor had 'opened his eyes to what really mattered'.

Counselling

- Requires skills developed through training and practice.
- Can be directive or non-directive.
- Aims to empower people to achieve their goals.
- Can help people adjust to a new situation or change behaviour.
- Involves communicating clearly about feelings and experiences.
- Depends upon being able to communicate genuinely and empathically.
- Helps people identify options and develop plans.
- Has been shown to be effective.

Adaptation, coping and control

It has frequently been suggested that there is a link between the manner of adaptation to, and coping with, the external environment and physical and mental health. It is, therefore, of considerable importance that we understand the way in which humans respond to external and internal stimuli.

Coping can mean any general adaptive process. It can also mean the mastery or control of major events. The behavioural sciences have developed two complementary ways of describing coping and adaptation – the first concerned with how people manage ordinary everyday things, the second with the way they deal with major life events. These two approaches have been brought together in what has been called the stress–coping paradigm.

The stress–coping paradigm

The stress–coping paradigm was originally developed by Lazarus (1980). Lazarus starts from the position that the social (and biological) worlds are ubiquitously stressful. People have to cope with and adapt to different things, large and small, all the time. The degree to which this produces stress is determined by the extent to which these external stimuli are perceived to exceed the ability of the person to deal with them and, therefore, to endanger well-being. People have to appraise the extent to which the stimuli do this. They then will act or react accordingly.

According to Lazarus, when confronted by a stimulus that is potentially stressful, an individual engages in two processes of appraisal. These are called primary and secondary appraisal. Primary appraisal is the means whereby the person determines whether a stimulus is dangerous or not. If that person decides it is not dangerous, they may conclude that it is irrelevant to them. Alternatively, they may view it as benign or positive. If the stimulus is appraised as irrelevant, or benign or positive, it is not regarded as a stressor (Fig. 1).

If a stimulus is regarded as stressful, this is because it is perceived to represent harm, or loss or threat (anticipated harm or loss). The secondary appraisal process is about mastering the conditions of harm or threat. This can take several forms: seeking out information; taking direct action to confront the stressor; doing nothing and attempting to ignore it; or worrying about it (see Fig. 1).

The importance of this model is that it recognizes that stimuli are not in themselves stressful. Stress arises as a consequence of the cognitive or thinking process which people bring to bear on particular stimuli (the appraisal processes) and on the extent to which they can control these stimuli by doing various things. It is when they are not able to control things, because they do not have the resources to do so, that stress arises. This approach emphasizes, therefore, the social context within which coping takes place.

Coping and illness

It has been argued that stress, and, by implication, the failure to cope or adapt, is responsible for the development of particular types of illness because certain biological responses in the individual lead to tissue damage (Seyle 1956). There is a good deal of research that focuses on

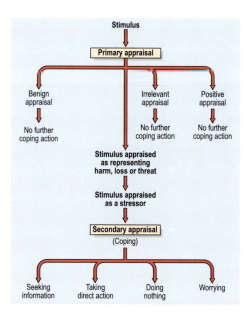

Fig. 1 **The stress–coping paradigm.** (Source: Kelly & Sullivan 1992)

specific illnesses that seem to follow stressful life events (Holmes and Rahe 1967, Fisher 1986, Hemingway and Marmot 1999).

While it is undoubtedly the case that exposure to external stimuli that are frightening and threatening may cause physiological changes in the human body, the question of the social environment in which this occurs is important. This is because coping is also related to the resources that people can bring to bear when they have difficult situations to deal with. Support of family and friends (a social network), and financial resources come into this category. These resources can and do have an important mediating effect on difficulties but cannot themselves prevent them. In the absence of social support, other life difficulties can be particularly damaging. A good deal of psychological morbidity can be accounted for in terms of combinations of low self-esteem, lack of financial resources and absence of social support (Brown et al 1975) (see pp 112–113).

Strategies of adapting to chronic illness

A number of typical strategies have been observed in the way people cope with, adapt to and try to gain some control over chronic illness. The responses are linked to the amount of threat their illness presents to them, and what they are able to do about the threat.

Normalizing

Here the patient acknowledges the symptoms, for example, of asthma, but redefines them as part of normal experience and hence as nothing to worry about. By defining something abnormal as normal, the patient is neutralizing the threat. This can present particularly difficult clinical management problems, because the more successful the patient is in neutralizing the symptoms, the more likely they may be not to comply with treatment (see pp. 92–93).

Denial

Here the patient denies the existence of the illness altogether. This may have profoundly beneficial effects, especially in the early stages of a very worrying or threatening diagnosis.

Case study

Childhood diabetes

It is important to avoid defining coping as either good or bad. The manner of people's response to stimuli will vary and in some cases people may draw certain psychological or social rewards from the way they cope, even though others may regard their manner of coping as dangerous or self-destructive. This is sometimes observed in long-term chronic illness.

In childhood-onset diabetes, for example, the family has to cope with illness and the difficulties presented by the symptoms and managing the self-medication and diet. However, it is perfectly possible for the young child to come to enjoy some of the benefits of being a sick person in the family: being spoiled and receiving special privileges in the family, for example. Also the family may come to adapt to the illness in ways that they too find rewarding. Parents may receive psychological rewards from taking on the role of carer. This may work quite well while the child is young, but as the child grows up and tries to free him/herself from the control of the parents, successful earlier coping may become highly maladaptive. The child's attempt to grow and be independent may be seen as a threat by the parents, who may insist on the adolescent remaining in the sick role. The diabetic may respond by taking dietary risks in an effort to cope with parental control. Particular dynamics become established within the family, and these in turn may produce other things with which the family has to cope.

 STOP THINK

■ While many disorders have been linked directly or indirectly to coping, the precise mechanisms whereby human behaviour in the face of stress produces psychological and biological consequences are very complex, and compared to many branches of medicine understanding of these mechanisms is limited. To what extent are coping and adaptation linked to psychological traits and psychosexual development on the one hand or to social factors, particularly availability of resources, on the other? Is it always going to be the case that what might be seen as maladaptive from a medical point of view would be bad for the patient?

about their life is their illness. Their whole being is consumed by their disease. They resign themselves to their fate. The illness is defined in such a way that instead of being something threatening, it grants certain psychological rewards. At certain times in a serious and grave illness, resignation may be an entirely appropriate way to respond. However, in many less serious conditions, total resignation leads to invalidism. The problem that this type of behaviour presents for the physician is that their best efforts to get the patient to attempt to take some control over their own life is resisted as the patient works hard to maintain their dependency on others.

Accommodation

Here the patient acknowledges and deals with the problems their illness produces – whether this is managing their symptom manifestations like pain, or managing a self-administered drug regime. The everyday work of handling the disease is seen as part of normal living. No attempt is made to build a special status out of the illness. Instead the person tries to deal with other people on the basis of his/her other characteristics, such as being a keen gardener, a football fan, a member of the church, and so on. They do not make their illness central to their life.

Denial may help the patient draw back, take stock and marshall help. In the longer run, however, denial prevents the patient from confronting the illness, will present particular difficulties for the treating doctor and may have considerable effects on the family or partner of the sufferer.

Avoidance

Patients who practise avoidance do not deny their problem. They set out to avoid those situations that might exacerbate their symptoms or lead to other problems. In this group of behaviours we find the person who suffers from claustrophobia and who therefore never lives or works anywhere where they may have to use a lift or get in an aeroplane. We find the reformed alcoholic who never goes to parties or social gatherings for fear that they might be tempted by the drink. We find the person with epilepsy who never applies for a job where they might have to reveal the fact of their illness. While individually each of these strategies is highly adaptive, they also contain within them certain maladaptive or potentially self-destructive elements. The person with claustrophobia or epilepsy may miss out on all sorts of opportunities, while the reformed alcoholic may be cut off from a great deal of social intercourse.

Resignation

In resignation we find the person who has totally embraced their illness and for whom the most important thing

Adaptation, coping and control

■ Adaptation and coping refer to behaviours that involve dealing with everyday problems as well as major life events.
■ It is the person who deals with these problems who defines them as everyday or major.
■ Coping and adaptation are linked to a range of psychological variables and social resources.
■ Stress results when the ability to deal with events is not equal to the events or stimuli.
■ Failure to cope and adapt may have serious health consequences at both a physical and a psychological level.
■ Some strategies of coping seem to be inherently unstable or potentially self-destructive.

Cognitive-behaviour therapy

Cognitive-behaviour therapy uses systematic techniques to enable people to think and act in a different way. It educates them to view themselves or their circumstances in a more adaptive way (see White 2001 for detailed guide to assessment and treatment).

Thoughts, mood and behaviour

The theory behind the approach is that patterns of thinking influence both mood and behaviour. A habit of thinking negatively may arise from attitudes and assumptions which developed in childhood, or from a major experience in adulthood. Many negative thoughts may arise from one basic assumption which colours all interpretation, e.g. 'I'm never any good at anything'. For some people, negative thoughts hinder healthy behaviour or prevent them from leading a full life (Fig. 1).

Applied to health problems, if people can change the way they think about themselves, they may change the way they behave: for example, cut down on drinking, alter eating habits, cope with pain, develop a social life or increase exercise.

What is the rationale behind cognitive-behaviour therapy?

Cognitive-behaviour therapy arose out of behaviour therapy, which had been shown to be effective in helping people change by means of classical and operant conditioning (see pp. 20–21). For example, people who are agoraphobic may be helped by building in rewards ('reinforcements') for venturing out a little farther each day. This would be an example of operant conditioning.

In medicine, an example would be a patient in hospital who will not take part in physiotherapy following a hip replacement, because it is painful and difficult. A similar system of self-reinforcement could be used for each small step towards recovery: she might plan to buy new clothes as soon as she could stand unassisted for 30 seconds; or go home for a weekend as soon as she could take three steps; or to go out for a meal when she could walk 10 metres with the aid of a walking stick. The use of goals and rewards helps us all to achieve difficult tasks.

The addition of cognitive elements to behaviour therapy came about because it was realized that sometimes people hold such strong negative beliefs that these beliefs prevent them from behaving in a way which would help their condition. In the above example, the patient may not even attempt to stand up because she thinks, 'I'm so weak, I'll never be able to stand'.

Date	Mood 0–10	Dysfunctional thought	Behaviour	Alternative thought	Mood 0–10
Tues. a.m.	2	I'll never be able to do the things I enjoyed – hillwalking, gardening, swimming. It's hopeless	Asked Mary how long it took her sister to recover who said it was about 2 months	I can't do a lot now, but I might be able to garden in 3 months' time	5

Fig. 2 **Thought diary showing the link between thought, mood and behaviour.**

The technique of cognitive-behaviour therapy

The answer is not to say to the sufferer 'Don't be silly, of course you'll be able to stand if you try,' as this may only antagonize. Instead, the aim is to lead the person to that conclusion by 'guided discovery'.

'You may be right, you may not be able to stand at the moment. Have you seen anyone else with a similar injury to yours? Have they made any progress? Is there any possibility that you might have the strength to do it? How can we test this out?'

The approach is collaborative: the patient is encouraged to gather evidence for and against particular beliefs and then to act on their conclusions in an experimental way. In this example data-gathering might include:

- attempting to stand for one second
- asking other patients with hip replacements how they felt at first and whether they made progress
- rating the probability in percentage terms of being able to walk again.

On the basis of results, she will revise her beliefs and will be asked to reflect on how she feels about the achievement. She learns actively about the role of negative thoughts in influencing both mood and behaviour.

Over time she will practise monitoring thoughts, challenging them, setting behavioural experiments and reviewing how these affect mood. Figure 2 shows a monitoring record. Work is carried out as 'homework' as well as within sessions. Having learned these skills, the patient is then in a position to be wary of negative thinking, to challenge it and to view circumstances and herself in a more objective way. Any basic assumptions which underlie negative thinking will also be elucidated and can themselves be challenged.

Cognitive-behaviour therapy and emotional disorders

Cognitive-behaviour therapy has been widely applied within the field of psychiatry, where it has been shown in clinical trials to be effective with many disorders.

Dysfunctional thoughts tend to lead to emotional difficulties and problems in behaviour: when depressed, someone may feel tired and lethargic and have difficulty concentrating. They may think that they are lazy, incompetent and not likeable. This leads to a worsening of low mood and inactivity. This in turn makes the person more likely to think negatively about themselves and the depression is maintained in a vicious circle (see Fig. 3) (see pp. 112–113).

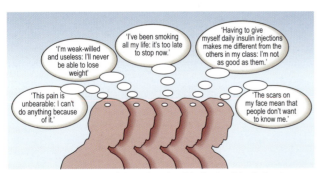

Fig. 1 **Some examples of thoughts that hinder healthy behaviour.**

'I'm weak-willed and useless: I'll never be able to lose weight'

'I've been smoking all my life: it's too late to stop now.'

'Having to give myself daily insulin injections makes me different from the others in my class: I'm not as good as them.'

'This pain is unbearable: I can't do anything because of it.'

'The scars on my face mean that people don't want to know me.'

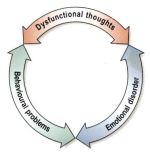

Fig. 3 **The link between dysfunctional thoughts, emotional disorder and behavioural problems.**

Cognitive-behaviour therapy and health problems

Cognitive-behaviour therapy has been used increasingly in all fields of medicine, where the same principles apply: the link between thought, mood and behaviour must be examined and any unhelpful aspects discussed critically. It has been shown to be effective in cardiac rehabilitation, the management of diabetes, asthma, chronic pain, epilepsy, irritable bowel syndrome and others. Pearce and Wardle (1989) outline a variety of applications.

Advantages and disadvantages

There are advantages in using cognitive-behaviour therapy rather than medication: it avoids problems of adverse reactions, side-effects and dependency. The effects of the treatment are long-lasting. The patient has learned how to tackle problems as they arise. The main disadvantage is the time taken by a member of staff to carry out the therapy, as this is comparatively expensive when compared with pills. In many cases this will be outweighed by the long-term benefits since the patient is less likely to come back for further treatment.

In clinical practice, although cognitive-behaviour therapy looks like common sense, and appears easy to apply, it takes much skill and there are pitfalls: one is 'Socratic questioning', i.e. the use of questions to lead someone to a different conclusion about themselves. This can easily turn into a seemingly aggressive cross-examination if the therapist is too persistent, or hasty, or selects inappropriate questions, or an inappropriate belief on which to target. Many people are trained in cognitive-behavioural techniques, including doctors, nurses, clinical psychologists and social workers, and it is likely that a patient with serious difficulties would be referred to one of these agencies for specialist help.

STOP THINK
- If you were working in your first week as a junior doctor and were very anxious, were not sure how to put up an intravenous drip properly, had made two mistakes writing up histories, had been humiliated by your consultant and doubted whether you were bright enough or competent enough ever to make it as a doctor, how might you apply cognitive-behaviour therapy to yourself?

How could you gather evidence for and against your suitability to be a doctor?

Case study

A 47-year-old van driver suffered a heart attack 5 months ago while driving home from work. He had stopped the car, and flagged down a passing motorist, who took him to hospital. On the day of his heart attack, he had felt unwell and had suffered chest pains when climbing stairs to make deliveries.

He made a full physical recovery and is not thought to be at great risk of another attack, but is now depressed, will not walk uphill or take much exercise at all, and thinks it unlikely that he will be able to return to work.

Figure 4 gives examples of the likely elements in the cognitive-behavioural cycle.

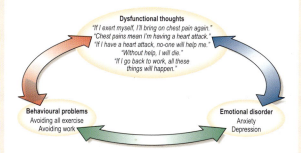

Fig. 4 **Dysfunctional thoughts: the vicious circle.**

How would you begin to tackle this man's difficulties? What questions would you ask to enable him to examine his dysfunctional thoughts? Suppose that he agreed to try some gentle exercise, and he did experience chest pain. Are there any possible psychological causes? (See pp. 144–145.)

Cognitive-behaviour therapy

- Cognitive-behaviour therapy proposes that dysfunctional thoughts influence both mood and behaviour.
- The predisposition to have such thoughts may be laid down in experience from early childhood where particular attitudes were learned, but they may also result from experience in later life.
- Congnitive-behaviour therapy aims to help a person to change dysfunctional beliefs so that they view circumstances more objectively, and as a consequence feel and behave differently.
- The methods of cognitive-behavioural therapy include education, collaboration, agreed goals, homework, and monitoring and evaluation of progress.

The role of carers

Doctors need to be aware of informal carers for two reasons: firstly, because caring for an elderly, chronically sick or disabled relative may affect the health of the carer and, secondly, because community care (see pp. 154–155) relies on families to take on the role of carer.

Caring has been divided into responsibility for the person (as may be the case, for example, when caring for an adult with schizophrenia) or carrying out of direct care tasks (as when caring for an elderly parent no longer able to care for him- or herself).

Role of carers

Different models of care give carers different roles. Twigg and Atkin (1991) have suggested four models: carers as a resource, as co-workers, as co-clients, and when superseded.

Carers as a resource

This is probably the most common view: that it is the natural order of things for a family to be responsible for the care of its members. This is the background against which current British community care policies are set. The focus of services is on the dependent person and the aim is to maximize the level of informal care. There is little concern for the well-being of carers, who are only doing their duty. The White Paper 'Caring for people – community care in the next decade and beyond' (1989) clearly states this policy:

> The government acknowledges that the great bulk of community care is provided by friends, family and neighbours. The decision to take on a caring role is never an easy one . . . However, many people make that choice and it is right that they should be able to play their part in looking after those close to them . . .
>
> (Paragraph 1.9)

Carers as co-workers

This model also aims to maintain and increase informal care, but acknowledges that to do so the needs of carers must be recognized – both psychological and physical needs such as domestic help, aids and time away, including holidays. Support for relatives may be provided along with education and advice, the latter aimed at making 'caring' more appropriate. This raises questions of how far relatives are being turned into quasi-professionals, and the appropriateness of this. In the mental-health field psycho-education groups for relatives of people with schizophrenia are popular. These give information, offer advice about coping and problem solving, and often aim to alter the emotional atmosphere of the family and thus reduce relapse (Lam 1991).

Carers as co-clients

Here the carer becomes an indirect client and is thus a legitimate focus for support and services. This may cause confusion in the health service, where the formal status of 'patient' is clear, but may prove less of a problem for social work, where the definition of 'client' is more accommodating. Thus carers may find it easier to get help and support in the social services than through the NHS unless such services can be seen to have a direct clinical outcome. Family therapy treats all members as 'patients' or 'clients'.

Superseded carers

The last model looks to the future of the dependent person, aiming to make him or her independent and thus not (or less) reliant on the support of the carer. This model may be most appropriate for those dependent on parents. Not only is it better for disabled persons to have greater independence for themselves, but it helps answer the question of who will look after them when their parents are themselves unable to cope.

Impact of caring on the family

The impact on the family is usually referred to as 'burden', being either objective (that which can be objectively measured and externally validated) or subjective (that which is perceived by the carer). It should be noted that objective burden and subjective burden are not necessarily correlated (Platt 1985).

Objective burden

Objective burden comprises the things that are externally observable and objectively quantifiable.

Financial problems include loss of earnings if the carer has to give up his or her job, as well as additional costs ranging from extra laundry or heating, to special aids and trips to hospital. The loss of employment not only affects finances, but also deprives the carer of outside contact and a role other than that of carer.

The disruption of household can be severe, particularly in terms of loss of freedom and privacy, which includes the difficulty couples may have in spending time alone together. Children may be affected through restrictions on their lives, particularly if they become carers for parents.

The tasks vary, depending on the needs of the person being cared for. For elderly dependants care may focus on physical tasks, and the drudgery of the unremitting tasks involved in caring for someone who can do little for him- or herself should not be underestimated. Where the dependent person has a mental illness, care may focus more on supervision and taking responsibility, perhaps for finances or medication. Behaviour that causes most concern to families is usually that which is socially disturbing or embarrassing, or which puts the person at risk.

The effect on the carer's health, both physical and mental, is both an objective burden and the consequence of objective and subjective burdens. Green (1988) reports that approximately two-thirds of carers are themselves in poor health, with about half at risk of a psychiatric illness (depression, anxiety). Many suffer physical injury, predominantly to their backs, from lifting. Social isolation is a problem both in terms of its own impact on the life of carers and because it contributes to other problems. The majority of carers receive no help from outside sources, and the amount of time spent caring can severely restrict the carers' involvement with the world outside the family.

Subjective burden

Subjective burden is difficult to measure objectively and is, to some extent, how the carer feels about caring. Thus social isolation is not just the absence of outside contacts, but the extent to which the carer feels isolated and withdrawn. Carers may feel their independence is eroded, together with their freedom and their sense of identity.

Case study

Mrs McLeod (65) lives alone with her son Alex (34), who has had schizophrenia since he was 19. He has always lived with his parents apart from a few short stays in hospital. Mr McLeod died 8 years ago. They are visited occasionally by Alex's sister, but an older brother has moved away and doesn't want any contact.

Alex hears voices, spends most of the day in bed and is up at night wandering round the house, smoking and playing music loudly. Mrs McLeod asks him to turn the sound down because of complaints from neighbours, but this leads to bitter arguments. At other times Alex gets very anxious and depressed and wakes his mother to talk to her. She gets very little sleep and is constantly tired. Although she had smoke alarms fitted Mrs McLeod still worries about the risk of fire, as Alex often leaves cigarettes burning. All the furniture has burn marks.

His only trips out of the house are to the clinic for medication and to buy cigarettes. He refuses to attend a day centre.

Mrs McLeod also rarely goes out as she does not like leaving Alex alone, both because she fears what might happen and because she feels guilty when he is alone. Because Alex doesn't like anyone coming into the house and because of his sometimes bizarre behaviour she has stopped inviting anyone. Her two great worries are whether she did anything that might have made Alex schizophrenic and what is going to happen when she dies.

- As a general practitioner, how does your responsibility to the ill or disabled person (the dependant) conflict with your responsibility to the carer (who may also be your patient)?
- Should relatives have the right to choose whether they care, or to what extent, for a dependent relative? What happens (and who pays) if they choose not to?

Stigma is experienced both by people with particular conditions (see pp 160–161) and by their carers, and reflects society's negative view. It may be a feature of being made to feel that they have contributed to the problem (e.g. a child's mental illness) or it otherwise reflects on them, as the following quotes suggest:

How can I tell anyone my husband's schizophrenic? They'll think there must be something wrong with me to have married him in the first place.

(Wife)

Sometimes I just want to kill us both. I'm getting on . . . can't go on like this much longer . . . what's to become of him? If I did it . . . we'd both be at peace.

(Mother)

The emotional impact includes everything from anxiety, depression, despair, hopelessness and helplessness, to resentment, frustration and anger. Stress results when the carer is unable to continue coping with the demands being made. This may be exacerbated by guilt and worry that they aren't doing enough or that they have somehow contributed to the problem. Concern about the future is

especially important for elderly carers, who worry about what will happen when they die.

Lastly, the role of carer has an impact as it changes the relationship between two people. For a woman, it is often expected and becomes an extension of the role she had been performing all her life, especially if caring for a child who has now grown into an adult. Roles are reversed when caring for parents, and when caring for a spouse the mutual support in the relationship may be lost. The role of carer usually falls on one person in a family, most commonly a woman.

Research has tended to concentrate on the negative aspects of caring and it is easy to ignore that caring for a loved one can bring rewards and pleasure as well as burdens and sorrow (Grant and Nolan 1993).

Carers' complaints

Not being recognized as providers of care is central to other problems such as lack of adequate services, support, and lack of information and advice. This may be particularly strong where people feel they had no choice in taking on the caring role.

Current position

Both social work and the health service now have to take account of carers' views when planning services. The Carers (Recognition and Services) Act 1995 gives carers their place in the provision of care. No new resources, however, have been forthcoming to implement the Act. The National Service Frameworks in both England and Wales, and Scotland set out standards for carers. The Clinical Standards Board for Scotland (2001) lays down seven essential criteria for judging services giving information and support to carers of people with schizophrenia (standard 7) (Table 1).

Table 1 **Information and standards for carers**
7.1 Carers are given information about schizophrenia and the services available both locally and nationally to support them and the person for whom they are caring.
7.2 Carers are offered the opportunity to meet with the staff supporting the person for whom they are caring, and are actively involved in the discussions about, and planning of, that person's care.
7.3 If a person who has a diagnosis of schizophrenia refuses to give consent for their carer to be given information and to be actively involved in discussions about their care, then this decision is discussed with the person and with their carer, and is recorded in the casenotes. A person's decision to either give or refuse consent is reviewed with them and with their carer on an ongoing basis.
7.4 Carers have access to an independent advocacy service.
7.5 When respite is required, the local social work services are advised of this need.
7.6 Carers have access to information and advice outwith normal working hours.
7.7 Carers are advised of their right to an independent assessment of their need by the local social work services.
Clinical Standards: Schizophrenia 2001. Clinical Standards Board for Scotland

The role of carers

- A relative is the first line of care for most people with chronic illness/disability.
- There are four models of care: carers as resources, co-workers, co-clients and superseded carers.
- Burden can be objective or subjective.
- Major problems are lack of recognition, lack of services and lack of information.

Self-help groups

No doctor or health professional can afford to ignore the rise of the self-help movement in the management of illness, disability and social problems. Self-help ranges from the large, national organizations, to small, unique, local groups. All have arisen from people wanting to take more control of their lives and responsibility for the management of their illness/disability. Probably the largest and most famous self-help organization is Alcoholics Anonymous (AA) (see pp. 78–79) with its 12-step programme (Table 1). This is a model followed by other organizations such as Gamblers Anonymous, Narcotics Anonymous and Overeaters Anonymous. The concepts behind the 12-step programme have been incorporated into some professionally run services.

Types of self-help groups

Self-help groups divide into two broad categories – those whose aim is to help members and those with a primarily campaigning role, aiming to change public attitudes and policy, although many include both aims.

In the health field, self-help groups exist for practically every condition whether defined as illness or some 'deviation from the norm'. There are groups for people with life-long conditions (e.g. Association of Cystic Fibrosis Adults), chronic medical conditions (e.g Ileostomy Association), mental-health problems (e.g. MIND), and people who define themselves as survivors – of the system (e.g. Survivors Speak Out) or of abuse (e.g. Incest Survivors Group). Groups exist for relatives (e.g. National Schizophrenia Fellowship, renamed 'Rethink' in July 2002). Other groups exist for those experiencing traumatic life events including bereavement (e.g. Compassionate Friends).

Functions of self-help groups

Support

The emotional support, acceptance and understanding that comes from others in a similar position cannot be overestimated and the importance of social support has been discussed elsewhere (pp. 124–125). For particularly stigmatized or disadvantaged groups their main source of social contact and friendship may come through such groups. Some people may feel more stigmatized by being expected to socialize with such people, or see it as a sign of weakness. Members of the British Council of Organizations of Disabled People (BCODP), who organize the 'Rights not Charity' demonstrations, are more likely to view themselves as political than those organizations who do not join.

Role models

Those who have overcome or learned to live with the problem provide a powerful model for others in the same position and can offer a hopeful and optimistic view of the future.

Information and advice about coping

Both patients and relatives complain of lack of information; this is collated and disseminated by self-help groups, and ranges from public lectures and specially written booklets (Fig. 1) to discussion groups. Information can shade into advice about coping, and even counselling. One study showed that as well as support, gaining information was the

Table 1 **Twelve steps of Alcoholics Anonymous**
1 – We admitted we were powerless over alcohol, that our lives had become unmanageable.
2 – Came to believe that a Power greater than ourselves could restore us to sanity.
3 – Made a decision to turn our will and our lives over to the care of God as we understood Him.
4 – Made a searching and fearless moral inventory of ourselves.
5 – Admitted to God, to ourselves and to another human being the exact nature of our wrongs.
6 – Were entirely ready to have God remove all these defects of character.
7 – Humbly asked Him to remove our shortcomings.
8 – Made a list of all persons we had harmed, and became willing to make amends to them all.
9 – Made direct amends to such people wherever possible, except when to do so would injure them or others.
10 – Continued to take personal inventory and when we were wrong promptly admitted it.
11 – Sought through prayer and meditation to improve our conscious contact with God as we understood Him, praying only for knowledge of His will for us and the power to carry that out.
12 – Having had a spiritual awakening as the result of these steps, we tried to carry this message to alcoholics and to practise these principles in all our affairs.

main reason women attended a Breast Cancer Support Group. They received information on specific and supplementary treatments, and general information on breast cancer (Stevenson and Coles 1993).

Coping strategies

Those with the problem usually have more to offer in the way of practical advice about day-to-day management of the disorder and general strategies for coping than do most professionals.

Ideology

Self-help groups have their own philosophies, with which members identify and which may or may not be in line with current professional thinking. When alternative views are put forward there is likely to be tension, if not hostility, between and within groups. People may seek out groups that support their position; thus it is suggested that carers' groups, such as

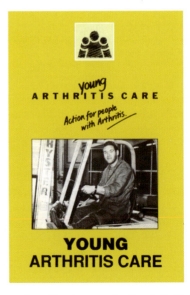

Fig. 1 **Booklet produced by the organization, Arthritis Care.**

the National Schizophrenia Fellowship (UK) and the National Alliance of the Mentally Ill (USA), focus on schizophrenia as a biological illness, whereas the users' organization MIND (UK) takes a more personal/social/political view of mental illness. The recognition of shared beliefs is an important part of support.

Mutual aid

In self-help groups, help is reciprocal and the giving as well as receiving of help is fundamental. Giving help has a range of benefits including: increased meaning and purpose to one's own life; increased feelings of self-worth and confidence; the positive reinforcement, both personal and social, that comes from helping; and even the rehearsal of coping strategies by advising others. AA is explicit about

■ The internet also offers an opportunity to promote non-standard approaches to conditions. There are websites that support anorexia nervosa as a lifestyle choice rather than an illness and offer advice on how to be anorexic. Concern over this has led some servers to deny access to such sites. What do you think about this? (pp. 82 83)

Case study

Rethink (formerly the National Schizophrenia Fellowship (NSF))

At its heart, the NSF is an organization that offers support to carers of people with schizophrenia, and 90% of its membership are carers. Local groups, usually run by a relative, meet regularly to share information, advice, problems, experiences and feelings, and to gain support, acceptance and help with coping. Professionals often give lectures and participate in discussion; although some groups have ongoing professional support to maintain them, the focus is on carer experience and control.

The organization has always had a campaigning role and, although not opposed to the closure of mental hospitals, it campaigns for this not to exceed the rate of replacement community services and also emphasizes the need for asylum. The NSF, both locally and nationally, responds to consultation documents and community care plans. It is frequently viewed as the voice of carers of the mentally ill, despite being predominantly white and middle class. It has always been active educationally, running local and national conferences for members and professionals, and in many areas carers speak to groups of nurses, social workers and doctors in training, giving their perspective on life with schizophrenia, the role of relatives as carers and their response to services.

Rethink is now firmly in the arena of service provision, running drop-in centres, employment projects, cafés, housing projects and respite care. The rapid expansion in service provision can be seen simply by looking at the accounts. In 1988–9 the turnover was £769,143, but by 1992–3 this had expanded by £6.1 million and incoming resources for 2000–2001 were £27,070,000.

The NSF has spawned similar organizations throughout the world, which meet together as the World Schizophrenia Fellowship. Founded in 1982, its membership includes Australia, Austria, Canada, Colombia, France, Germany, Great Britain, India, Indonesia, Ireland, Israel, Japan, Malaysia, Netherlands, New Zealand, South Africa, USA and Uruguay.

www.rethink.org

this reciprocal help, its twelfth step requiring members to take the message to other alcoholics (Table 1).

Most self-help groups engage in face-to-face contact, although the number of support groups springing up on the Internet suggests this is not always necessary (Klemm et al 1998). The Internet offers the opportunity for support outside one's immediate area, anonymity for those who feel stigmatized and important contact for those with mobility problems or in rural areas.

Empowerment

Patients frequently feel powerless in the face of both their illness and the medical profession. Self-help groups foster empowerment in two ways. One is through information, education and advice about the illness and coping, thus giving the individual some sense of mastery and control. Secondly, self-help groups may seek to influence service delivery and policy both nationally and locally, and educate the public with the aim of changing public attitudes. This can be seen as a more consumer-oriented approach to empowerment. Some groups specifically challenge the media portrayal of their disability. Disability rights groups, for example, picket the 'Children in Need' appeal to make people aware of their views and their objection to charity.

Self-help and service provision

Small, local self-help groups that aim to do nothing more than offer support and advice within the group will continue to flourish, although individual groups may wax and wane, dependent largely on the health of those who run them. In Britain as elsewhere, the development of community care (see pp 154–155) has pushed many self-help groups to become service providers. Groups have gained grants to provide services directly (to client groups rather than just members) and the distinction between self-help groups and voluntary organizations is sometimes not clear. In some areas, particularly mental health and physical disability, the user movement is strong and overlaps with self-help groups.

Although this has positive aspects, as services are more likely to be tailored to users' needs and those most involved have a say in the running of services, it can also have some less desirable consequences. Self-help projects usually suffer from insecure, short-term funding and can be used to plug gaps in services rather than adequately resourcing statutory agencies. Groups may lose their 'mutual aid' orientation, and the centrality of the user's experience may be diminished as staff are brought in to run the organization and its services. In the chase after money to fund services some of the campaigning and more 'political' aspects of the group may be lost in an attempt not to offend potential funders.

■ What can professionals gain from being involved with a self-help group?
■ Is there a danger that self-help could be seen as a 'cheap alternative' to other services?

Self-help groups
- Provide an alternative to the traditional approach.
- Value personal experience.
- Seek to empower members.
- Have roles as service providers and campaigners as well as offering support.

Palliative care

Development of palliative care

The main pioneer of the hospice (palliative care) movement in Britain was Dame Cicely Saunders, who worked as both a volunteer nurse and a social worker, and later as a doctor, at two of the first London Hospices, St Joseph's and St Luke's. This experience made her aware of the need for a place of care that would specialize in pain and symptom control in the terminal stages of disease, but that would also provide an environment that would allow people to adjust emotionally and spiritually to their approaching death (Saunders and Sykes 1993). Her subsequent foundation of St Christopher's Hospice in London as a centre of excellence in palliative care provided the cornerstone of the modern hospice movement in both Europe and America (Clark et al 2000). Its rapid expansion over the past three decades has been accompanied by the recognition of palliative medicine as a medical specialty.

Defining palliative care

In 1990 the World Health Organization defined palliative care as 'the active care of patients whose disease is not responsive to curative treatment'. It also developed guiding principles for practitioners (WHO 1990), which stated that palliative care:

- affirms life and regards dying as a normal process
- neither hastens nor postpones death
- provides relief from pain and other distressing symptoms
- integrates the psychological and spiritual aspects of patient care
- offers a support system to help patients live as actively as possible until death
- offers a support system to help the family cope during the patient's illness and their own bereavement.

Although the advent of hospice care has dramatically improved the care of terminally ill people, particularly in the area of pain and symptom control, evidence suggests that these goals are still not being met in every setting in which palliative care is provided. There is, therefore, an increasing drive to make hospice standards of care available for all dying patients and not an exception for a small minority. New definitions now distinguish different levels of palliative care according to the setting in which it is provided and the expertise of staff delivering the care. 'The Palliative Care Approach' aims to promote both physical and psychosocial well-being as an integral part of all clinical practice, whatever the illness or stage, through a knowledge and practice of palliative care principles (National Council for Hospice and Specialist Palliative Care Services 1997). At the other end of the spectrum, 'Specialist Palliative Care is the active total care of patients with progressive far-advanced disease and limited prognosis, and their families, by a multi-professional team who have undergone recognized specialist palliative care training' (National Council for Hospice and Specialist Palliative Care Services 2000). The words 'palliative' and 'terminal' care are often used interchangeably, but should be differentiated. 'Terminal care' refers to the management of patients during their last few days, weeks or even months of life from a point when it becomes clear that the patient is in a progressive state of decline (National Council for Hospice and Specialist Palliative Care Services 2000).

Beyond the hospice

In the past, hospice care has largely been confined to those patients who were dying from cancer, because most were funded by charitable contributions. An important consequence of the expansion of the hospice movement, however, has been the spread of its principles and goals to other places of care, and to patients with progressive non-malignant disease. Palliative care services now exist in a wide variety of forms ranging from autonomous in-patient units, day centres where patients can attend for medical or social care, to multi-disciplinary hospital support teams that provide specialist palliative care advice to patients in large acute hospitals (Hospice Information Directory 2002). In addition, specialist palliative home-care teams can assist general practitioners in caring for patients being cared for at home.

Total pain

The philosophy of the hospice movement is the alleviation of total pain and the affirmation of the quality of life remaining. This means tackling not only physical pain (pp 144–145), but also any emotional, psychological, social or spiritual problems the patient has that might contribute to the patient's total distress.

Figure 1 shows that the extent of a patient's pain may be affected by a whole range of physical, psychological, social and situational factors that may influence his/her ability to cope with it. Physical effects of the disease process and treatment, for example, radiotherapy or surgery, may therefore be exacerbated or precipitated by other complications of the illness. These may include anger at medical staff over unnecessary delays in diagnosis, lack of communication from them or failure to provide a cure, anxiety about other family members, finances or prognosis, or depression or loss of hope resulting from the loss of job, role, or function, due to illness.

The degree to which individuals are free from total pain will therefore depend on the ability of their professional carers to understand and solve its many causes.

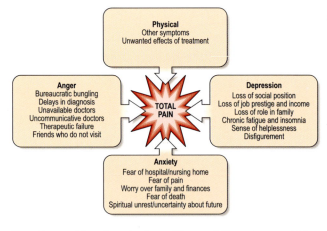

Fig. 1 **Composition of total pain, and factors influencing sensitivity.** (Source: Twycross 1994)

The multidisciplinary team

The need for multidisciplinary teams of health professionals who work together is essential to tackling total pain (Twycross 1999). Core members will include medical and nursing staff, social workers, chaplains, physiotherapists and occupational therapists. However, the individual needs of the patient and his/her family will dictate which member of the team plays a central role. For example, in the case of a patient with persistent nausea it may be the doctor who directs the patient's care. On the other hand, a patient who is facing severe financial difficulties due to loss of work as a result of the illness may need most help from the social worker. A patient who has difficulty in coping may benefit from consultations with a psychologist. The team should delegate tasks amongst its members to ensure that its resources are mobilized effectively and care prioritized in order to meet each individual's needs as efficiently as possible.

The effectiveness of the team will largely depend on good communication between its members, and between itself and other health professionals, as well as with patients and their families.

Measuring palliative care

As with every other medical specialty, practitioners of palliative care are increasingly having to be accountable for the care they provide. Standards and guidelines are now being developed to enable professionals to deliver and audit the process and outcome of the care they provide (National Council for Hospice and Specialist Palliative Care 1997, Higginson 1993). Quality of life (QoL) scales can be used to measure and monitor outcomes that go beyond the traditional end-points of tumour size, side effects of treatment, and survival (pp 38–39). QoL scales are multi-

- Consider the case study and write down how you think Jane's daughters felt when initially they were not told of the seriousness of her condition.
- Think of how you would go about breaking down the barriers to communication between the family. Imagine that you were the GP in this situation, and plan what you would say to Jane and Adam.
- Think how you might negotiate between them and Sara and Louise.

dimensional instruments that measure the physical, psychosocial and spiritual needs of patients. Such measures can enable doctors and researchers to evaluate the care patients receive more holistically and allow comparisons of care to be made across settings, between patients with different types of cancer, and between patients at different stages of the disease process.

Palliative care

- The provision of terminal care has been revolutionized by the modern hospice movement, particularly in the area of pain control.
- With the growth of the hospice movement has come the recognition of the care of the dying as a medical specialty known as palliative medicine.
- The philosophy of the hospice movement emphasizes the alleviation of total pain, and the patient and his/her carer as a unit of care.
- Palliative care is provided by a multidisciplinary team of health professionals including doctors and nurses, physiotherapists and occupational therapists, social workers, psychologists, pastoral staff and nurses specifically trained to be advisors in palliative care
- Quality-of-life measures are now being developed to enable doctors and researchers to measure and evaluate the physical and psychosocial well-being of patients. These conceptualize patients' needs in multi-dimensional instruments and provide outcomes of care that allow comparisons to be made across settings and between patients with different types of cancer and at different stages.

www.hospice-spc-council.org.uk; www.hospiceinformation.info.

Case study

Jane was a 49-year-old woman with cancer of the breast and bony metastasis. She was married to Adam, a lawyer, and had two teenage daughters, Sara and Louise. Her prognosis was poor and after receiving a course of palliative radiotherapy, she had come home to spend her remaining time with her family. Neither daughter knew how serious their mother's condition was, though both suspected that it was not good because of the number of health professionals constantly visiting the house. Both Jane and her husband thought that in protecting their daughters from the truth they were shielding them from unnecessary anxiety and grief. As a result, relationships in the family were strained and both girls were doing badly at school. Jane was experiencing uncontrolled pain and nausea, which prevented her from sleeping and eating properly. At this point the general practitioner, after consulting the district nurse, decided to refer Jane to a specialist nurse for advice on pain control and help with improving communications among the family. As her visits to the family progressed, Jane and Adam were encouraged to share their knowledge of Jane's prognosis with their daughters. Both learned that instead of protecting their daughters they were in fact alienating them, causing them to feel confused and isolated. Gradually, through open communication, Louise and Sara came to accept that their mother was dying, but that as a family they could still make the most of the time that was left. Jane was also given a different form of pain relief: a syringe driver which administered analgesia continuously while allowing her to remain as mobile and unrestricted as possible. In the end Jane died peacefully and comfortably at home surrounded by Adam and her daughters.

Complementary therapies

'Complementary therapies' is the term used to include complementary and alternative medicine (CAM). The Cochrane Collaboration defines CAM as 'a broad domain of healing resources that encompasses all health systems, modalities, and practices and their accompanying theories and beliefs, other than those intrinsic to the politically dominant health systems of a particular society or culture in a given historical period.' Complementary therapies are usually, if not invariably, complementary to conventional medical treatment and so the term alternative is less appropriate. They may be described as being in the folk sector of medicine (pp. 98–99)

The use of complementary therapies

The use of complementary therapies has become very popular in recent years. In a survey of over 1200 British adults, 20% had used CAM in the previous 12 months, of which 34% had used herbal medicine (Ernst and White 2000). Sales of CAM-related products in the UK are predicted to rise to over £125 m by 2002 (House of Lords 2000). A survey of first-year medical students found that 37% had had previous experience of CAM and, of those that used it, 82% said that they had found it helpful (Greenfield et al 2002).

Patients may ask doctors and other health professionals about the wisdom of trying complementary therapies or may conceal their interest because of a fear of disapproval. An open discussion of the costs and benefits is essential so that the practitioner is aware of other therapies that the patient may be having. Many have no adverse effect but some may interact with conventional therapy (see Case study). It is possible that the efficacy of some complementary therapies may occur because of the placebo effect (pp. 90–91).

The popularity of CAM is increasing across the Westernized world. Increased concern over ecological and environmental issues may have helped to fuel interest in 'natural' healing systems. Astin (1998) identifies key points in society that represent this shift towards alternative medicine,

which are linked to holistic beliefs in perceiving the body, mind and spirit in an integrative manner. This is totally different from conventional medicine, where disease is treated by looking specifically at organs or tissue of the body. Other identifiable reasons for this movement are related to patients' rights, a more active role in consumer health, self-care and fitness, and dissatisfaction with conventional medicine (Cassileth 1998). Many people seek complementary therapy because: they want to use all options in health care; they want a cure without side effects or pain; they are disappointed with the traditional orthodox consultation; they believe in holistic care; they perceive conventional medicine to be ineffective; or they may be concerned about the side effect of powerful drugs (Vincent and Furnham 1997).

Consultations are generally longer and concentrate on a person's overall well-being and own subjective experience. Complementary therapists undoubtedly have well-developed communication skills (see pp. 94–95). They are often active listeners and are perceived as being 'low tech' (Fig. 1). In Britain, more general practitioners are becoming trained in complementary therapies such as homeopathy and hypnotherapy.

Types of complementary therapies

The House of Lords Select Committee on Science and Technology (House of Lords 2000) published a report on CAM and grouped the different kinds of complementary therapy into three:

- Group 1 included the disciplines of osteopathy, chiropractic, acupuncture, herbal medicine and homeopathy. These are sometimes known as the big five, and Acts of parliament regulate osteopathy and chiropractic in their professional activity and education.
- Group 2 includes therapies used to complement conventional medicine and do not claim to diagnose. They include aromatherapy and reflexology.
- Group 3 includes therapies that claim to diagnose as well as treat and generally have a different paradigm of the causes of disease. It includes traditional

Chinese medicine, crystal therapy and iridology.

There are many others not mentioned here but conventional medical or health practitioners may encounter the following:

Group 1

■ *Acupuncture*
One of the oldest therapies, originating in China over 2000 years ago. Small needles are inserted into specific points in the body. It is assumed that vital energy 'qi' travels along meridians, and if yin and yang are unbalanced the energy becomes blocked

■ *Chiropractic*
This manipulates the joints and uses massage to treat musculo-skeletal complaints, particularly in the back. It assumes that nerves that control posture and movement become irritated, which leads to referred pain

■ *Herbal medicine or phytotherapy*
Remedies derived from plants and plant extracts are used to treat complaints. They are traditional pharmaceuticals, but consist of many chemical constituents and are usually unstandardized

■ *Homeopathy*
Homeopathy is a therapy that treats like with like. Patients are given a small dose of a substance that is thought to produce the same symptoms in a healthy person if given in a higher dose. The remedies are highly diluted so that not even a single molecule may be left in the solution. The patient's constitution is also assessed.

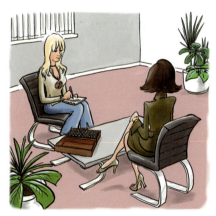

Fig. 1

■ *Osteopathy*
The therapy involves manipulation of the spine. It assumes that the blood supply is impaired. It may be used together with chiropractic.

Group 2

■ *Aromatherapy*
Essential oils extracted from aromatic plants and diluted in vegetable oils are applied to the skin. Small quantities are absorbed through the skin or by inhalation. Essential oils also have mood-altering effects via the limbic olfaction system.

■ *Reflexology*
This is massage of the foot, which assumes that there are zones in the body so that each organ has a corresponding location in the foot. It produces feelings of relaxation.

Group 3

■ *Traditional Chinese medicine*
If the two types of energy (or 'qi'), yin and yang, are in imbalance, disease may occur. Traditional Chinese medicine restores the balance and may use herbs, massage or acupuncture.

■ *Crystal therapy*
Crystals are placed in patterns around the body to adjust the energy field or person's 'aura'.

■ *Iridology*
The iris's pigmentation reflects the health status enabling diagnosis.

The effectiveness of therapies outside the current mainstream of medicine may occur through a variety of methods, which may include conventional biochemical routes, by the effect of the therapeutic interaction, or in ways as yet not understood. Research on the efficacy of these therapies has been difficult to carry out using conventional research designs but there is increasing pressure to evaluate complementary therapies and to provide an evidence base (Lewith et al 2002)

STOP THINK
■ Complementary therapies are often considered to be risk free.
■ Why might there be more risks or side effects with herbal medicine than homeopathy?
■ Balance the costs and benefits of consulting an osteopath to a patient with chronic low back pain.

Case study

St John's wort (Hypericum perforatum) (Fig. 2)

Extracts of this herb have long been used in folk medicine. In Germany it is licensed for use in anxiety, depression and sleep disorders. It has been shown to be an effective antidepressant for mild or moderate depression (Williams 2000, Woelk 2000). The extracts contain many different chemical classes, so the 'active agent' is a matter of uncertainty. It may be hypericin or hyperforin (Fig.3) (Kingston 2001). It may be preferred to conventional antidepressants because of their perceived side effects. However, there may be herb–drug interactions. St John's wort interacts with oral contraceptives and may lead to reduced blood levels with a risk of breakthrough bleeding and unplanned pregnancy.

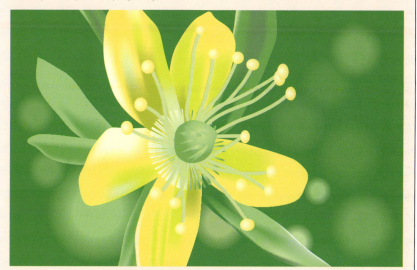

Fig. 2 **St John's wort flower.**

	R
Hypericin	H
Pseudohypericin	OH

Hyperforin

Fig. 3 **Diagram of molecules of hypericin and hyperforin.** (Source: adapted from Mills and Bone 2000)

Complementary therapies

■ Complementary therapies and alternative medicine are growing in popularity.
■ Therapies have been grouped on the basis of evidence and regulation.
■ The evidence for their efficacy is sparse, but there is a high level of patient satisfaction.

The management of pain

Pain is defined by the International Association for the Study of Pain as: 'An unpleasant sensory and emotional experience associated with actual or potential tissue damage, or described in terms of such damage'. It is important that we recognize that the experience of pain is subjective and dependent on past experiences of injury. Note that the definition includes the emotional experience, indicating that the pain perception is not just sensory. We often associate pain with an acute injury or event that is assumed to signal harm or damage. This may be an appropriate interpretation where pain has an obvious cause and is of recent onset. However, many people's experience of pain is a more chronic picture. Chronic pain may present in a variety of ways and is estimated to have a prevalence of 10% in the population. Chronic back pain is one of the commonest causes of sickness from work and contributes to escalating figures for disability benefits.

Neurophysiology of pain

Research on the neurophysiology of pain in recent years has provided some remarkable insights into pain mechanisms. We now know about the development of neural plasticity, where damaged pathways reconnect and pain signals are present outside an expected dermatomal distribution. Central sensitization can occur, which causes a 'wind-up' phenomenon of increased firing of nerve pathways. 'Pain memory' is a neural imprint of past pain experiences. These developments have built on the earlier concepts of a gate-control mechanism described by Melzack and Wall (1999). This model clarified that the experience of pain is also modulated by downward neural pathways, i.e. from the brain.

The way forward – a biopsychosocial approach

The developments in understanding pain mechanisms have allowed us much greater understanding of how to provide a multi-disciplinary approach to pain. It is no longer appropriate to dismiss pain as being 'all in the mind' if investigations show nothing to account for the cause of pain. The neurophysiology of pain now allows

much more complex understanding. However, management of pain is also complex. Psychological and social factors contribute significantly to the way in which pain is perceived and managed. It is very important that good practice in the management of pain begins early on and that consistent approaches are taken in both primary and secondary care.

Why psychosocial factors are important

Continuing pain can lead to many adverse psychological consequences. Significant losses may occur, such as an inability to work, medical retirement, financial restrictions, an inability to continue with normal activities; all of which may in turn lead to relationship difficulties and reduced quality of life. This may result in the development of depression, hopelessness and reduced sense of control. Constant pain may make it difficult to sleep, reduce ability to concentrate, and, subsequently, increase irritability and friction. Sexual activity may be reduced and thoughts of suicide are not uncommon.

Health beliefs and misconceptions

Health beliefs can powerfully influence an individual's response to their symptoms and expectations of treatment (pp. 146–147). If someone with chronic pain believes that their pain is a signal of harm and damage, then they are likely to avoid doing things that will bring on pain. This usually leads to a gradual reduction in physical mobility and can result in secondary problems, such as postural changes, stiffness in joints or the lack of use of an affected limb. Individuals may be fearful of exercise and less compliant with advice. This kind of health belief can lead to anxiety and significant unhelpful behavioural changes.

Cognitive-behavioural approaches to management of pain

There are three linked components to the management of pain: dealing with unhelpful patterns of thinking, which can then lead to changes in behaviour and subsequent improvement in mood (pp. 134–135). These psychological

principles can be applied by all clinicians who have contact with pain patients. A more integrated and intensive approach is commonly used in pain-management programmes.

Changes in cognitions

- Identify and help to reshape misconceptions about pain (Box 1). The basis of this is to ensure that the patient has a good understanding of the principles of pain mechanisms early on.
- People are often fearful of exercise and activity in case this flares up pain, which will then be attributed to having caused harm and damage. Fear-avoidance can lead to a decrease in mobility and to lower levels of fitness
- Help patients to recognize and reframe unhelpful patterns of negative thoughts, e.g. 'I used to be able to decorate my house in no time – now I'm useless – there's no point in trying.' . . . 'If I get some help with the heavy bits, I could do this decorating in chunks of half an hour. It may take me longer but it means I will have done it without having to rely on others'.

Changes in behaviour

Pain often leads to behaviour that is shaped by operant conditioning (pp. 20–21).

- 'Good days' often lead to doing too much and trying to catch up. This usually results in 'bad days', when little can be done while waiting for the pain to settle. Mood is then often low, and frustration and anxiety high.
- This cycle can be broken by setting behavioural goals where a level of activity is found that does not flare up pain. The level is then gradually increased, which reduces the 'wind-up' effect of pain and helps improve mood and confidence. This can apply to exercise as well as other activities such as housework, gardening, sports, concentration tasks, social activity and hobbies.
- Setting levels of activity as goals that are achieveable helps to increase the likelihood of positive results, which in turn helps to increase a sense of control and positive thinking.
- Learning relaxation techniques can greatly improve a sense of being in

Box 1 Common misconceptions about pain

- I've been told my X-rays show wear and tear. This must mean that my bones are wearing away. I had better not do too much in case I wear things away even further.
- If you have pain it means that you have damaged and harmed something. I had better not do anything that gives me pain in case I harm myself.
- The doctor said my bones are degenerating.
- It's best to avoid getting dependent on medication, so I'll go as long as possible without taking anything.

control of pain. With regular relaxation practice, it is possible to alter the vicious cycle where pain causes increasing frustration and irritability, raised adrenaline levels, increased spasm, all of which lead to changes in pain threshold. Relaxation skills can also help improve sleep.

Changes in mood and sense of control or self-efficacy

- As people accumulate skills and strategies to build up activity, this can help to provide evidence of ways of regaining some of what was felt to be lost, and so reduces frustration and improves mood.
- Correcting misconceptions and helping people to reframe negative patterns of thinking provides a basis for improvement in sense of control and mood.

What is the evidence?

Waddell (1998) has synthesized the evidence on treatment of back pain and concluded that most medical specialist services are inappropriate and may be harmful for patients with simple backache, who need a biopsychosocial approach to early mobilization and to address issues of misconceptions and psychological distress. A systematic review of pain treatments by McQuay et al (1997) found large and sustainable improvements in outcomes using a psychological approach. A meta-analysis and systematic review of randomized controlled trials for cognitive-behaviour therapy for chronic pain by Morley et al (1999) found cognitive-behavioural treatments associated with significant effects on pain experience, measures of coping, and behavioural expression of pain.

The New Zealand National Health Committee have described a 'yellow flags' approach to back pain, where psychosocial indicators predicted poor outcome in terms of increased pain, disability and work loss. A comprehensive account of an interdisciplinary approach to chronic pain is found in Main and Spanswick (2000).

STOP THINK

- Why is bed rest no longer recommended for people with back pain?

Case study

John is a 43-year-old ex-policeman who has had back and neck pain for the last 4 years. He had an RTA with minor whiplash 7 years ago. He has had intermittent time off work with pain that became progressively more troublesome and he was medically retired 1 year ago. He tried lighter duties, but sitting, driving and walking were all too difficult. MRI scan shows some degenerative changes, but no indications for surgery.

John now has disturbed sleep, poor concentration and increasing irritability with his wife and family. His wife works full time. He feels very guilty that he is not working or able to do much with his family. He tends to push himself as he thinks he shouldn't give in to pain, then has to recover for the rest of the week. He has given up golf, rarely sees friends, his sex life is non-existent, his mood is very low and he gets angry with himself and withdraws. His marriage is under strain. He is fearful of exercise in case he causes harm and this has led to weight gain.

He was assessed in a multi-disciplinary pain clinic and given explanations about chronic pain and its effect on physical and psychological state. His worries about pain leading to more degeneration were addressed so that he was clear that there was not ongoing damage from pain. He could readily identify with the overactivity/rest cycle described to him, and driven patterns of thoughts. He and his wife were helped to see that irritability and low mood were linked to these patterns and losses of role.

John began a pain-management programme and initially found it difficult to shift from his pattern of overactivity. However, with regular setting of activity and exercise goals he was able to gradually increase what he could do, and felt less anxious about harm, which lead to increasing confidence. He initially found relaxation difficult, but gradually built up skills, resulting in less irritability and he was more able to enjoy things with his family. He began some voluntary work and felt less guilty about not working, having had help to recognize negative patterns of thinking and their effect on mood. Six months later he still had the same degree of pain, but was feeling fitter, more confident about activity, was walking and swimming regularly, his mood and his sex life had improved, and he was more able to contribute to his family.

The management of pain

- Lack of findings on investigation doesn't mean pain is not genuine.
- The mind/body split (i.e. all physical or all psychological) is incorrect and (sorry!) not a helpful way to conceptualize pain.
- Injuries from accidents can lead to post-traumatic stress disorder or similar symptoms, which are frequently missed and contribute to the maintenance of pain and disability.
- There is good evidence that a cognitive-behavioural approach is effective in managing pain.
- Identify and correct patients' misconceptions.
- Help patients to reframe negative thinking.
- Help patients set achievable goals.
- Affirm patients' progress and improvements in their sense of control and self-efficacy of progress.

Health beliefs, motivation and behaviour

If we can identify 'cognitions' such as beliefs, attitudes and intentions that distinguish between people who do and do not undertake health-related actions then we may be able to change these cognitions and so promote health behaviours amongst the general population. Research in this area focuses on individual differences in what people think but these differences often reflect social, that is family and cultural, differences.

The health belief model

In the 1950s US public health researchers began to investigate which beliefs were associated with health behaviour. The resulting model focused on people's beliefs about the threat of ill health and the costs and benefits of health behaviour (see Fig. 1). Threat perception involved perceived susceptibility to illness or health breakdown (e.g., 'How likely am I to suffer from breathing difficulties or contract lung cancer if I smoke?') and the anticipated severity of the consequences of illness (e.g. 'How bad would it be if I suffered from breathing difficulties or contracted lung cancer?'). The model also included beliefs concerning the benefits or effectiveness of a recommended health behaviour (e.g. 'If I give up smoking what will I gain?') and the costs or barriers associated with the behaviour (e.g. 'How difficult will it be to give up smoking and what will I lose?'). Two other factors were included. Cues to action that trigger health behaviour when people are aware of a health threat and convinced of the effectiveness of action (e.g. advice from a doctor) and general health motivation (i.e. how highly a person values good health).

How useful is the health belief model?

Reviews of research into the health belief model (e.g. Janz and Becker 1984, Harrison et al 1992) confirm that measures of the beliefs highlighted by the model provide useful predictors of a range of preventive behaviours (e.g. breast self-examination) and sick-role behaviours (e.g. taking medication). However, these reviews also suggest that the beliefs included in the model are not strong predictors of future behaviour. This implies that other cognition differences may help distinguish between those who do and do not take health-related action.

Implications of the health belief model

Reviews have shown that perceived costs or barriers are especially important, suggesting that minimizing the degree to which health behaviours are thought to be painful, time consuming, expensive or embarrassing will help promote them. Perceived severity has been shown to be less important in relation to prevention than responses to symptoms or medical advice. Thus stressing susceptibility to future health problems is likely to be more effective in promoting preventive health behaviour than emphasizing severity (pp 92–93).

The theory of planned behaviour

King (1982) extended the health belief model in a study of hypertension screening. She designed a questionnaire that included measures of intentions. Her model correctly predicted whether people did or did not attend later screening in 82% of cases. Measures of intention were found to be the most powerful predictors of attendance. A number of cognitive models have proposed that intentions are important indicators of whether or not people will take action. The most popular of these models is the 'theory of planned behaviour' (Ajzen 1991, see Fig. 2). Ajzen (1991) notes that '. . . intentions are assumed to capture the motivational factors that influence a behavior; they are indications of how hard people are willing to try, of how much of an effort they are planning to exert, in order to perform a behavior' (p. 181).

The theory of planned behaviour has been shown to predict a range of behaviours (Ajzen 1991, Armitage and Conner 2001). It proposes that 'perceived control' is an important determinant of intention. Perceived control refers to the person's assessment of their ability to undertake an action or sequence of actions and includes awareness of barriers to performing actions. Perceived control affects our intentions because we do not usually intend to undertake the impossible. However, perceived control can also affect performance because those who believe in their ability are more persistent and devote more effort to trying to succeed (Bandura 1997).

The theory of planned behaviour proposes that intentions are also determined by our attitudes towards the action and by our subjective

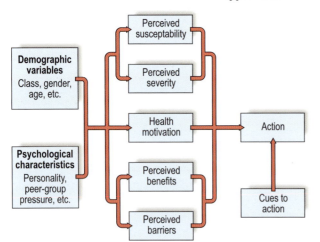

Fig. 1 **The health belief model.** (Based on Becker et al 1977)

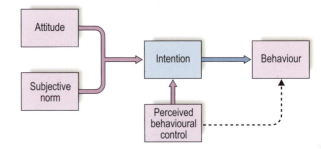

Fig. 2 **The theory of planned behaviour.** (Adapted from Ajzen 1991 *Organizational Behaviour and Human Decision Processes*)

norms. Attitudes refer to our overall evaluation of an action and encompass many of the health beliefs included in the health belief model. For example, if a smoker believes that giving up smoking will reduce her chances of contracting a serious illness then we will evaluate this action positively. However, if she also believes that she is more likely to feel more positive and relaxed when smoking and highly values such mood control, she may accept the increased chances of lung cancer, while acknowledging that this outcome would be disastrous. A person's subjective norm refers to his or her beliefs about others' approval of the action in question. When we value others' approval and know that they have strong views about what we do (e.g. 'Do my friends think I should not smoke?' or 'Does my partner think we should use a condom during intercourse?') this can have an important impact on our decisions.

The theory of planned behaviour has three advantages over the health belief model. First, the research-supported proposal that beliefs have their effects on behaviour through intentions provides an explanation of how many (frequently contradictory) beliefs culminate in a decision to act. Secondly, the focus on action-specific cognitive measures shifts attention away from general representations of illness to representations of particular actions and enhances behavioural prediction. Thirdly, the theory acknowledges the impact of social influence on individual behaviour.

Implications of cognitive models for health promotion

Davies (1968) found that 44% of patients who had not followed their doctor's advice had in fact not intended to do so and only 8% of those who had not intended to follow the advice actually did so. These findings strongly suggest that people's intentions provide an important indication of whether or not they will perform preventive and sick-role behaviours. Doctors might enhance the effectiveness of their advice by finding out what their patients' intentions are and promoting health-related intentions.

A person is more likely to intend to take action and actually act when when they believe:

1. their health is important
2. they are susceptible to a health threat which could have serious consequences
3. the proposed action will be effective and does not have too many costs
4. others who are important to the person approve of the action
5. they can successfully carry out the action.

Perceived control can be increased by: (1) teaching someone how to do something (e.g. explaining how to take the progestogen-only oral contraceptive so as to maximize its reliability), (2) encouraging someone to believe in their own abilities (e.g. by discussing how someone gave up cigarettes successfully in the past), (3) modelling a behaviour so that the person can watch a successful performance (e.g. seeing someone use an inhaler correctly on video), and (4) encouraging practice of preparatory behaviours (e.g. discussing condom use with sexual partners).

STOP THINK

- Mr Davidson is a 48-year-old lorry driver who has seen his GP about a series of illnesses over the past 6 months. He always complains of stress and overwork and his GP thinks he needs to take more rest and exercise, and reduce his working hours.
- List some helpful remarks that his GP could make to help Mr Davidson's view of his health.

Case study

Health beliefs and condom use

John and Mary are heterosexual teenagers. They are motivated to protect their health. They acknowledge the potential seriousness of sexually transmitted diseases and know that condoms offer good protection. However, John believes that only gay men and drug injectors are at any appreciable risk of HIV infection and that other sexually transmitted diseases are not very serious. He has never used a condom and believes that they may reduce intimacy and sensation during intercourse. Consequently, he does not buy or carry condoms.

Mary takes oral contraceptives. She is concerned about her susceptibility to HIV and chlamydia infection, and has consistently used condoms with her last two partners. She does not find them off-putting and thinks they provide good protection against infection. Mary no longer has a regular sexual partner and does not carry condoms because she is worried that if she is seen carrying them her girlfriends and boyfriends will think she is regularly seeking casual sex and question her morals.

John and Mary become attracted to each other in a club and go back to John's home because his parents are away. When Mary mentions condoms John rejects the implication that he is infected and declares that he 'never' uses condoms. In fact, he does not have any and is unsure about using them. Mary is very attracted to him and decides to take a risk rather than lose John's affection. The next day Mary has a hangover and is worried about the risk of infection. John also has a hangover but he is not worried and intends to go 'clubbing' again that night.

Health beliefs, motivation and behaviour

- By identifying beliefs associated with health-related behaviour and seeking to change those beliefs it is possible to promote health-related behaviour.
- The health belief model highlights the importance of perceived susceptibility and severity, perceived costs and benefits of health behaviours, general health motivation and cues to action.
- The theory of planned behaviour highlights the importance of intentions as predictors of future behaviour and also the impact that others' approval may have on intention formation.
- In addition to attitudes and subjective norms, high perceived control or self-efficacy promotes intention formation and makes successful performance more likely.
- Health beliefs can be targeted in individual consultations and mass-media campaigns to increase patient adherence.

Organizing and funding health care

The organization and funding of health care affects patients as well as health-care providers. Doctors, as health-care providers, might be restricted in their actions owing to the existing organization of health care, or they might feel that their patients' access to certain expensive tests or interventions is restricted.

- In what ways is government of your country involved in the provision of health care?

Health-care systems all over the world seem to be facing a funding crisis. The main issue is the allocation of scarce resources. This is not simply a question of money but also of political decision-making and priorities. In order to understand the current organization and funding of health care, we have to look at historical developments and the underlying political decision-making process.

We concentrate on three countries, the UK (with a predominantly state-run welfare system), the USA (with a predominantly free-market system), and Germany (with a mixed health economy), representing the major ways health care is organized and funded (see Case study 1). Total expenditure on health (including private and public health expenditure) in these three countries differs considerably, as does the proportion of the gross national product spent on health care.

United Kingdom

All citizens of the UK are included in the NHS. The NHS is a universal, tax-funded health-care system. Doctors, nurses and hospitals are paid by the state. The NHS requires some additional payments from patients, for example, for prescriptions and dental check-ups, but the overwhelming majority of care provision is free of charge. Treatment is decided on (mostly) by doctors. General practitioners are gate-keepers in this system, selecting patients and referring patients to the appropriate specialist. Medical care is available to all, and is therefore without stigma to the poor. However, there is a problem of waiting lists in certain areas (see pp 152–153). This has stimulated an increase in the small (14.6% in early 1996), but growing private health-care sector, which is often provided by the same doctors in the same hospitals as the standard NHS care.

USA

The system in the USA is predominantly commercial insurance-based (Navarro 1989). Most people take out their own private health insurance. These insurance companies reimburse doctors, hospitals, and others, for care provided. Most people have the freedom to go to the medical professional or hospital of their choice. A limited number of people are covered by state-organized schemes, such as Medicaid, which provides health care for the poor, but eligibility is incomplete and coverage usually excludes dental services and prescribed drugs, and Medicare, for all people over 65, which provides limited coverage. Over 40 million people are not insured or are seriously under-insured.

Germany

Of the German population, 88% are insured by one of nearly 500 sick funds, which are funded by income-related contributions and are self-governing and self-financing institutions. The average contribution rate is approximately 13.5% of an employee's gross income. Half of the contributions are paid by the employers and the other half by the employees. Self-employed persons and employees earning over a certain ceiling are allowed to opt out of the statutory insurance scheme and join one of the 60 (approximately) private health-insurance companies. As in the UK, family doctors are gate-keepers, selecting and referring patients to the appropriate specialist. Patients receive comprehensive coverage, which entitles them to unlimited primary and hospital care. The sick funds reimburse the doctors, hospitals and pharmacists for delivery of their services. Privately insured people pay the doctor or pharmacist and their insurance company reimburses the patient. Legal restrictions and government regulations limit the freedom of the sick funds to control cost, prices and the quantities and range of provisions.

What are the advantages of each system?

The German national-insurance-funded and the British tax-funded systems have many similarities as predominantly universal and comprehensive systems. The two are more similar to each other than either is to the American system. Therefore the European collective system will be compared with the American private system.

Table 1 lists some of the main

- What are the main differences in the way health care is organized in the USA, Germany and the UK?

Case study 1

Three different ways of funding and organizing health–care provision

United Kingdom
- State-run national health service funded mainly through taxation
- Every citizen covered
- Per capita spending on health US$ 1391
- 6.8% of GNP spent on health services.

United States of America
- Mainly private health-insurance system with market-based health-care provision
- 10% population not covered
- Per capita spending on health US$ 3912
- 13.4% of GNP spent on health services.

Germany
- National health-insurance-based system with a market-based health-care system
- Every citizen covered
- Per capita spending on health US$ 2364
- 10.7% of GNP spent on health services.

Table 1 **Collective systems of health care: advantages and disadvantages**	
Advantages	**Disadvantages**
■ Social citizenship/cohesion	■ Reduces individual responsibility
■ Combats the Inverse Care Law[1]	■ Increases deference towards the doctor
■ No fee results in less over-doctoring	■ Free care encourages trivial complaints
■ More scope for coordinated planning	■ Impedes search for market-solutions
■ Bargaining-power economies of scale	■ Vote-catching discourages quality
■ Tax revenue is cheap to collect	■ Higher public spending
■ Easier to meet emergencies, e.g. AIDS, war	■ Makes health a political football

[1]The Inverse Care Law argues that the provision of health care in a market economy is inversely related to the need for it; in other words poor facilities are to be found in depressed areas characterized by high morbidity, and better facilities in affluent areas characterized by low morbidity (Tudor Hart 1971: 405).

Table 2 **Advantages and disadvantages of private systems of health care**	
Advantages	**Disadvantages**
■ Liberal citizenship/choice	■ Choice only for those who can pay
■ Market: best mechanism for regulating any distribution	■ Health insurance market does not equate health care market
■ Similar quality care for low price; better care for higher price	■ Many cannot afford the higher price
■ Direct service and short waiting lists	■ Inverse Care Law: services concentrated
■ Improvements stimulated by market	■ Improvement stimulated by profit, not need
■ Patients = consumers, i.e. know their rights	■ Patients still depend on doctors' opinion

advantages and disadvantages of collective health-care systems. Some of the listed issues are political, others more clearly medical. For example, the first advantage is obviously political: it expresses ideals of shared citizenship and enhances social cohesiveness in society. The issue that 'free care encourages trivial complaints' has a direct impact on the doctor. If care is free for the patients we might expect that more people will come forward with relatively minor complaints.

Table 2 shows some of the main advantages and disadvantages of private health care. For example, in the first advantage, 'liberal citizenship/choice', Americans have the freedom to shop around for their health care; they can decide to have an all-inclusive insurance or only insure for hospital treatment. They are not told by the state what they must do; this is a very political argument. The first disadvantage, 'choice for only those who can pay', refers to the fact that many Americans do not have access to proper health care, and therefore no choice at all. In the USA, only people with enough money or a good health insurance scheme can buy the best available medical care. Consequently, people who have a good medical insurance cover have little incentive to seek lower prices for health care. This is one of the reasons why the system is so expensive. Finally, an issue concerning doctors directly is the extent to which patients have a choice. For example, whether they opt for brain surgery, chiropractic or psychiatric treatment is not completely a free choice, since most patients will be unable to judge the quality and the usefulness of the services on offer. Furthermore, the increase in patients' complaints and litigation indicates that patients are dissatisfied with the services provided. However, this is not completely a problem of private medicine, since the number of complaints and court cases in the UK is also on the increase.

Paying the doctor

These are observations of imperfections in the different ways of organizing health care, not judgements about these systems. Take the remuneration of the doctor's fees. There is no right way of fixing the doctor's payment. Every method has significant disadvantages: a fee-for-service payment may have the effect of encouraging some doctors to advise more treatment than is really necessary, whereas payment on a capitation basis, i.e. number of patients on the roll, may mean that doctors are in too much of a hurry to give adequate individual attention to each patient.

Convergence

There appears to be a tendency for the different models of health-care provision to converge. In the 1990s the Clinton administration pushed for reforms in the health-care system that would increase the role of the state, while in countries with a national health-care system (e.g. the UK) or national health-insurance system (e.g. Germany), governments are trying to increase the role of the market (see Case study 2).

Case study 2

In 2000 the UK Secretary of State for Health signed an official concordat with the private health-care sector. The arrangement meant that Regional Health Authorities/Boards were, for the first time, able to make local contracts with the private health-care sector. In this way NHS patients could benefit from spare capacity in the private sector (see pp. 152–153).

Organizing and funding health care

■ The organization of a nation's health-care system is closely related to the way it is funded.
■ Public and private health-care and health-funding systems both have specific advantages and disadvantages
■ It seems as if the different health-care systems are converging.

www.heritage.org/library/lecture/h/711.html

Assessing needs

The health services are constantly in a state of flux due to alterations at the supply side of care, for example, the appearance of new drugs, the introduction of new medical technology, and attempts to make services more efficient and effective. Health services are also changing through alterations in demand, for example, the changing composition of the population (more people live longer), the appearance of new diseases (HIV/AIDS) and changing preferences and expectations among consumers for certain kinds of treatment. Somewhere in this pool of potentially conflicting interests we have to establish the needs of individuals, communities and populations whilst ensuring that each receives maximum benefit within the limits of available resources, such as staff, buildings and funding (see web pages).[1]

Different kinds of need

The first distinction to make is the difference between 1) the need for health and 2) the need for health care. The former refers to the WHO definition of health: 'all aspects of physical and mental well-being'. The latter refers to the ability to benefit from health care or prevention services. It is, therefore, more specific and, as such, will depend on the health care and preventive services (potentially) available.

The need for 'needs' assessment

Why does a service provider, a policy-maker, a doctor or a hospital manager set about identifying the needs of people? Providers of health care need to know (a) what users need in the way of health care and (b) what is needed in a particular area, in order to achieve an improvement in the health of the population. These two objectives are not the same. What potential or actual service users feel they need (Fig. 1) might only partially overlap with what policymakers consider to be the best possible range of services in an area that can improve the health of the people there ('normative needs'). Both types have to be distinguished from 'expressed needs', the actual use or demand for a service, and 'comparative needs', which compares services across similar communities or client groups, for example, comparing the services available to people with HIV and those with cancer, or comparing services available in the West of London with those in the East End. Thus need is not a unified concept.

Needs-assessment

It is difficult to assess all needs at the same time, since needs-assessment exercises require funding and can be time consuming like any other piece of research. Consequently, needs assessments usually focus on a specific illness and a limited area of care, thus assessing the needs of a particular group of (potential) patients in order to determine how their need might be met. When we consider the needs of the population in a given area we also have to ask questions such as: 'Whose needs do we take into consideration?' and 'Are we looking at the present needs of people currently ill or the potential future needs of the total population?'. The assessment of the needs of the local population also should be performed on a regular basis, since a population changes over time, and their actual or perceived needs might change. Planning health-care provision takes time, whether it be training of doctors and nurses or building hospitals. Changing funding from one type of health service to another, such as the transformation from hospital care to community-based services, is also time consuming.

Thus one of the main issues is: 'How do we firstly define, and secondly measure, *need*?'. The next main questions are: 'Who should perform a needs assessment?' and 'Whose definition of 'needs' is it to be based on: (a) lay people; (b) professionals; (c) researchers; (d) politicians; (e) managers; or (f) a combination of groups?'

One main issue in needs-assessment exercises is the way one measures health needs. We can focus on all people (healthy or unhealthy), or only on those with the specific disease or illness. The former is the most equal way of assessing the overall need in a population, whilst the latter ensures that those who know what it is to have a particular illness help to establish an overview of the needs of its sufferers. Both approaches also have drawbacks. Asking a sample of *all* people to identify needs will result in highlighting the need for provisions

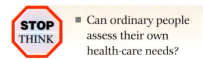

STOP THINK
- Can ordinary people assess their own health-care needs?

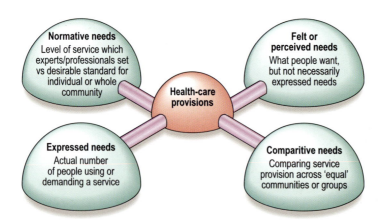

Fig. 1 **Types of needs in health care provision.** (Source: Bradshaw 1972)

Diagram labels:
- **Normative needs** — Level of service which experts/professionals set vs desirable standard for individual or whole community
- **Felt or perceived needs** — What people want, but not necessarily expressed needs
- **Health-care provisions**
- **Expressed needs** — Actual number of people using or demanding a service
- **Comparitive needs** — Comparing service provision across 'equal' communities or groups

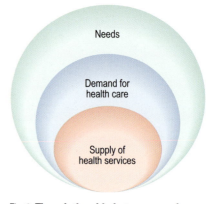

Diagram labels:
- Needs
- Demand for health care
- Supply of health services

Fig. 2 **The relationship between needs, demand and supply.**

related to more common illnesses and related health services, and will under-represent specific needs for people with 'rarer' or less 'acceptable' conditions (Hopton and Dlugolecka 1995). Conducting a needs assessment among people with specific conditions will highlight needs that might be specific to them only, but not to the general population or to people with other conditions. Thus, although previous users are likely to have a bias towards existing services, non-users are likely to lack experience and knowledge of the topic and will generally opt for provision for more common conditions.

The way a needs assessment is conducted can have an influence on its outcome. An uncritical social marketing approach may lead to more service for the general population, at the expense of specific services for those most in distress.

The Case study shows that the needs as assessed by different people all have a role to play in the provision of health services.

It is important to remember that a prediction of more pregnancies in a certain area does not automatically mean that more hospital beds and doctors are needed to cope with the increase in deliveries. Different illnesses require different approaches to service provision, and the needs assessment itself might vary according to the illness in question. It is likely that service users have less input in a needs assessment of hospital-based orthopaedic surgery than in one of community-based mental-health care.

Unmet and unlimited needs

There is a potential problem of unmet needs, as well as unlimited needs. The former issue refers to missing out people in assessing needs, whilst the latter refers to whether we will be able to fulfil the needs we identify in a needs-assessment exercise. Asking people about their health problems in order to identify unmet needs might raise expectations about the service they expect to receive, but which we cannot provide.

In Figure 2 three circles represent needs, demand and supply. Demand in this figure can be seen as the 'expressed needs' mentioned above. Figure 1 indicates that there might be needs that are not as such recognized by those who have them. This implies that people other than the users have conducted the needs assessment.

The realization that health needs are far more than

demands from patients presented to the medical profession gave rise to the idea of a *clinical iceberg* or *iceberg of disease*. From a social science perspective the concept of an iceberg of disease is an indication that different perceived needs in different groups of people can lead to different reactions; some will result in seeking medical help while others will lead to self-medication or are simply ignored (see pp. 86–87).

Needs-assessment and users

Needs-assessment cannot be left completely to users: for example, recreational drug users might not feel that they have a drugs problem, so a needs-assessment exercise conducted among this group would indicate that there is no need for a problem drug service. However, a small proportion of these recreational drug users will develop problems in the near future, leading to a need for specific drug services. Furthermore, needs assessment has to be linked to the provision of services. If needs assessments are conducted in different health and social services areas, we (society as a whole, i.e. our politicians) have to decide which of those needs have priority over others.

 STOP THINK

- Considering the Case study on the organization of maternity care, what would you think will be the main needs identified by the following groups:

  – general practitioners in the community
  – obstetricians in the regional hospital
  – regional health administrators
  – local politicians
  – community midwives
  – pregnant women
  – women of childbearing age but not currently pregnant?

Remember to have another look at pages 2–3.

Assessing needs

- There is a difference between the need for health and the need for health services.
- There are four ways of defining need: normative need, felt need, expressed need and comparative need.
- Needs assessment should include the views of users, as well as lay public, professionals, managers, politicians and researchers.
- Needs assessment runs the risk of raising people's expectations and of not having the resources to meet them.

www.htm-treasury.gov.uk/mediastore/otherfiles/chap3.pdf

Case study

The organization of maternity care

Epidemiologists and policymakers can establish the likely number of healthy babies that will be born in a city, region or any other area. This estimate will be based on (1) the number of women of childbearing age in the area and (2) the birth rate for that area, subtracting the likely number of mothers and babies needing specialist obstetric care before, during or after the delivery.

This information in itself will not be sufficient to predict the need for maternity services in the area. We need to ask women and their partners how and where they want the maternity services to provide health care. Do women want a predominantly midwife-led care, or do they want general practitioner (GP) maternity care, or do they want shared care between doctors and midwives, or shared care between obstetricians and GPs? A further set of questions is: Where should these maternity services be delivered – at home, in a GP maternity unit, in a midwifery unit, or in a specialist obstetric hospital?

Setting priorities and rationing

The medical profession often has to prioritize treatment and ration services at a patient level. Any practising doctor can tell a personal story of having to choose between patients because resources are limited – whether staff, money, theatres or organ donors.

Rationing of health care has always taken place, however wealthy the country, but until recently it was done implicitly, was often invisible and often inequitable (see pp. 148–149). As spending on health services has increased in most countries, discussion about priorities and rationing has become more explicit. Thus, the question is not, 'Will we have rationing?', but 'How will we organize rationing?'

SECRET SUMMIT PLANS RATIONING FOR NHS:
TOP DOCTORS TOLD PRIORITY SETTING IS
INEVITABLE

This headline in the newspaper *The Guardian* (27–11–1995) indicates that rationing is regarded by some as (a) unavoidable and (b) neither popular nor desirable, hence the secrecy.

Setting priorities

Setting priorities implies choosing a limited number of options from a wider range and ranking these in order of importance. Following on from priority setting is a process of rationing. Rationing is often defined as allocating scarce resources by some criteria other than the price mechanism. This does not mean that the price is not an important consideration, but that the price (or cost, which may not be the same as price) of a service, say a hip replacement, is not the only factor in the decision whether or not a patient who is in need of such surgery will receive treatment. Priority setting is a dynamic process, and in every budget cycle new technologies and information on health outcomes are taken into consideration in setting new priorities.

Forms of rationing

Rationing is a trade-off between providing all services to a limited number of people, or providing a limited number of services to all people. Rationing often involves a limitation of both the range and the volume of service provision (example below from the British Medical Journal). Decisions regarding rationing also have to be made at different levels: at an individual, local/regional and national level.

A variety of rationing mechanisms have been identified (Klein et al 1996):

- **Denial:** for example, refusing to treat people over 70 years of age for certain conditions.
- **Deterrence:** putting up social, economic or psychological barriers.
- **Dilution:** prescribing cheaper non-brand-name drugs, or reducing length of stay in hospital.
- **Delay:** hospital waiting lists.
- **Deflection:** having GPs as gatekeepers; or referring an elderly person for local authority services rather than keeping him/her in hospital.

Neonatal care may become too expensive: Doctors at Sheffield's main maternity unit have been told that if demand for neonatal services continues to rise an 'arbitrary ban' may have to be introduced according to Panorama, a British television documentary programme. This could mean that babies born more than 15 weeks prematurely could be refused treatment.

This cutting from the British Medical Journal (1994: 309, p. 282) highlights limited availability of resources and the ever growing demand for medical services.

Free-market provision of care is often not regarded as a form of rationing. Everybody who has enough money can buy any treatment, e.g. expensive operations, privately. However, many will not have the money either to buy the service directly or to take out comprehensive private insurance. Hence, practically, the effect is similar to rationing.

Rationing: underlying principles

We now consider some of the principles that underpin rationing. The key principle is generally considered to be 'equity' but a number of other principles are also important (see Harrison and Hunter 1994):

- **Equity:** ideally everyone should have a fair opportunity to attain their full health potential and, more pragmatically, no one should be disadvantaged from achieving their potential if it can be avoided. Equity could refer to access to health care, but also to healthy living conditions or equity of autonomy.
- **Needs:** the British NHS was introduced on the principle that people should receive health services on the basis of their health and medical need rather than their 'ability to pay', but 'need' is not a simple, clear concept (see pp 150–151).
- **Equality:** all individuals have an equal access to health care. Should a 70-year-old smoker and heavy drinker have the same chance of getting the next available donor kidney as a 21-year-old non-smoker and non-drinker?
- **Effectiveness:** the ability of an intervention to achieve its intended effect in those to whom it is offered (i.e. does it work?).
- **Cost-effectiveness (efficiency):** the effectiveness of an intervention in relation to the resources used (e.g. time, labour, equipment and materials).
- **Quality-adjusted life years (QALYs):** a technique for estimating the extra years of life gained from particular inter-

---

- What principles should guide a decision to spend more money on either (a) clinical psychology services for people with depression, or (b) hip replacement surgery, both of which have 6-month waiting lists? What information would you need to help you make a decision between them?
- What effect would using different principles have on the decision?

ventions, adjusted for the quality of the extra years. They are often combined with costs to give a 'cost per additional QALY', but there are many assumptions built into their calculation (see also pp 38–39).

Decision-making

In a democracy, we have to establish who should set priorities and ration services. Should it be doctors, administrators, politicians, service users, pressure groups, courts or some sort of consensus group?

Case study 1

During World War II penicillin was scarce on the battlefields. Doctors had to make decisions on which soldiers would be treated and which not. The recovery rate of getting the soldiers back to the front was considerably higher among with those with a STI (sexually transmitted infection) rather than those with serious shot and shrapnel wounds. However, medical considerations (i.e. the highest recovery rate) were overruled by political (what people at home might think) and ethical considerations, such as 'soldiers with a STI are less deserving than those with bullet wounds'.

Commissioning is one of the growing fields in health care, where decisions have to be made by the purchasers of health care regarding the range, the quantity and the quality of health services bought for a specific population at a specific time. Local NHS health-care trusts and health authorities are effectively taking decisions on the rationing of services. This is a case where decision-making about priority setting and rationing lies predominantly with the health-care managers and, to a lesser extent, the medical profession, but certainly not the services users.

Since 1999 the National Institute for Clinical Effectiveness (NICE) has started analyzing the effectiveness of drugs and medical technology in the UK. NICE is trying to balance clinical effectiveness and cost effectiveness.

Consultation of users

The appeal of the Oregon experiment (see Case study 2) lies partly in its explicit approach to rationing and partly in community participation in priority setting. It is interesting to note that prevention comes high on the priority list.

Figure 1 shows the main different forms of rationing, whereby medical and economic considerations are taken in to account. The bottom left-hand corner is the situation often found in the UK, the top right-hand corner is a serious possibility in countries with private medicine working for profit.

Case study 2

The Oregon experiment

The American state of Oregon pioneered a system for prioritizing health care in an attempt to address the widespread problem of the growing number of people who are without private health insurance and who are not eligible for federal assistance programmes. Most controversial of the reforms is the use by the legislature of a priority list of health services to determine benefit levels for the insurance programmes. In addition, Oregon aimed to bring cover for the rationed services to everyone in the population. Priorities were set by a Health Services Commission, initially on the basis of a technical methodology similar to 'cost per QALY', and, subsequently, on broad-based consensus through public consultation. The Commission came up with the following priorities:

- acute, fatal conditions where treatment prevents death and leads to full recovery
- maternity care
- acute, fatal conditions where treatment prevents death, but does not lead to full recovery
- preventive care for children
- chronic, fatal conditions where treatment prolongs life and improves quality of care
- comfort or palliative care.

The next step was for the politicians to determine how much could be funded from existing and additional sources. This clearly brought the provision of health care to the centre of the political arena, since an increase in the health budget meant an increase in taxation or a decrease in the provision of other state provisions, for example, in education. Thus the Oregon experiment introduced a rational plan for expanding services to the entire population of the state, while acknowledging the limitations of funding resources.

(Based on Kitzhaber 1993)

Fig. 1 **Overview of medical and economic considerations in decision-making.**

Setting priorities and rationing

- All health-care systems have some in-built form of rationing.
- Rationing takes different forms.
- The key principles of rationing care are equity, equality, effectiveness and cost effectiveness. Needs and value are also important but difficult to operationalize.
- Much rationing and setting of priorities takes place implicitly. Explicit rationing forces people to make difficult choices. Who makes these choices and decisions is another key issue.

Community care

For over a decade, community care has been a cornerstone in the development of health services, and in the future many doctors who previously spent their lives in hospitals will increasingly be based in community settings. Community care is a concept embraced by people of all professions and political persuasions.

At its broadest, community care involves service delivery, economic policy, political rhetoric and philosophical ideology. It can be seen as a way of delivering services, a way of enhancing quality of life or a way of reducing spending by an out-of-control welfare state. It has come from the New Right in both Britain and the USA, and from a Marxist background in Italy. The development of community care throughout developed countries has come about through a variety of clinical, social and political influences (see Fig. 1).

The most numerous group within community care is the elderly, but it also covers people with mental-health problems, and people with learning, physical or sensory disabilities. Some of the problems in discussing community care come from translating what is a generic policy to services appropriate for different patient and client groups. Guiding users through a variety of different agencies and organizations, all of which should cooperate and inter-relate (Fig. 2), adds to the problem.

Influences on community care

The community

There are two powerful beliefs at work here. The first is that there is a community that cares and that will accept its old, its ill and its disabled people and treat them as equal and valued members of that community. The second is that living in the community is, by definition, better than living in an institution. For those who receive good care and support, have appropriate housing and a good social network, living in the community empowers them to make choices over their lives, freed from the restrictions of institutions. For those who are ignored by their neighbours, with a very low income from benefits and little support from services, living in the community can be a nightmare existence of loneliness and poverty.

Anti-institutions

Institutions are visibly expensive and can be dehumanizing and lead to loss of abilities, apathy and dependency (Goffman 1968b). As the population of long-stay psychiatric patients, mainly people with schizophrenia, diminished, their place was taken by the growing number of elderly people with dementia. The true meaning of asylum as sanctuary has been forgotten and, as the number of beds are cut, it can be difficult to admit patients in acute crisis.

Consumerism

The political right supports the view that market forces should dictate services are thus needs led not service led. Consumers (formerly patients) are to be consulted about service delivery. The left supports consumerism more from a position of advocacy and empowerment.

Welfare pluralism

There is a move from the welfare state (in Britain, for example) towards a mixed economy of care, in which services are provided by statutory agencies, voluntary organizations and the private sector. This can incorporate means testing for certain kinds of care.

Cost-cutting

The growing elderly population means that the cost of residential care is escalating for welfare-state countries. Community care is a way of capping this cost by restricting residential care and moving costs to families. This has also involved trying to make the divide between health care and social care more distinct. In continuing care of elderly people in England and Wales, distinctions are made between medical care, which requires hospitalization, and nursing care, which can take place in nursing homes and thus is not part of free health care. In Scotland this distinction has been removed and personal care for the elderly is funded.

Family values

A return to traditional family values has been a major political theme for conservative governments in both Britain and North America for the last decade. The family is promoted as the front line of care, and services are directed at helping families care rather than replacing that care with state or private facilities (see pp 136–137).

User-movement

Although this can be linked to consumerism it has more to do with advocacy, the promotion of patients' rights and often

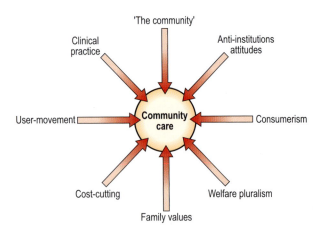

Fig. 1 **Influences on community care.**

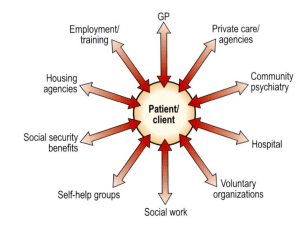

Fig. 2 **Agencies with whom the patient/client may be involved.**

an anti-medical, anti-psychiatry model of mental-health problems (see pp 138–139).

Clinical practice

From the 1950s onwards new advances in treatment, including the introduction of phenothiazines, behaviour therapy, rehabilitation and psychosocial therapies, meant that custodial care for groups such as those with mental-health problems became less relevant.

Underlying problems

Coherence of vision

Community care requires multidisciplinary cooperation at all levels; staff and policy in housing, social work, benefits, medicine, nursing, occupational and physiotherapy, psychology and employment are all involved. Current policy requires joint planning and working between health and social services to provide 'seamless' services to community care clients. Different professional views and priorities can cause practical problems. In mental illness, for example, the bio-medical versus the social–environmental view requires radically different approaches to clients and services. A bio-psychosocial approach brings these together and is advocated by many. The reality of service delivery, however, can be difficult as many agencies that have to cooperate have different views and priorities.

The role of women

By and large women relatives and friends are expected to fill the gaps left by the shortage of public service resources and provide informal care at home (see pp 136–137). Community services tend to be staffed by low-paid, predominantly female workers with poor conditions and terms of employment.

'Them' and 'us'

The well-known NIMBY syndrome (not in my back yard) means that the community is often not willing to accept people with problems. Plans to develop hostels or sheltered housing are frequently met with local opposition.

Treatment model of community care

As well as seeing the community as a more appropriate place for people to live than hospitals, research has looked at how well people do who are discharged from long-term care. One long-term study by TAPS (Team Assessment of Psychiatric Services) has followed the closure of Friern and Claybury hospitals in London, demonstrating the success of the project (Trieman et al 1999). Not all studies are completely positive and, although people live in the community, they may not show improvements in daily living or social skills (Donnelly et al 1996). MIND, however, conducted a survey of users' views that was overwhelmingly positive, with users feeling generally more independent and active, and having greater control over their lives with more choices open to them (Rogers et al 1993).

Community care in the UK

Community care in Britain has been both defined and limited by the NHS and Community Care Act 1990, which came into operation on April 1st 1993.

Whereas previously patients were fitted into established services, now patients are to be assessed as to their 'needs',

---

Case study

Tom was born with cerebral palsy and, until he was 21, had been cared for by his mother. When she became too old and frail to look after him, he was taken into a large psychiatric hospital (although he was not intellectually impaired), where he was put in a wheelchair and became dependent for help from staff who had many others to tend to and who worked to fairly fixed timetables. There were few opportunities for privacy and when (25 years later) he met a woman (with learning disabilities) he wanted to marry, they would have had to sleep apart.

He and his wife chose to leave hospital and live in a flat in a newly built block of 50, which included two other flats for disabled people. Support was provided by a care worker, who also lived in the block, and agency staff, who covered the care worker when she was off. Over the subsequent 10 years, Tom has experienced some problems with his health and has had to spend time in hospital, but he is still adamant that living in the community has given him control over his own life and a far higher quality of life than he had experienced in hospital.

---

with services being designed and provided to meet these needs (see pp 150–151). This ties in with who provides services. Health boards and social work departments now buy-in services from the mixed economy rather than provide them themselves. Many residential establishments for the elderly, or sheltered housing for those with mental-health problems, are expected to be provided by private companies or voluntary organizations rather than social work departments.

The impact of this for patients is that there is no longer free-at-point-of-delivery care by the NHS, but means-tested care through social work. Services are targeted to 'concentrate on those with greatest needs'; they should 'allow for a range of options', 'respond flexibly and sensitively to the needs of individuals and carers', and, above all, 'intervene no more than is necessary to foster independence'. Key objectives for service delivery:

- to promote the development of domiciliary, day and respite services to enable people to live in their own homes wherever feasible and sensible
- to ensure that service providers make practical support for carers a high priority
- to make proper assessment of need and good case management the cornerstones of high-quality care
- to promote the development of a flourishing independent sector alongside good-quality public services
- to clarify the responsibilities of agencies and so make it easier to hold them to account for their performance
- to secure better value for tax-payers' money by introducing a new funding structure for social care.

- Is the community willing and able to accept everyone with a problem?
- Is there a role for institutions/asylums?

Community care

- Is a generic policy.
- Is a needs-led service.
- Places care outside institutions.
- Is both inter- and multidisciplinary.
- Relies on care by families.

Medical students' experience

Wherever you train to be a doctor, there are some experiences common to all medical students. These set you apart from the rest of the undergraduate population. Thinking about how you solve problems during this time should enable you to see how you might tackle challenges in the future. It will also facilitate an understanding of how other people (including patients) deal with their own difficulties.

There have been a number of studies of the process of becoming a doctor from 'Boys in White' (Becker 1961) to Allen's UK study (1994). Research into students' experience of UK medical education began in the early 1980s (Firth 2001, Firth-Cozens 1986) and continued into the early 1990s (Miller 1994, Guthrie et al 1998, McManus et al 1999), but this impetus has not been been sustained through the years of major UK curriculum reform following the publication of 'Tomorrow's Doctors' (General Medical Council 1993), and the overall research-based picture has developed only a little over the last 10 years.

What is different about medicine?

Many of the pressures on medical students are not qualitatively different from those on other students: they worry about coursework, exams, money, relationships, but the workload is heavier and the length of the course potentially increases the burden of financial debt. The new developments of problem-based, self-directed learning and earlier clinical contact have been positively received by students and supervisors (Jones et al 2002), although they require some adjustment and the time spent in preparation is not substantially less than the time spent rote-learning.

Family background may add to the pressure, since parents may have high expectations of medical student offspring. There is evidence that where this is the case, it adds to the stress experienced throughout the medical career (Brewin and Firth-Cozens 1997, Firth-Cozens 1998). This may operate by setting up specific personal beliefs about the need for high achievement. These then influence both feelings and behaviour, and in some individuals can lead to excessive self-criticism, which has been found to be a strong predictor of subsequent stress and depression (Firth-Cozens 2001).

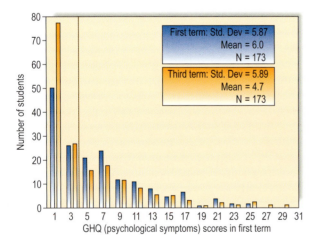

Fig. 1 **Proportion of students above the GHQ threshold in first and third term. Dotted vertical line indicates threshold for significant psychological symptoms.** (Data reproduced by permission of P Miller.)

Personality influences a student's reactions to the medical course. One factor is the student's ability to tolerate ambiguity and uncertainty. Medical students are all excellent at science, but people, including patients, are often seemingly irrational and unpredictable. The realization of this fact can cause distress in students, and there is evidence that this influences career choice. Those most intolerant of ambiguity tend to choose specialties such as pathology, anaesthesiology, radiology and surgery: those with greater tolerance go into general practice and psychiatry, where they have closer contact with people.

Adjustment to university and medical school takes time. The first term seems to be stressful, as it is for many other students. Miller (1994) surveyed a complete class cohort of first-year students at a medical school in the UK. He found that in the first term, nearly half the class scored above the threshold on a screening device (the General Health Questionnaire) for psychological distress. By the summer term, only one-third showed these levels of distress (see Fig. 1). Learning to balance social relationships and activities with heavy academic commitments was particularly stressful.

In the more traditional courses, the sources of stress change with clinical experience. Firth-Cozens (1986) found the item most commonly reported as 'particularly stressful' in fourth-year students in the UK was 'relationships with consultants'. A common complaint is that some senior staff teach by humiliation rather than encouragement (Moss and McManus 1992, Allen 1994), and some students can become so anxious that they fail to attend ward rounds. Any objective assessment of teaching would recognize this as not only grossly inappropriate and unfair, but a very poor teaching method. Reporting such incidents through a formal feedback mechanism, anonymously if necessary, would help to stop it. Discussing them with others could reduce distress. It is to be hoped that earlier introduction to clinical experience, better educational training of clinical teachers and more community-based clinical teaching have reduced these complaints but there is, as yet, no research evidence to support such a belief. Indeed, Radcliffe and Lester (2003) recently found that it was still a major concern amongst fourth-year students, though things improved in the fifth year, when they reported being more appreciated by senior clinical staff, particularly if they were made to feel part of a team.

Coping strategies

There are some well-known maladaptive responses. One is avoidance, for example, by putting off work that is difficult. Similarly, denial and dismissal of a negative event have been found to be coping strategies that increase stress levels, not reduce them. Alcohol abuse is another poor coping strategy. Alcohol consumption amongst university students has been rising, and consumption by medical students has followed this trend (Newbury-Birch et al 2000). This study reported that 49% of men and 43% of women were drinking above the 'low-risk' level of alcohol (respectively: <21 units/week and <14 units/week). Alcohol use was also strongly correlated with cannabis use. In a related study, Newbury-Birch et al (2001) report that, contrary to expectation, mean alcohol consumption, and drinking above the recommended safe limits, had increased in a cohort of medical students as they

- There is evidence that levels of anxiety and depression in students are, to some extent, predetermined by personality, but it has also been shown that teaching stress management to medical students enables them to control the symptoms of stress. Another view is that some experience of anxiety and depression may not be a bad thing anyway, since doctors who score more highly on these symptoms are more empathetic and approachable.

Given these various findings, and that lack of support from senior staff is a common complaint, should more be done for students – stress-management courses, regular meetings with members of staff, or support groups across years? Or is it the case that 'If you can't stand the stress, you should get out of the medical school?'

progressed from second year to final year and into their pre-registration year. Whilst there was a negative relationship between alcohol use and anxiety levels at all 3 years, and no association between alcohol use and depression, qualified doctors have a higher than average risk of developing alcohol problems, and these student studies suggest that the habit may be established early in their medical careers.

Tackling stress can be done on all levels (see pp 124–125). Try to deal with the source of the stress:

- Manage the workload. Prioritize what you are doing, then delegate, delay, or drop things that are not urgent.
- Seek support. Talk to others. If you are worried, listen to someone else's point of view.
- Look at your thinking style. If you think that you may set unrealistic standards for yourself, try to challenge this (see pp 134–136). Ask yourself what you would say to a friend in a similar situation, then take your own advice.
- Relax. Trying to work all the time leads to tiredness and inefficiency. Set aside time to switch off by doing something else: sport, yoga, music or seeing friends.

In the competitive environment of a medical school, students can sometimes feel inadequate. Classmates may enjoy demonstrating their knowledge and skills. Remember that the requirements for being a good doctor are diverse and not necessarily based on being the first to display textbook knowledge. For example, giving an immediate diagnosis on the basis of the initial information given by a patient can be faulty. Research on students has shown that many of them start off with a wide-ranging interview style (being unsure of possible diagnoses). They explore all possibilities. Over the course of medical school, however, they gradually use increased medical knowledge to home in early on a diagnosis. They may fail to investigate the other possibilities. In this situation, a more open-minded approach would be more appropriate.

In the early experience of clinical work, remember that you arc still a student. Set realistic standards for yourself. If you have persistent thoughts about leaving medicine, it is important to talk this over with someone. You may feel great pressure from your family or a medical member of staff. It may be helpful to talk to an outsider. Most universities have

counsellors or those who can offer careers guidance. It is important that the decision is yours and not dominated by feelings of duty or consideration of how much you have invested already. Remember that there are many branches of medicine that you may not have considered: the choice is not limited to general practice versus hospital medicine.

Satisfaction

Despite the demanding conditions of medical training, there are many rewards in the practice of medicine. Students and young doctors can have experience of different specialties and are likely to settle eventually in one that suits their personality and abilities. Those who derive most interest from the science can move towards laboratory research and those who enjoy the 'art' of medicine will go into specialties that include closer contact with patients. Although very different, both types of career can bring enormous personal satisfaction.

Case study

Ian, a third-year medical student, appeared before a faculty committee appealing to stay on, despite having twice failed an exam in paediatrics. He said that he had fallen behind in studying, but assured the committee that he would not do so again.

When asked whether there were any relevant circumstances, he described a catalogue of misfortune. During his third year he had been off for several weeks with abdominal pain that eventually proved to be appendicitis and resulted in an appendectomy. Just before Christmas, his parents separated, and he kept going home at weekends to help his depressed mother. In the spring, his landlord evicted him because a drunken flatmate had smashed furniture. By the summer term, he was camping out in friends' flats, trying to study and missing many days on clinical attachments. He was extremely anxious and unable to sleep or concentrate. Having failed the exam, he attempted to revise over the summer, but had to earn money by working in a bar and made little progress.

The committee took a sympathetic view of his circumstances, but criticized him for not discussing his difficulties with a tutor and arranging to have time off officially, especially when he was ill. He was permitted to repeat his third year, but strongly advised to make contact with the accommodation service, the counselling service, and with his tutor. He did this and scraped through his repeated year. In subsequent years, he maintained reasonable passes and graduated successfully.

Medical students' experience

- Medical students' experience of stress is different from other students: at first in terms of the amount of work, then later in terms of clinical contact.
- Adaptation to medical school is influenced by family background and personality: these factors also influence career choice.
- Relationships with senior medical staff are often stressful in the clinical years.
- Students' use of alcohol to relieve stress may establish a habit that puts them at risk of becoming doctors with alcohol problems.
- If you have doubts about medicine as a career, talk it over with someone, and make your own decision.

Being a junior doctor

After graduating from a university course in medicine comes the reality of working with the patient population. In most countries, this period of training is tough. The hours are long and the knowledge to be gained is substantial. At the same time, the pressure of carving out a career path impinges on daily work. New doctors often feel that clinical supervision and support is inadequate, and the responsibility for patients can seem overwhelming. Yet this is also a time when new graduates can realize how useful and effective they can be in dealing with health problems and this experience is satisfying.

Sources of stress for young doctors

Hours
Young doctors are affected by the long hours that they work. Cognitive performance on medical tasks and standard psychological tests is worse after a night on call; mood is also affected (Lingenfelser et al 1994). In the past, junior doctors have been known to work very long hours. These long hours over a working week were associated with increased psychosomatic symptoms (e.g. feeling ill, feeling run down, pains in the head) and poorer social functioning (e.g. taking longer over things, inability to make decisions) (Baldwin et al 1997). Whilst research since new guidelines has shown a reduction in hours and an improvement in induction and supervision, there is still concern that too many doctors find their first year of doctoring excessively stressful and distressing (Bligh 2002). Sleep deprivation, overwork and too little personal time are still perceived to be major causes of stress (Paice et al 2002).

Feeling overwhelmed
Despite the relationship between hours worked and somatic symptoms and social dysfunction, long hours were not associated with a feeling of being overwhelmed or of making minor mistakes (Baldwin et al 1997). Feeling overwhelmed was, however, associated with the number of emergency admissions, and the number of deaths in the past week, and fetching equipment. Feeling overwhelmed was strongly related to anxiety, depression,

somatic symptoms, social dysfunction and physical illness. Similarly, Paice et al (2002) also found that long hours on their own were not a major cause of distress, but overwork underlay many descriptions of distressing incidents.

Other sources of stress
Other sources of stress for young doctors have been studied systematically. In the UK, Firth-Cozens (1987) found that the most stressful aspects of the first postgraduate year were 'overwork', 'talking to distressed relatives', 'effects of work on your personal life', and 'serious treatment failures'. Similar results were found for young doctors in the USA, but because they completed other degrees before they started medical education and were therefore older, for them marriage appeared to buffer the effects of these stressors (Butterfield 1988).

Table 1 details the main categories of stressful incidents reported by 1321 junior doctors working in 336 hospitals in the UK, and shows that facing responsibilities beyond their competence or experience was the most commonly reported incident and was associated with high mean scores on the General Health Questionnaire (GHQ). In 133 of the 'interpersonal' incidents, the difficult relationship was with senior medical colleagues who were 'critical, unreasonably demanding, incompetent or uncaring' (Paice et al 2002). Whilst dealing with dying people and their relatives was often mentioned as a difficult event, it was not so often associated with high GHQ scores. 'Self' incidents involved making a mistake, or loss of self-esteem or difficult career choices, and although they were not that common, they were associated with high GHQ scores.

Table 1 Categories of reported incidents and mean GHQ-12 scores.		
Category	Number (%)	Mean GHQ-12
Responsibility	444 (33.6)	13.1
Interpersonal	392 (29.7)	12.5
Overwork	225 (17.0)	12.0
Death and disease	172 (13.0)	11.3
Self	88 (6.7)	13.6
Total	**1321 (100)**	
(Adapted from Paice et al 2002)		

Mistakes
In medicine, it is inevitable that doctors will sometimes make mistakes, whatever their grade. The majority of serious mistakes made by young doctors are made through ignorance or inexperience; less common are mistakes through lack of information or poor communication, and tiredness. The most common types of mistake are misdiagnosis (including underestimating the severity of a condition) and procedural errors. The fear of making mistakes is an important source of stress for young doctors and this is exacerbated by the fear of litigation, which is becoming increasingly common.

Where there is doubt about clinical management, it is always wise to get another opinion. Despite what has been said above, in general, senior staff would prefer this to the increased risk of mistakes, no matter how irritable or unapproachable they may appear. Apart from any legal worries associated with making mistakes, there are always emotional effects. Junior doctors, in particular, experience feelings of remorse and guilt, even when they were not responsible for a mistake. In good teams, the incident will be discussed so that feelings of remorse can be shared, put into perspective and lessons learned. Often junior doctors have a distorted perception of the incident, believing themselves to be wholly to blame when, in fact, they were only partly, or not at all, responsible. In most cases, the prevention of similar incidents in the future lies in good organizational and teamwork practice and support, rather than in the hands of the individual young doctor.

How can you prepare to cope in the early years?
You can approach this stressful situation in the same way as other difficulties (see pp 124–125). Looking at three different aspects may help you: these are cognitions, feelings and behaviour.

Cognitions
- Put the situation in perspective: this period of training is limited and conditions will improve within a few years.
- Focus on what you have achieved on a

STOP THINK

■ How do you think you will react to your first job? Can you predict what will give you satisfaction, and what you will find most difficult?

Although medical students may be aware that the first postgraduate year is tough, many of them seem surprised by the high demands of the early years. When asked: 'What is different about medicine from what you thought when applying to university?', a class cohort of British junior doctors in 1994 wrote comments that were grouped into the following factors:

- the hours are even longer than expected (40%)
- the work is more demanding/stressful (25%)
- there is little respect from patients, or care from other staff (21%)
- inadequate training for the job (13%)
- lack of support/supervision by senior medical staff (13%)
- frequent mundane, routine, non-clinical work (10%)

(Baldwin, Dodd and Wrate 1997)

At the same time, a survey of attitudes to work amongst these same doctors showed that despite these conditions, 88% believed that they were useful most of the time; 87% thought that they were developing new skills, and most were satisfied with their choice of medicine as a career.

day-to-day basis. Junior doctors are highly skilled and learning all the time. The part they play is vital to the clinical team.

- Some mistakes are inevitable: what is important is to learn from them and to assess them objectively. It will help to discuss them with other people.
- Think about what you want from a career: is it to have a varied job, to be an eminent specialist, to enjoy a balanced work and personal life, or to work part-time? Make choices that fit in with your own needs.

Feelings

- Discuss feelings with others in a similar situation, whether these are feelings of pleasure, fatigue, disillusionment, guilt, incompetence, pride or anger.
- Discuss feelings with friends, partner or family. They may not know what it is like, but they can still empathize with you and it may help them to understand your situation.

Behaviour

- Look after your health. Try to rest when you can and to eat properly whenever possible. If you are ill, despite the culture of working through illness, take time off and see a doctor if necessary.
- Find good ways to unwind: going away, going out, taking exercise, reading, watching television, socializing. Do whatever works for you.
- Seek support from others: junior medical staff at work, friends and family at home.

Case study

Being a junior doctor

Debbie was in her first job in a teaching hospital, intending to go into paediatrics. Her boyfriend, Peter, was training in surgery 350 miles away. On one of their rare weekends together, Peter was very bitter and depressed, and expressed doubts about medicine as a career.

Debbie returned after the weekend and was herself then very low. She worked a 72-hour week during which she contracted tonsillitis. One night she admitted an elderly man but did not realize the severity of his unstable angina. He was not treated and died in the early hours of the morning. Although a more senior member of staff said that this was likely to have happened even with appropriate treatment, her consultant implied that she was negligent, and said so in front of nursing staff. She was devastated and decided to give up hospital medicine and go into general practice, where she would be away from hospitals and able to be nearer Peter. On telephoning him, she learned that he had decided to leave surgery. Being now less concerned about her consultant's reference, she took time off to recover from tonsillitis. She then went to stay with Peter for the weekend and told him what had happened on the ward. He was sympathetic and helped put the incident in perspective.

A year later, Debbie was in another teaching hospital in paediatrics, and despite regularly working long hours, was enjoying good clinical supervision and had resumed her original career plans. Peter was in medical publishing and only 60 miles away.

Several factors had helped her to get through her crisis: the temporary relief of knowing that she could leave hospital medicine if she wanted to; taking time off to recover from illness; catching up on sleep; and talking about her misery had been enough help at a critical period. Her next job was one with better senior support and this was enough to sustain her in working towards her career in paediatrics.

Being a junior doctor

- Long hours have been shown to affect young doctors' cognitive performance, mood, general health and functioning.
- Stressful factors reported by young doctors are long hours, the effects on personal life and concern about making mistakes.
- Mistakes happen most often through ignorance and inexperience. It is important to seek help, however uncomfortable this may be.
- Most junior doctors feel useful and are satisfied with their choice of medicine as a career.
- Stress-management techniques can be helpful: focus on cognitions, feelings and behaviour.

The profession of medicine

Being a medical student means learning about the discipline of medicine. However, more is learnt that is not part of the official medical curriculum. Implicit in medical training is showing students how to behave and act as doctors. Your medical education is a socialization into medicine. Socialization refers to a new recruit being exposed to the predominant norms (expected ways of behaving) and values of an occupation, and gradually absorbing these ideas until they become 'natural'. Students, for example, learn to take decisions, to deal or cope with cutting up bodies in pathology practicals, but also to adhere to a dress code on the wards, or to talk to patients and staff in a certain way. In other words, one learns to become a medical professional, as much as a medical doctor.

The nature of professions

Professions are an important element in the organization of medical care and the structure of society. The former refers to the position that the medical profession has in the health services; the latter refers to the way professions are regarded as special occupations in society. We could ask: 'What do professionals such as doctors, clergy, and lawyers have in common?' or 'What is the difference between doctors and rubbish collectors, two occupations we cannot really do without?' (Fig. 1).

  ■ What makes medicine a 'profession' rather than just an 'occupation'?

There are two main perspectives on the origin and nature of professions. Professions, in the older of the two perspectives, represent the institutionalization of altruistic values, since the professions are seen as committed to providing services for the common good. Thus, stockbrokers and company directors differ from teachers, lawyers and doctors in that the former occupations consist of people working for an immediate personal gain, be it money, prestige, or promotion. The latter occupations consist of people who are motivated not only by personal interest or by financial gains. Those engaged in a profession are often said to have a 'vocation', or a 'calling'. Sociologists who studied professions in the 1950s drew up lists of characteristics of professions as opposed to other occupations. Greenwood (1957) developed one such list:

1. systematic theory
2. authority recognized by its clientele
3. broader community sanction
4. code of ethics
5. professional culture sustained by formal sanctions.

The medical profession incorporates all the above features: (1) it has a theoretical basis; (2) patients come to doctors for advice/help, and also governments come to the medical profession for advice/help; (3) no one is allowed to practise medicine without a licence; (4) the Hippocratic oath and the Declaration of Geneva are its code of ethics and (5) it has strong professional organizations that guard

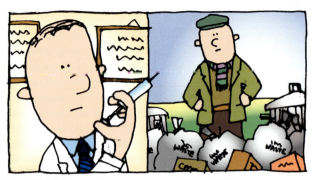

Fig. 1 'Which is more important for public health?'.

the quality of the work done by its members, leaving it relatively free of lay evaluation or legal contracts.

Continuous professional development, the doctor's obligation to keep up to date in both skills and knowledge, is part of this professional culture.

Professions and competition

More recent thinking approaches professions from the notion of 'autonomy', which is based on the profession being able to exercise power and control over, for example, other occupations. policy makers, and clients (Turner 1995). Such approaches emphasize competition between different occupations. For example, the crucial feature of the division

  ■ How altruistic is medicine as a profession?

The World Medical Association Declaration of Geneva: Physician's Oath

At the time of being admitted as a member of the medical profession:

I solemnly pledge to consecrate my life to the service of humanity;

I will give to my teachers the respect and gratitude which they are due;

I will practise my profession with conscience and dignity; the health of my patients will be my first consideration;

I will maintain by all means of power the honour and the noble traditions of the medical profession; my colleagues will be my brothers;

I will not permit considerations of religion, nationality, race, party politics or social standing to intervene between my duty and my patient;

I will maintain the utmost respect of human life from the time of conception, even under threat; I will not use my medical knowledge contrary to the laws of humanity;

I make these promises solemnly, freely and upon my honour.

of labour in health care is the control that doctors exercise over their own work and that of allied occupations. The original function of nursing, for example, was to serve the doctor. Today nursing has developed to a more autonomous profession with its own education (with professors of nursing in many universities), field of knowledge, control over its members and some power to exclude other occupations from its area of expertise. The maintenance of the medical profession requires the continuing exercise of dominance over allied and competing occupations. As a result the medical profession can be seen to possess an officially approved monopoly of the right to define health and illness, and to treat illness. For example, in many countries it is illegal to practise medicine without a licence.

Depending on which approach one takes, a profession is defined as either an altruistic occupation serving the common good or a particularly successful competitor in the occupational arena. Perhaps we can see elements of both approaches at different times or in different types of doctors.

■ What does it mean to be a 'professional'?

In many countries doctors belong to the best-paid categories of professionals. One way of being able to guarantee jobs for medical graduates is to limit the intake of students. Matching the supply of and demand for doctors maintains a sense of exclusiveness and enables the medical profession to claim a high remuneration.

Professions can be seen as occupations that somehow reduce risk and uncertainty in our lives. The priest, the lawyer and the doctor look after our soul, our well-being, and/or our body. Some have argued that this factor gives these occupations a higher status in society.

The organization of the medical profession

Doctors in nearly every country have a strong professional organization, which acts both as an advisory body to governments and the public and as a trade union. The medical view is often aired in prestigious medical journals,

which are in themselves part of the organization of the profession. More significantly, such medical journals are regarded as important by the general population and government officials, which makes them highly influential. The importance and influence of professions is not so much based on their claims, as on society's reaction to these claims. Aromatherapists, clinical psychologists, kinesiologists and faith healers make claims that are often not dissimilar to those made by doctors, but most people in industrialized societies put their faith most of the time in the medical profession and not in the other healers.

Challenges to medical autonomy

The medical profession is self-regulating in many countries, and in Britain it is regulated by the General Medical Council. Doctors often argue that the only person who can evaluate the work of a doctor is a fellow doctor. However, medical autonomy has been increasingly challenged and eroded in recent years:

- The state has varying degrees of control over professionals, such as regulating their income, training or the right to practice.
- Hospital administrators/managers and health-insurance companies have a certain amount of control over doctors. Managers can direct funding from one medical specialty to another, or from hospital- to community-based practitioners, while insurance companies can influence the kind and amount of medical interventions conducted.
- Challenges have also come from the professionalization of other 'paramedical' occupations, particularly nursing.
- Within medicine, there have been attempts to change the hierarchical structure of the profession and to embrace 'complementary' therapies such as homeopathy and acupuncture.
- Consumers (and patients) have begun to question the kind of services they receive. In Britain the introduction of the Patient Charter has changed the balance towards the lay public.
- The effectiveness of medical treatments has been challenged and the number of complaints against doctors has increased, and the number of court cases against doctors, especially in the USA, has made indemnity insurance very costly. The consequence of all these societal factors is that doctors have increasingly limited autonomy over medical issues.
- Negative media publicity has also led to calls for more control over the medical profession (pp 50–51).

Case study

The development of the medical profession in Britain

It was only as the 19th century progressed that doctors became the dominant group in treating illness. The British Medical Association was founded in 1832, and one role of the BMA was to transform the status of medicine into a profession ranking with other learned professions.

After 15 unsuccessful attempts to convince Parliament that doctors could be trusted with monopoly powers, the 1858 Medical Act unified the profession, combining surgeons, physicians and apothecaries, and created the General Medical Council, which was empowered to keep a register of qualified practitioners. As a result, employment positions were increasingly open only to registered doctors, particularly those posts controlled by the state's Poor Law hospitals and by the mutual Friendly Societies that provided insurance protection and medical care to working-class patients, often through trade unions. In 1911, again after successful political lobbying, the National Insurance Act brought the control of these Friendly Societies under local health committees with strong medical representation, thereby reducing the degree of external and lay control over these doctors' activities.

The profession of medicine

- Professionals are said to work towards professional standards, which are higher than the standards to which other occupations work.
- Professional standards combine an element of altruism with a well-developed system of quality control.
- Students are socialized into the profession.
- The state is the most limiting factor on professional freedom.
- The rise in importance of managers, other health practitioners and patients has eroded the professional power of doctors.

References

Abraham C, Sheeran P 2003 Acting on intentions: the role of anticipated regret. British Journal of Social Psychology 42: 495–511

Abraham-Van der Mark E (ed.) 1993 Successful home birth and midwifery: the Dutch model. Bergin & Garvey, Westport, CT, USA

Acheson D 1998 Independent inquiry into inequalities in health. The Stationery Office, London

Ahmedzai S 1982 Dying in hospital: the residents' viewpoint. British Medical Journal 285: 712–714

Ajzen I 1991 The theory of planned behavior. Organisational Behaviour and Human Decision Processes 50: 179–211

Albrecht GL, Devlieger PJ 1999 The disability paradox: high quality of life against all odds. Social Science and Medicine 48: 977–988

Alder EM 2002 How to assess quality of life: problems and methodology. In: Schneider HPG (ed.) Hormone replacement therapy and quality of life. Parthenon Publishing, Lancaster

Allbutt H, Amos A, Cunningham-Burley S 1995 The social image of smoking among young people in Scotland. Health Education Research 10: 443–454

Allen I 1994 Doctors and their careers: a new generation. Policy Studies Institute, London

Alonzo AA, Reynolds NR 1995 Stigma, HIV, and AIDS: an exploration and elaboration of a stigma trajectory. Social Science and Medicine 41: 303–35

American Psychiatric Association 2000 Diagnostic and statistical manual of mental disorders IV – text revision (DSM-IV-TR). American Psychiatric Association, Washington

Amos A, Cunningham-Burley S, Kerr EA 1998 The social and cultural impact of the new genetics. ESRC Risk and human behaviour programme, Grant No. L21125003

Anderson EA 1987 Preoperative preparation for cardiac surgery facilitates recovery, reduces psychological distress and reduces the incidence of acute postoperative hypertension. Journal of Consulting and Clinical Psychology 55: 513–520

Anionwu EN 1993 Sickle cell and thalassaemia: community experiences and official response. In: Ahmad W (ed.) 'Race' and health in contemporary Britain. Open University Press, Buckingham

Armitage CJ, Conner M 2001 Efficacy of the theory of planned behaviour: a meta-analytic review. British Journal of Social Psychology 40: 471–495

Armstrong D 1994 An outline of sociology as applied to medicine. Butterworth/Heinemann, London

ASH 2001a Smoking statistics: illness and death – fact sheet 2. ASH, London

ASH 2001b Smoking statistics: who smokes and how much – fact sheet 1. ASH, London

ASH 2002 Smoking and economics – basic facts 3. ASH, London

Ashton CH, Kamali F 1995 Personality, lifestyles, alcohol and drug consumption in a sample of British medical students. Medical Education 29: 187–192

Astin J 1998 Why patients use alternative medicine: results of a national study. Journal of the American Medical Association 279: 1548–1553

Baldwin PJ, Dodd M, Wrate RM 1997 Young doctors' health: attitudes health and behaviour. Social Science and Medicine 45: 35–40

Bancroft J 1989 Human sexuality and its problems. Churchill Livingstone, Edinburgh

Bandura A 1997 Self-efficacy: the exercise of control. Freeman, New York

Barsky AJ, Saintfort R, Rogers MP, Borus JF 2002 Nonspecific medication side effects and the nocebo phenomenon. Journal of the American Medical Association 287: 622–627

Bartley M, Blane D, Davey Smith G 1998 The sociology of health inequalities. Blackwell, Oxford

Batchelor S, Kitzinger J 1999 Teenage sexuality in the media. Health Education Board for Scotland, Edinburgh

Bates I 2001 The supply and consumption of over-the-counter drugs. In: Taylor K, Harding G (eds) Pharmacy practice. Taylor and Francis, London

Beale N, Nethercott S 1985 The health of industrial employees four years after compulsory redundancy. Journal of the Royal College of General Practitioners 37: 390–394

de Beauvoir S 1960 The second sex. Four Square Books Ltd, London

Becker HS 1961 Boys in white: student culture in medical school. University of Chicago Press, Chicago

Becker HM, Heafner DP, Kasl SV, Kirscht JP, Maiman LA, Rosenstock IM 1977 Selected psychosocial models and correlates of individual health-related behaviours. Medical Care 15 (suppl.): 27–46

Benzeval M, Dilnot A, Judge K, Taylor J 2001 'Putting the picture together: prosperity, redistribution, health and welfare'. In: Graham H (ed.) Understanding health inequalities. Open University Press, Buckingham

Berkman LF, Breslow L 1983 Health and ways of living: the Alameda County Study. Oxford University Press, Oxford

Bibace R, Walsh ME 1980 Development of children's concepts of illness. Pediatrics 66: 912–917

Biener L, Harris JE, Hamilton W 2000 Impact of the Massachusetts tobacco control programme: population based trend analysis. BMJ 321: 351–354

Biggs S 1999 The mature imagination: dynamics of identity in middlife and beyond. Open University Press, Buckingham

Birkhead JS on behalf of the Joint Audit Committee of the British Cardiac Society and a Cardiology Committee of the Royal College of Physicians of London 1992 Time delays in provision of thrombolytic treatment in six district hospitals. British Medical Journal 305: 445–448

Blackburn IM, Bishop S, Glen IM, Whalley LJ, Christie JE 1981 The efficacy of cognitive therapy in depression: a treatment trial using cognitive therapy and pharmacotherapy, each alone and in combination. British Journal of Psychiatry 139: 181–189

Blaxter M 1987 Self reported health. In: Cox, BD (ed.) The Health and Life style Survey. Health Promotion Trust, London

Blaxter M 1990 Health and lifestyles. Tavistock Routledge, London

Blaxter M, Paterson E 1982 Mothers and daughters: a three-generation study of health attitudes and behaviour. Heinemann, London

Bligh J 2002 The first year of doctoring: still a survival exercise. Medical Education 36: 2–3

Bloor M, McKeganey NP, Finlay A, Barnard MA 1992 The inappropriateness of psycho-social models of risk behaviour for understanding HIV-related risk practices among Glasgow male prostitutes. Aids Care 4: 131–137

BMA 1995 Alcohol: guidelines on sensible drinking. British Medical Association, London

Boakes RA, Popplewell DA, Burton M 1987 Eating habits. John Wiley, Chichester

Bond J, Coleman P 1990 Ageing in society: an introduction to social gerontology. Sage, London

Bosley CM, Fosbury JA, Cochrane GM 1995 The psychological factors associated with poor compliance with treatment in asthma. European Respiratory Journal 8: 899–904

Bower TGR 1977 A primer of infant development. WH Freeman, San Francisco

Bowlby J 1998 Attachment and loss, Vol 3. Loss, sadness and depression. Pimlico, London

Bowling A 1995a Measuring disease: A review of disease-specific quality of life measurement scales. Open University Press, Buckingham

Bowling A 1995b What things are important in people's lives? A survey of the public's judgements to inform scales of health related quality of life. Social Science and Medicine 41: 1447–1462

Bowling A 1997 Measuring health: A review of quality of life measurement scales. Open University Press, Buckingham

Bowling A 2002 Research methods in health, 2nd edn. Open University Press, Buckingham

Bradshaw J 1972 A taxonomy of social need. In McLachlan G (ed.) Problems and progress in medical care, 7th series. Oxford University Press, Oxford

Bramley G, Doogan K, Leather P et al (eds) 1987 Homelessness and the London housing market. School for Advanced Urban Studies, Bristol

Brandstater J, Greive W 1994 The ageing self: stabilising and protective processes. Developmental Review 14: 52–80

Brenner MH, Mooney A 1983 Unemployment and health: the context of economic change. Social Science and Medicine 17: 1125–1138

Brewin CR 2001 A cognitive neuroscience account of posttraumatic stress disorder and its treatment. Behaviour Research and Therapy 39: 373–393

Brewin CR, Firth-Cozens J 1997 Dependency and self-criticism as predicting depression in junior doctors. Journal of Occupational Health 2: 242–246

Bromley DB 1990 Behavioural gerontology: central issues in the psychology of ageing. Wiley, London

Brown GW 1978 Depression. In: Tuckett D, Kaufert JM (eds) Basic readings in medical sociology. Tavistock, London

Brown G, Davison S 1978 Social class, psychiatric disorder of mother and accidents to children. Lancet 1, 368–380

Brown GW, Harris T 1978 Social origins of depression. Tavistock Publications, London

Brown GW, Moran P 1994 Clinical and psychological origins of chronic depression episodes I: a community survey. British Journal of Psychiatry 165: 447–456

Brown G, Brolchain M, Harris T 1975 Social class and psychiatric disturbance among women in an urban population. Sociology 9: 225–254

Bruner JS 1983 Child's talk. Norton, New York

Buckman R 1994 How to break bad news. Pan Macmillan, London

Bunton R, Burrows R 1995 Consumption and health in the 'epidemiological' clinic of late modern medicine. In: Bunton R, Nettleton S, Burrows R (eds) The sociology of health promotion. Routledge, London

Burgess C, O'Donohoe A, Gill M 2000 Agony and ecstasy: a review of MDMA effects and toxicity. European Psychiatry 15: 287–294

Butterfield PS 1988 The stress of residency. Archives of Internal Medicine 148: 1428–1435

Buxton M 1985 Costs and benefits of the heart transplant programme at the Harefield and Papworth hospitals. HMSO, London

Bytheway B 1995 Ageism. Open University Press, Buckingham

Cairns E, Wilson R 1984 The impact of political violence on mild psychiatric morbidity in Northern Ireland. British Journal of Psychiatry 145: 631–635

Calman KC 1984 Quality of life in cancer patients – an hypothesis. Journal of Medical Ethics 10: 124–127

Campbell DA, Yellowlees PM, McLennan G et al 1995 Psychiatric and medical features of near fatal asthma. Thorax 50: 254–259

Campbell J, Elton RA 1994 Consultation, waiting, prescribing and referral patterns: some methodological considerations. Family Practice 11: 182–186

Campbell NC, Thain J, Deans HG, Ritchie LD, Rawles JM, Squair JL 1998 Secondary prevention clinics for coronary heart disease: randomised trial of effect on health. British Medical Journal 316: 1434–1437

Carlat DJ, Camargo CA, Herzog DB 1997 Eating disorders in males: a report on 135 patients. American Journal of Psychiatry 154: 1127–1132

Carpenter PA, Just MA, Shell P 1990 What one intelligence test measures: a theoretical account of the processing in the Raven Progressive Matrices Test. Psychological Bulletin 97: 404–431

Carson AJ, Ringbauer B, MacKenzie L, Warlow C, Sharpe M 2000 Neurological disease, emotional disorder and disability: they are related. A study of 300 consecutive new referrals to a neurology outpatient department. Journal of Neurology, Neurosurgery and Psychiatry 68: 202–206

Cartwright A 1982 The role of the general practitioner in helping the elderly widowed. Journal of the Royal College of General Practitioners 32: 215–227

Cassileth B 1998 The social implications of questionable cancer therapies. Cancer 63: 1247–1250

Cattell RB 1971 Abilities: their structure, growth and action. Houghton Mifflin, Boston

Cegala DJ, McGee DS, McNeilis KS 1996 Components of patients' and doctors' perceptions of communication competence during a primary care medical interview. Health Communication 8 (1): 1–27

Chadwick DJ, Gillat DA, Gingell JC 1991 Medical or surgical orchidectomy: the patients' choice. British Medical Journal 302: 572

Chaiken S 1980 Heuristic versus systematic information processing and the use of source versus message cues in persuasion. Journal of Personality and Social Psychology 37: 1397

Champion VL 1994 Strategies to increase mammography utilization. Medical Care 32: 118–129

Chappell AL, Goodley D, Lawthorn R 2001 Making connections: the relevance of the social model of disability for people with learning difficulties. British Journal of Learning Disabilities 29: 45–50

Clark D, Seymour J 1999 Reflections on palliative care. Open University Press, Buckingham

Clark D, Have H, Janssen R 2000 Common threads? Palliative care service developments in seven European countries. Palliative Medicine 14: 479–490

Clarke A 1995 Population screening for genetic susceptibility to disease. British Medical Journal 311: 35–38

Clarke V, Lovegrove H, Williams A, Macpherson M 2000 Unrealistic optimism and the health belief model. Journal of Behavioral Medicine 23: 367–376

Clement S 1995 Diabetes self-management education. Diabetes Care 18: 1204–1214

Coburn D 2000 Income inequality, social cohesion and the health status of populations: the role of neo-liberalism. Social Science and Medicine 51: 135–146

Cohen S, Herbert TB 1996 Health psychology: psychological factors and physical disease from the perspective of psychoneuroimmunology. Annual Review of Psychology 47: 113–142

Coker N (ed.) 2002 Understanding race and racism. Racism in medicine. An agenda for change. King's Fund Publishing, London

Coleman J, Hendry L 1999 The nature of adolescence, 3rd edn. Routledge, London

Coleman P, Bond J, Peace S 1993 Ageing in the twentieth century. In: Bond J, Coleman P, Peace S (eds) Ageing in society: an introduction to social gerontology, 2nd edn. Sage, London

Committee on Health Promotion 1996 Women and coronary heart disease (Guidelines for Health Promotion No. 45). Faculty of Public Health Medicine, London

Common Services Agency 1994 Scottish health statistics 1994. HMSO, Edinburgh

Conger JJ 1991 Adolescence and youth. Psychological development in a changing world, 4th edn. Harper Collins, New York

Cornwell J 1984 Hard-earned lives: accounts of health and illness from East London. Tavistock, London

Coupland N, Coupland J, Giles H 1991 Language, society and the elderly. Blackwell, Oxford

Cox J 1986 Postnatal depression. A guide for health professionals. Churchill Livingstone, Edinburgh

Cox T 1995 Coping and physical health. In: Broome A, Llewelyn S (eds) Health psychology: processes and applications. Chapman & Hall, London

Cox T, Griffiths A, Barlowe C, Randall R, Thomson L, Rial-Gonzalez E 2000 Organisational interventions for work stress: a risk management approach. HMSO, Norwich. Retrieved from www.hse.gov.uk/research/crr_htm/2000/crr00286.htm

Crawford R 1987 Cultural influences on prevention and emergence of a new health consciousness. In: Weinstein N (ed.) Taking care: understanding and encouraging self-protective behaviour. Cambridge University Press, Cambridge

Cromarty I 1996 What do patients think about during their consultations? A qualitative study. British Journal of General Practice 46: 525–528

Cunningham-Burley S, Boulton M 2000 The social context of the new genetics. In: Albrecht G, Fitzpatrick R, Scrimshaw C (eds) Handbook of social studies in health and medicine. Sage, London

Cunningham-Burley S, Irvine S 1987 'And have you done anything so far?' An examination of lay treatment of childrens' symptoms. British Medical Journal 295: 700–702

Cunningham–Burley S, Maclean U 1987 The role of the chemist in primary health care for children with minor complaints. Social Science and Medicine 24 (4): 371–377

Cunningham-Burley S, Maclean U 1991 Dealing with children's illness: mothers' dilemmas. In: Wyke S, Hewison J (eds) Child health matters. Open University Press, Milton Keynes

Cunningham-Burley S, Milburn K 1995 Health, health promotion and middle age. SOHHD Grant No. K/OPR/212/D64

Cunningham-Burley S, Irvine DA, Maclean U 1983–85 The cultural context of children's illnesses. SHHD

Davey Smith G, Shipley M, Rose G 1990 The magnitude and causes of socioeconomic differentials in mortality: further evidence from the Whitehall Study. Journal of Epidemiology and Community Health 285: 265–270

Davey Smith G, Shaw M, Mitchell R, Dorling D, Gordon D 2000 Inequalities in health continue to grow despite government's pledges. British Medical Journal 320: 582

Davidson RJ, Ekman P, Saron CD, Senulis JA, Friesen WV 1990 Approach-withdrawal and cerebral asymmetry: emotion expression and brain physiology 1. Journal of Personality and Social Psychology 58: 330–341

Davis MS 1968 Physiologic, psychological and demographic factors in patient compliance with doctor's orders. Medical Care 5: 115–122

Davison C, Davey Smith G, Frankel S 1991 Lay epidemiology and the prevention paradox: the implications of coronary candidacy for health education. Sociology of Health and Illness, 13: 1–19

Davison G, Neale JM 2001 Abnormal psychology, 8th edn. Wiley & Sons, London

DCCT Research Group 1993 The effect of intensive treatment of diabetes on the development and progression of long-term complications in insulin-dependent diabetes mellitus. New England Journal of Medicine 329: 977–986

Dennehy A, Smith L, Harker P 1997 Not to be ignored: young people, poverty and health. Child Poverty Action Group, London

Dennis M, Barbor TF, Roebuck MC, Donaldson J 2002 Changing the focus: the case for recognizing the treatment of cannabis use disorders. Addiction 97(suppl. 1): 4–15

Department of Health 1991 Drug misuse and dependence: guidelines on clinical management. HMSO, London

Department of Health 2001 Valuing people: a new strategy for learning disability for the 21st century (Cm 5086). The Stationery Office, London

Deutsch FM, Le Baron D, Fryer MN 1987 What is in a smile? Psychology of Women Quarterly 11: 341–352

Dingemans AE, Bruna MJ, van Furth EF 2002 Binge-eating disorder: a review. International Journal of Obesity 26: 299–307

Ditton J, Hammersley R 1996 A very greedy drug: cocaine in context. Harwood, Reading

Doll R, Peto R 1981 The causes of cancer. Oxford Medical Publications, Oxford University Press, Oxford

Donaldson LT, Donaldson RJ 2000 Essential public health, 2nd edn. Petroc Press, Newbury

Donaldson M 1978 Children's minds. Fontana, London

Donaldson ML, Elliot AS 1990 Children's explanations. In Grieve R, Hughes M (eds) Understanding children. Blackwell, Oxford

Donnelly M, McGilloway S, Mays N, Knapp M, Kavanagh S, Beecham J, Fenyo A 1996 Leaving hospital: one and two-year outcomes of long-stay psychiatric patients discharged to the community. Journal of Mental Health 5: 245–255

Donovan JL, Blake DR 1992 Patient non-compliance: deviance or reasoned decision-making. Social Science and Medicine 34: 507–513

Doyle D, Hanks GWC et al 1993 Oxford textbook of palliative medicine. Oxford University Press, Oxford

Drever F, Whitehead M (eds) 1997 Health inequalities: decennial supplement, DS 11. HMSO, London

Drever F, Whitehead M, Roden M 1996 Current patterns and trends in male mortality by social class (based on occupation). Population Trends No. 86, HMSO, London

Drewett RF, Young B, Wright P (1998) From feeds to meals: the development of hunger and food intake in infants and young children. In: Niven C A & Walker A (eds) The psychology of reproduction Vol. 3 Butterworth Heinemann pp. 204–217

Dye L, Blundell JE 1997 Menstrual cycle and appetite control: implications for weight regulation. Human Reproduction 12: 1142–1151

Eaker ED, Pinsky J, Castelli WP 1992 Myocardial infarction and coronary death among women: psychosocial predictors from a 20-year follow-up of women in the Framingham Study. American Journal of Epidemiology 135: 854–864

Ebbeling CB, Pawlak DB, Ludwig DS 2002 Childhood obesity: public-health crisis, common sense cure. The Lancet 360: 473–482

Edwards G 2000 Alcohol: the ambiguous molecule. Penguin, London

Egan G 1990 The skilled helper: a systematic approach to effective helping, 4th edn. Books/Cole, California

Egbert LD, Battit GE, Welch CE, Bartlett MK 1964 Reduction of post-operative pain by encouragement and instruction of patients. New England Journal of Medicine 270: 825–827

Egeland JA, Hotstetter AM 1983 Amish study, 1: affective disorders among the Amish, 1976–1980. American Journal of Psychiatry 140: 56–61

Eiser C, Havermans T, Casas R 1993 Healthy children's understanding of their blood: implications for explaining leukaemia to children. British Journal of Educational Psychology 63: 528–537

Ekman P 1993 Facial expression and emotion. American Psychology 48: 384–392

Ellershaw J, Ward C 2003 Care of the dying patient: the last hours or days of life. British Medical Journal 326: 30 34

Emerson E, Hatton C 1994 Moving out: relocation from hospital to community. HMSO, London

Erikson EH 1968 Identity: youth and crisis. Norton, New York

Erikson KT 1976 Loss of communality at Buffalo Creek. American Journal of Psychiatry 133: 302–305

Ernst E, White A 2000 The BBC survey of complementary medicine use in the UK. Complementary Therapies in Medicine 8: 32–36

European Bureau for Action on Smoking Prevention 1993 The labelling of tobacco products in the European Union. European Bureau for Action on Smoking Prevention, Brussels

Evans J, Heron J, Francomb H, Oke S, Golding J 2001 Cohort study of depressed mood during pregnancy and after childbirth. BMJ 323: 257–260

Eyer J 1977 Prosperity as a cause of death. International Journal of Health Services 7: 1

Eysenck HJ 1992 Psychosocial factors, cancer, and ischaemic heart disease. British Medical Journal 305: 457–459

Eysenck M 1996 Simply psychology. Psychology Press, Hove, pp. 115–131

Fagin L, Little M 1984 The forsaken families. Penguin, Harmondsworth

Fallowfield L 1990 The quality of life. The missing measurement in health care. Souvenir Press, London

Farrell M, Boys A, Bebbington P et al 2002 Psychosis and drug dependence: results from a national survey of prisoners. British Journal of Psychiatry 181: 393–398

Faulkner A 1995 Working with bereaved people. Churchill Livingstone, Edinburgh

Faulkner A et al 1994 Breaking bad news – a flow diagram. Palliative Medicine 8: 145–151

Ferguson E 2001 Personality and coping trials: a joint factor analysis. British Journal of Health Psychology 6: 311–325

Festinger L 1957 A theory of cognitive dissonance. Row Peterson, Evanston, Illinois

Fhanér G, Hane M 1979 Seat-belts: opinion effects of law-induced use. Journal of Applied Psychology 64: 205–212

File SE, Fluck E, Leahy A 2001 Nicotine has calming effects on stress-induced mood changes in females, but enhances aggressive mood in males. International Journal of Neuropsychopharmacology 4 (4): 371–376

Fiore MC, Bailey WC, Cohen SJ et al 1996 Smoking cessation. Agency for Health Care Policy and Research, US Department of Health and Human Services (clinical practice guideline No. 18, publication No. 96–0692), Rockville, MD

Field TM, Woodson R, Greenberg R, Cohen D 1982 Discrimination and imitation of facial expression by neonates. Science 218: 179–181

Firth S 1993 Cultural issues in terminal care. In: Clark D (ed.) The future for palliative care. Issues of policy and practice. Open University Press, Buckingham, pp. 98–110

Firth S 2001 Wider horizons. Care of the dying in a multicultural society. National Council for Hospice and Specialist Palliative Care Services, London

Firth-Cozens J 1986 Levels and sources of stress in medical students. British Medical Journal 292: 1177–1180

Firth-Cozens J 1987 Emotional distress in junior house officers. British Medical Journal 295: 533–536

Firth-Cozens J 1996 Stress in doctors: a longitudinal study. Unpublished report for the Department of Health, Research and Development Division

Firth-Cozens J 1998 Individual and organisational predictors of depression in general practitioners. British Journal of General Practice 48: 1647–1651

Firth-Cozens J 2001 Interventions to improve physicians' well-being and patient care. Social Science and Medicine 52: 215–222

Fisher K, Johnston M 1996 Experimental manipulation of perceived control and its effect on disability. Psychology and Health 11: 657–669

Fisher S 1986 Stress and strategy. Lawrence Erlbaum, London

Fitzpatrick R 1994 Health needs assessment, chronic illness and the social. In: Popay J, Williams G (eds) Researching the people's health. Routledge, London

Flynn JR 1987 Massive IQ gains in 14 nations: what IQ tests really measure. Psychological Bulletin 101: 171–191

Foster GD, Sarwer DB, Wadeen TA 1997 Psychological effects of weight-cycling in obese persons: a review and research agenda. Obesity Research 5: 474–488

Foxwell M, Alder E 1993 More information equals less anxiety. Anxiety and screening: an intervention by nurses. Professional Nurse 9: 322–336

Frankel S, Ebrahim S, Davey Smith G 2000 The limits to demand for health care. British Medical Journal 321: 40–44

Frasure-Smith N, Lesperance F, Talajic M 1995 Coronary heart disease/myocardial infarction: depression and 18-month prognosis after myocardial infarction. Circulation 91: 999–1005

Freeman GK, Horder JP, Howie JGR, Hungin AP, Hill AP, Shah NC, Wilson A 2002 Evolving general practice consultations in Britain: issues of length and context. British Medical Journal 324: 880–882

Freidson E 1975 Profession of medicine – a study of the sociology of applied knowledge. University of Chicago Press, London

Friedman M, Thoresen CE, Gill JJ et al 1986 Alteration of type A behavior and its effect on cardiac recurrences in post myocardial infarction patients: summary results of the Recurrent Coronary Prevention Project. American Heart Journal 112: 653–665

Fulder SJ, Munro R 1982 The status of complementary medicine in the United Kingdom. Threshold Foundation, London

Gannon L 2000 Psychological well-being in aging women. In: Usher JM (ed.) Women's health. Contemporary international perspectives. BPS Books, Leicester, pp. 476–484

Gardner H 2001 Intelligence reframed: multiple intelligences for the 21st century. Basic Books

General Medical Council 1993 Tomorrow's doctors. GMC, London

General Medical Council 2002 http://www.gmc-uk.org/med_ed/tomdoc.htm

General Medical Council (UK) 1995 Duties of a doctor. GMC, London

Gillon R 1994 Principles of health care ethics. Wiley, Chichester

Gill P, de Wildt G 2002 Housing and health: the role of primary care. Radcliffe Medical Press, Oxford

Glasgow RE, La Chance P, Toobert DJ, Brown J, Hampson SE, Riddle MC 1997 Long term effects and costs of brief behavioural dietary intervention delivered in the medical office. Patient Education and Counseling 32: 175–184

Goffman E 1968a Stigma. Penguin, London

Goffman E 1968b Asylums. Penguin, Harmondsworth

Goldberg EM, Morrison SL 1963 Schizophrenia and social class. British Journal of Psychiatry 109: 785

Gollwitzer PM 1993 Goal achievement: the role of intentions. European Review of Social Psychology 4: 142–185

Gollwitzer PM 1999 Implementation intentions: strong effects of simple plans. American Psychologist, 54: 493–503

Gordon RA 1990 Anorexia and bulimia. Blackwell, Oxford

Gorwood P, Bouvard M, Mouren-Simeoni MC, Kipman A, Ades J 1998 Genetics of anorexia nervosa: a review of candidate genes. Psychiatric Genetics 8: 1–12

Gossarth-Maticek R, Schmidt P, Vetter H, Arndt S 1984 Psychotherapy research in oncology. In: Steptoe A, Mathews A (eds) Health care and human behaviour. Academic Press, London

Gotzsche PC, Olsen O 2000 Is screening for breast cancer with mammography justified? The Lancet 355: 129–134

Graham H 1984 Women, health and the family, Harvester Wheatsheaf, Hemel Hempstead

Graham H (ed.) 2000 Understanding health inequalities. Open University Press, Milton Keynes

Grant L 1998 Remind me who I am, again. Granta Books, London

Grant G, Nolan M 1993 Informal carers: sources and concomitants of satisfaction. Health and Social Care in the Community 1: 147–159

Green H 1988 Informal carers: agenda for action. A report to the Secretary of State for Social Services. HMSO, London

Greenfield S 2000 Brain story. BBC Worldwide Ltd, London

Greenfield SM, Innes MA, Allan TF, Wearn A 2002 First year medical student's perceptions and use of complementary and alternative medicines. Complementary Therapies in Medicine 10: 27–32

Greenwood 1957 Attributes of a profession. Social Work 2: 45–55

Greer S, Morris TE, Pettingale KW 1979 Psychological responses to breast cancer: effect on outcome. Lancet ii: 785–787

Griffiths R 1989 Community care: agenda for action. HMSO, London (The Griffiths Report)

Guildford JP 1967 The nature of intelligence. McGraw Hill, New York

Hallowell N 2000 Doing the right thing: genetic risk and responsibility. In: Conrad P, Gabe J (eds) Sociological perspectives on the new genetics. Blackwell Publishers, Oxford

Hammen C 1997 Depression. Psychology Press Ltd, Hove

Hammersley R, Reid M 2002 Why the pervasive addiction myth is still believed. Addiction Research and Theory 10: 7–30

Hankin BL, Abramson LY 1999 Development of gender differences in depression: description and possible explanations. Annals of Medicine 31: 372–379

Hannay D 1979 The symptom iceberg – a study of community health. Routledge and Kegan Paul, London

Harding S et al 1997 Office for National Statistics, The Stationery Office, London

Harrison JA, Mullen PD, Green LW 1992 A meta-analysis of studies of the health belief model with adults. Health Education Research 7: 107–116

Harrison S, Hunter DJ 1994 Rationing health care. Institute for Public Policy Research, London.

Hassell K, Rodgers A, Noyce P, Nicolaas G 1998 Advice provided in British community pharmacies: what people want and what they get. Journal of Health Services Research and Policy 3: 219–225

Hassell K, Rodgers A, Noyce P 2000 Community pharmacy as a primary health and self-care resource: a framework for understanding pharmacy utilization. Health and Social Care in the Community 8: 40–49

Haster F 1991 The international year of disabled people. Disability Now, January

Hawton K, Salkovskis PM, Kirk J, Clark DM 1989 Cognitive behaviour therapy for psychiatric problems: a practical guide. Oxford Medical Publications, Oxford

Health and Care Group 1999 The future of health and care of older people: the best is yet to come. Age Concern, London

Health and Safety Executive 2000a Revitalising health and safety. HSE, Suffolk

Health and Safety Executive 2000b Securing health together. HSE, Suffolk

Health Committee 1992 Maternity services second report. Vol 1 (Winterton Report), HMSO, London

Heather N, Robinson I 1983 Controlled drinking. Routledge, London

Heather N, Robinson I 1996 Let's drink to your health! Routledge, Oxford

HEBS/ASH Scotland 2001 Helping smokers to stop and stay stopped – a guide for health professionals. HEBS/ASH Scotland, Edinburgh

Hemingway H, Marmot M 1999 Evidence based cardiology: psychosocial factors in the aetiology and prognosis of coronary heart disease: systematic review of prospective cohort studies. British Medical Journal 318: 1460–1467

Henderson L, Kitzinger J 1999 The human drama of genetics: 'hard' and 'soft' media representations of inherited breast cancer. Sociology of Health and Illness 21: 560–578

Henderson L, Kitzinger J, Green J 2000 Representing infant feeding: content analysis of British media portrayals of bottle feeding and breastfeeding. British Medical Journal 321: 1196–1198

Hepworth M 1995 Images of old age. In: Nussbaum JF, Coupland J (eds) Handbook of communication and ageing research. Lawrence Erlbaum, Mahwah, NJ

Herbert JD, Lilienfeld SO, Lohr JM, Montgomery RW, O'Donohue WT, Rosen GM, Tolin DF 2000 Science and pseudoscience in the development of eye movement desensitisation and reprocessing: implications for clinical psychology. Clinical Psychology Review 20: 945–971

Higginson I 1993 Clinical audit in palliative care. Radcliffe Medical Press, Oxford

Hill MJ, Harrison RH, Talbot V 1973 Men out of work. Cambridge University Press, Cambridge

Hilton S, Sibbald B, Anderson HR, Freeling P 1986 Controlled evaluations of the effects of patient education on asthma morbidity in general practice. The Lancet 1: 26–29

Hilts PJ 1995 Memory's ghost. Simon & Schuster, New York

Holland M, Youngs C 1990 Mental handicap. In: Primary care for people with a mental handicap. Occasional paper 47. Royal College of General Practitioners, London

Holman H, Lorig K 2000 Patients as partners in managing chronic disease. British Medical Journal 320: 526–527

Holmes TH, Rahe RH 1967 The social readjustment scale. Journal of Psychosomatic Research 11: 213–218

Hopton JL, Dlugolecka M 1995 Patients' perceptions of need for primary health care services: useful for priority setting? British Medical Journal 310: 1237–1240

Horne R, James D, Petrie K, Weinman J, Vincent R 2000 Patients' interpretation of symptoms as a cause of delay in reaching hospital during myocardial infarction. Heart 83: 388–393

House of Lords 2000 Select Committee on Science and Technology, Sixth Report. Stationery Office, London

Howe MJA 1997 IQ in question: the truth about intelligence. Sage, London

Howells G 1991 Mental handicap – care in the community. British Journal of General Practitioners 41: 2–4

Howie JGR, Porter AMD, Heaney DJ, Hopton JL 1991 Long to short consultation ratio: a proxy measure of quality of care for general practice. British Journal of General Practice 41: 48–54

Howie JGR, Hopton JL, Heaney DJ, Porter AMD 1992 Attitudes to medical care, the organisation of work, and stress among general practitioners. British Journal of General Practice 42: 181–185

Howie JGR, Heaney D, Maxwell M, Walker J 1998 A comparison of a patient enablement instrument (PEI) against two established patient satisfaction scales as an outcome measure of primary care consultations. Family Practice 15: 165–171

Hunt S 1997 Housing-related disorders. In: Charlton J, Murphy M (eds) The health of adult Britain 1841–1994. Vol 1. Office for National Statistics. Decennial supplement No 12, The Stationery Office, London. Chapter 10, pp 156–170

Hunter M 1993 Counselling in obstetrics and gynaecology. BPS Books, Leicester

Illsley R 1986 Occupational class, selection and inequalities in health. Quarterly Journal of Social Affairs 2: 151–165

Ineichen B 1987 Measuring the rising tide: how many dementia cases will there be by 2001? British Journal of Psychiatry 150: 193–200

Information and Statistics Division 1996 Scottish Health Statistics 1995. Common Services Agency, Edinburgh

Innes NJ, Reid A, Halstead J, Watkin SW, Harrison BD 1998 Psychosocial risk factors in near-fatal asthma and in asthma deaths. Journal of the Royal College of Physicians London 32: 430–434

Irvine S, Cunningham-Burley S 1991 Mothers' concepts of normality, behavioural change and illness in their children. British Journal of General Practice 42: 371–374

James W 1884 What is an emotion. Mind 9: 188–205

Janis LL 1958 Psychological stress. Wiley, New York

Janssen I, Hanssen M, Bak M, Bijl RV, De Graaf R, Vollergh W 2003 Discrimination and delusional ideation. British Journal of Psychiatry 182: 71–76

Janz NK, Becker HM 1984 The health belief model: a decade later. Health Education Quarterly 11: 1–47

Jerram KL, Coleman PS 1999 The big five personality traits and reporting of health problems and health behaviour in old age. British Journal of Health Psychology 4: 181–192

Jerrome D 1992 Good company: an anthropological study of old people in groups. Edinburgh University Press, Edinburgh

Johnston G, Abraham C 2000 Managing awareness: negotiating and coping with a terminal prognosis. International Journal of Palliative Nursing 6: 485–494

Johnston M 1980 Anxiety in surgical patients. Psychological Medicine 10: 145–152

Johnston M 1987 Emotions and cognitive aspects of anxiety in surgical patients. British Journal of Clinical Psychology 21: 255–261

Johnston M 1988 Impending surgery. In: Fisher S, Reason J (eds) Handbook of life stress, cognition and health. Wiley, London, pp. 79–100

Johnson M 2003 Ethnic diversity in social context. In: Kai J (ed.) Ethnicity, health and primary care. Oxford University Press, Oxford

Johnston M, Vogele C 1993 Benefits of psychological preparation for surgery: a meta-analysis. Annals of Behavioral Medicine 15: 245–256

Johnston M, Wright S, Weinman J 1995 Measures in health psychology: a user's portfolio. NFER-Nelson, Windsor

Jones A, McArdle PJ, O'Neill PA 2002 Perceptions of how well graduates are prepared for the role of pre-registration house officer: a comparison of outcomes from a traditional and an integrated PBL curriculum. Medical Education 36: 16–25

Jones PK, Jones SL, Katz J 1987 Improving compliance for asthmatic patients visiting the emergency department using a health belief model intervention. Journal of Asthma 24: 199–206

Judge K, Paterson I 2001 Poverty, income, inequality and health. Treasury Working Paper 01/29 The Treasury, Wellington

Kai J, Bhopal R 2003 Ethnic diversity in health and disease. In: Kai J (ed.) Ethnicity, health and primary care. Oxford University Press, Oxford

Karasek RA 1979 Job demands, job decisions latitude and mental strain: implications for job design. Administrative Science Quarterly 24: 285–308

Katz AH, Bender EI (eds) 1976 The strength in us: self-help groups in the modern world. Franklin Watts, New York

Kaye P 1996 Breaking bad news (pocket book). EPL Publications, Northampton

Kelleher D 1994 Self-help groups and their relationship to medicine. In: Gabe J, Kelleher D, Williams G 1994 Changing medicine. Routledge, London, pp. 104–117

Kelly M 1991 Coping with an ileostomy. Social Science and Medicine 33: 115–125

Kelly M 1992 Colitis. Routledge, London

Kelly MP, Sullivan F 1992 The productive use of threat in primary care: behavioural responses to health promotion. Family Practice 9: 476–480

Kessler RC, Sonnega A, Bromet E, Hughes M, Nelson CB 1995 Posttraumatic stress disorder in the National Comorbidity Survey. Archives of General Psychiatry 52: 1048–1060

Kiecolt-Glaser JK, Garner W, Speicher CE, Penn GM, Holliday J, Glaser R 1994 Psychosocial modifiers of immunocompetence in medical students. Psychosomatic Medicine 46: 7–14

Kiecolt-Glaser JK, Marucha PT, Marlakey WB, Mercado AM, Glaser R 1995 Slowing of wound healing by psychological stress. The Lancet 346: 1194–1196

King JB 1982 The impact of patients' perceptions of high blood pressure on attendance at screening. An extension of the health belief model. Social Science and Medicine 16: 1079–1091

Kingston R 2001 It's only natural. Chemistry in Britain January: 18–21

Kinmonth A, Woodcock A, Griffin S, Spiegal N, Campbell N 1998 Randomised controlled trial of patient centred care of diabetes in general practice: impact on current well-being and future disease risk. British Medical Journal 317: 1202–1208

Kinnersley P, Stott N, Peters T, Harvey I 1999 The patient-centredness of consultations and outcome in primary care. British Journal of General Practice 49: 711–716

Kister MC, Patterson CJ 1980 Children's conceptions of the causes of illness: understanding of contagion and use of immanent justice. Child Development 51: 839–846

Kitwood T 1997 Dementia reconsidered: the person comes first. Open University Press, Buckingham

Kitzhaber JA 1993 'Prioritising health services in an era of limits: the Oregon experience'. British Medical Journal 307: 373–376

Kitzinger J 1995 'The face of AIDS'. In: Markova I, Farr R (eds) Representations of health and illness. Harwood Academic Publishers, Newark

Kitzinger J 2001 Transformations of public and private knowledge: audience reception, feminism and the experience of childhood sexual abuse. Feminist Media Studies 1: 91–104

Klee H, Morris J 1997 Amphetamine misuse: the effects of social context on injection related risk behaviour. Addiction Research 4: 329–342

Klein R, Day P, Redmayne S 1996 Managing scarcity. Open University Press, Buckingham

Kleinman A 1985 Indigenous systems of healing: questions for professional, popular and folk care. In: Salmon J (ed.) Alternative medicines: popular and policy perspectives. Tavistock, London

Klemm P, Repperty K, Lori V 1998 A non-traditional cancer support group: the internet. Computers in Nursing 16: 31–36

Korsch BM, Gozzi EK, Francis V 1968 Gaps in doctor–patient communication: 1. Doctor–patient interaction and patient satisfaction. Pediatrics 42: 855–871

Kubler-Ross E 1970 On death and dying. Tavistock Publications, London

Kury SP, Rodrigue JR 1995 Concepts of illness causality in a pediatric sample. Clinical Pediatrics 34: 178–182

Lader D, Meltzer H 2001 Drinking: adults' behaviour and knowledge in 2000. Office for National Statistics, London

Lam DH 1991 Psychosocial family intervention in schizophrenia: a review of empirical studies. Psychological Medicine 21: 423–441

Langrish M 1981 Assertiveness training. In: Cooper CL (ed.) Improving interpersonal relations. Gower Press, Epping

Lazarus R 1980 Stress and coping paradigm. In: Bond L, Rosen J (eds) Competence and coping during adulthood. University Press of New England, Hanover, NH

Lazarus RS 1991 Cognition and motivation in emotion. American Psychologist 46: 352–367

Leatherman S, Berwick DM 2000 The NHS through American eyes. British Medical Journal 321: 1545–1546

Leeson J, Gray L 1978 Women and health. Tavistock, London

Leff J, Trieman N, Gooch C 1996 The TAPS Project 33: Prospective follow-up of long stay patients discharged from two psychiatric hospitals. American Journal of Psychiatry 153: 1318–1324

Lemert E 1951 Social pathology. McGraw Hill, New York

Leventhal H 1971 Fear appeals and persuasion: the differentiation of a motivational construct. American Journal of Public Health 61: 1208–1224

Leventhal H, Benyamini Y, Brownlee S, Diefenbach M, Leventhal EA, Patrick-Miller L, Robitaille C 1997 Illness representations: theoretical foundations. In: Petrie KJ, Weinman J (eds) Perceptions of health and illness: current research and applications. Harwood Academic, Amsterdam, pp. 19–45

Levine JD, Gordon NC, Fields H L 1978 The mechanisms of placebo analgesia. The Lancet 2(8091): 654–57

Levine M 1988 An analysis of medical assistance. American Journal of Community Psychology 16: 167–188

Levinson DJ, Darrow DN, Klein EB, Levinson MH, McKee B 1978 The seasons of a man's Life. Knopf, New York

Levy LH, Derby JF 1992 Bereavement support groups: who joins; who does not; and why? American Journal of Community Psychology 20: 649–662

Lewis G, Sloggett A 1998 Suicide, deprivation and unemployment: record linkage study. British Medical Journal 317: 1283–1286

Lewith G, Jones WB, Wlach H 2002 Clinical research in complementary therapies. Churchill Livingstone, Edinburgh

Ley P 1997 Communicating with patients; improving communication, satisfaction and compliance. Stanley Thornes Publishers, Cheltenham

Ley P, Llewelyn S 1995 Improving patients' understanding, recall, satisfaction, and compliance. In: Broome AK (ed.) Health psychology: processes and applications. Chapman and Hall, London

Ley P, Whitworth MA, Woodward R, Pinsent RJFH, Pike LA, Clarkson M E, Clark PB 1976 Improving doctor–patient communication in general practice. Journal of the Royal College of General Practitioners 26: 720–724

Leydon GM, Boulton M, Moynihan C, Jones A, Mossman J, Boudioni M, McPherson K 2000 Cancer patients' information needs and information seeking behaviour: in depth interview study. British Medical Journal 320: 909–913

Lingenfelser T, Kaschel R, Weber A, Zaiser-Kapel H, Jakober B, Kuper J 1994 Young hospital doctors after night duty: their task specific cognitive status and emotional condition. Medical Education 28: 566–572

Little P, Everitt H, Williamson I et al 2001 Preferences of patients for patient centred approach to consultation in primary care: observational study. British Medical Journal 322: 468–472

Lock P et al 1985 Action on smoking at work. ASH, London

Low JTS, Payne S 1996 The good and bad death perceptions of health professionals in palliative care. European Journal of Cancer Care 5: 237–241

Luck M, Bamford M, Williamson P 2000 Men's health: perspectives, diversity and paradox. Blackwell Sciences, Oxford

Lydeard S, Jones R 1989 Factors affecting the decision to consult with dyspepsia: comparison of consulters and non-consulters. Journal of the Royal College of General Practitioners 39: 495–498

MacDonald ML, Butler AK 1974 Reversal of helplessness: producing walking behaviour in nursing home wheelchair residents using behavior modification procedures. Journal of Gerontology 29: 97–101

Mackay J, Eriksen M 2002 The tobacco atlas. WHO, Geneva

MacLeod S 1981 The art of starvation. Virago, London

Macpherson W 1999 The Stephen Lawrence inquiry report. The Stationery Office, London

Maguire P, Fairbairn S, Fletcher C 1986 Consultation skills of young doctors. British Medical Journal 292: 1573–1578

Main C, Spanswick C, Bond M 1999 Pain management. Churchill Livingstone, Edinburgh

Manuck SB, Kaplan JR, Clarkson TB 1983 Social instability and coronary artery atherosclerosis in cynomolgus monkeys. Neuroscience and Behavioural Reviews 7: 485–491

Marks IM 1986 Genetics of fear and anxiety disorders. British Journal of Psychiatry 149: 406–418

Marmot M, Wilkinson RG (eds) 1999 Social determinants of health. Oxford University Press, Oxford

Marmot M, Adelstein AM, Bulusu L, Shukla V 1984 Immigrant mortality in England and Wales 1970–78 (OPCS Studies on Population and Medical Subjects: No. 47). HMSO, London

Marteau TM 1989 Psychological costs of screening. British Medical Journal 299: 527

Marteau TM 1993 Health related screening: psychological predictors of uptake and impact. In: Maes S, Leventhal H, Johnston M (eds) International review of health psychology. Wiley, Chichester

Marteau T, Anionwu E 1996 Evaluating carrier testing: objectives and outcomes. In: Marteau T, Richards M (eds) The troubled helix. Cambridge University Press, Cambridge

Martin et al 1988 – reference incomplete to be completed by MarieJohnston

Martin M, Block JE, Sanchez SD, Arnaud CD, Beyene Y 1993 Menopause without symptoms: the endocrinology of menopause among rural Mayan Indians. American Journal of Obstetrics and Gynecology 168: 1839–1845

Mathews A, Ridgeway V 1984 Psychological preparation for surgery. In: Steptoe A, Mathews A (eds) Health care and human behaviour. Academic Press, London

McDonald IG et al 1996 Opening Pandora's box: the unpredictability of reassurance by a normal test result. British Medical Journal 313: 329–332

McGee HM, O'Boyle CA, Hickery A, O'Malley K, Joyce CR 1991 Assessing the quality of life of the individual: the SEIQoL with a health and gastroenterology unit population. Psychological Medicine 21: 749–759

McGuffin P, Katz R, Watkins S, Rutherford J 1996 A hospital-based twin register of the heritability of DSM-IV unipolar depression. Archives of General Psychiatry 53: 129–136

McKeown T 1979 The role of medicine: dream, mirage or nemesis? Blackwell, Oxford

McKinlay JB 1973 Social networks, lay consultation and help seeking behaviour. Social Forces 51: 279–292

McKinnis KJ 2000 Exercise and obesity. Coronary Artery Disease 11: 111–116

McLauchlan CAJ 1990 Handling distressed relatives and breaking bad news. British Medical Journal 301: 1145–1149

McManus IC, Richards P, Winder BC 1999 Intercalated degrees, learning styles, and career preferences: prospective longitudinal study of UK medical students. British Medical Journal 319: 542–546

McNally RJ, Steketee GS 1985 The etiology and maintenance of severe animal phobia. Behavior Research and Therapy 23: 431–436

McQuay HJ, Moore RA, Eccleston C, Morley S, Williams AC 1997 Systematic review of outpatient services for chronic pain control. Health Technology Assessment 1(6): i–iv, 1–135

McWhinney I 1989 The need for a transformed clinical method. In: Steward M, Roter D (eds) Communicating with medical patients. Sage, London

Mead N, Bower P 2000 Patient-centredness: a conceptual framework and review of the empirical literature. Social Science and Medicine 51: 1087–1110

Mead N, Bower P, Hann M 2002 The impact of general practitioners' patient-centredness on patients' post-consultation satisfaction and enablement. Social Science and Medicine 55: 283–299

Mehler PS 2001 Diagnosis and care of patients with anorexia nervosa in primary care settings. Annals of Internal Medicine 134: 1048–1059

Melzack R 1987 The short form McGill pain questionnaire. Pain 20: 191–197

Melzack R, Wall PD. The textbook of pain, 4th edn. Churchill Livingstone, 1999

Miles A 1991 Women, health and medicine. Open University Press, Buckingham

Milgram S 1963 Behavioural study of obedience. Journal of Abnormal and Social Psychology 67: 371–378

Milgram S 1974 Obedience to authority. Tavistock, London

Miller D, Kitzinger J, Eilliams K, Beharrell P 1998 The circuit of mass communication: media strategies, representation and audience reception in the AIDS crisis. Sage, London

Miller PMcC 1994 The first year at medical school: some findings and student perceptions. Medical Education 28: 5–7

Miller TQ, Smith TW, Turner CW, Guijarro ML, Hallet AJ 1996 A meta-analytic review of research on hostility and physical health. Psychological Bulletin 119: 322–348

Miller WR, Rollnick S 1991 Motivational interviewing: preparing people to change addictive behaviour. Guilford Press, London

Miller WR, Sanchez-Craig M 1996 How to have a high success rate in alcohol treatment. Addiction 91: 779–785

Mills S, Bone K 2000 Principles and practice of phytotherapy. Modern herbal medicine. Churchill Livingstone, Edinburgh, p. 544

Mischel W 1968 Personality assessment. Wiley, New York

Molfino NA, Nannini LJ, Rebuck AS, Slutsky AS 1992 The fatality-prone asthmatic patient. Follow-up study after near-fatal attacks. Chest 101: 621–623

Morgan A, Whent H, Sayers M 1991 Smoking. Health Education Authority, London

Morisky DE, Green LW, Levine DM 1986 Concurrent and predictive validity of a self-report measure of medication adherence. Medical Care 24: 67–74

Morley S, Eccleston C, Williams A 1999 Systematic review and meta-analysis of RCT trials of cognitive behaviour therapy and behaviour therapy for chronic pain. Pain 80: 1–13

Morris JK, Cook DG, Shaper AG 1994 Loss of employment and mortality. British Medical Journal 308: 1135–1139

Moser KA, Fox AJ, Jones DR 1984 Unemployment and mortality in the OPCS longitudinal study. The Lancet ii: 1324–1329

Moss F, McManus C 1992 The anxieties of new clinical students. Medical Education 26: 17–20

Muldoon MF, Barger S, Flory JD, Manuck AQ 1998 What are quality of life measurements measuring? British Medical Journal 16: 542–545

Mullen K 1993 A healthy balance: Glaswegian men talking about health, tobacco and alcohol. Avebury, Aldershot

Mullen P D 1997 Compliance becomes concordance. British Medical Journal 314: 691–692

Myers F 1982 Nonbehavioural testing of the newborn infant. Clinics in Perinatology 9: 191–214

Myers LB, Midence K 1998 Concepts and issues in adherence. In: Myers LB, Midence K (eds) Adherence to treatment in medical conditions. Harwood Academic Publishers, Amsterdam, pp. 1–24

National Center for Health Statistics 1995 Health, United States 1994.

Public Health Service, Hyattsville MD: Table 77

National Council for Hospice and Specialist Palliative Care Services 1997 Making palliative care better. Quality improvement, multiprofessional audit and standards. Occasional Paper, 12 March 1997

National Council for Hospice and Specialist Palliative Care Services 2000 Specialist palliative care. Palliative care 2000. Commissioning through partnership

Navarro V 1989 Why some countries have national health insurance, others have national health services, and the US has neither. Social Science and Medicine 28: 887–898

Naysmith A, O'Neill W 1989 Hospice. In: Sherr L (ed.) Death, dying and bereavement. Blackwell Scientific Publications, Oxford, pp. 1–16

Neale J 2002 Drug users in society. Palgrave, London

Neisser U et al 1996 Intelligence: knowns and unknowns. American Psychologist 51: 77–101

Nerenz DR, Leventhal H, Love RR 1982 Factors contributing to emotional distress during chemotherapy. Cancer 50: 1020–1027

Newbury-Birch D, White M, Kamali F 2000 Factors influencing alcohol and illicit drug use amongst medical students. Drug and Alcohol Dependence 59: 125–130

Newbury-Birch D, Walshaw D, Kamali F 2001 Drink and drugs: from medical students to doctors. Drug and Alcohol Dependence 64: 265–270

Newcomb MD 1995 Identifying high-risk youth: prevalence and patterns of adolescent drug abuse. In: Rahdert E, Czechowicz D (eds) Adolescent drug abuse: clinical assessment and therapeutic interventions. NIDA Research Monograph 156, National Institute on Drug Abuse, Rockville MD

Nicolson P 1998 Postnatal depression: psychology, science and the transition to motherhood. Routledge, London

Nuffield Council on Bioethics 1993 Genetic screening. Ethical issues. Nuffield Council on Bioethics, London

Office for National Statistics 1997 Living in Britain 1995. HMSO, London

Orbell S, Hodgkins S, Sheeran P 1997 Implementation intentions and the theory of planned behaviour.

Personality and Social Psychology Bulletin 23: 953–962

Orford J 2000 Excessive appetites: a psychological view of addiction, 2nd edn. Wiley, Chichester

Osman L 1998 Health habits and illness behaviour: social factors in patient self-management. Respiratory Medicine 92: 150–155

Osman LM, Russell IT, Friend JA, Legge JS, Douglas JG 1993 Predicting patient attitudes to asthma medication. Thorax 48: 827–830

Osman LM, Calder C, Godeen DJ, Friend JAR, Legge JS, Douglas JG 2002 A randomised trial of self management planning for adult patients admitted to hospital with acute asthma. Thorax 57: 869–874

Ostrowski J 1989 Thinking about drug legalization. Cato Institute Paper No. 121. Cato Institute, Washington DC

Paice E, Rutter H, Wetherall M, Winder B, McManus IC 2002 Stressful incidents, stress and coping strategies in the pre-registration house officer year. Medical Education 36: 56–65

Palmore E 1997 Facts on aging: a short quiz. The Gerontologist Magazine

Parkes CM 1975 Bereavement. Studies of grief in adult life. Penguin Books, Harmondsworth

Parkes CM 1980 Bereavement counselling: does it work? British Medical Journal 281: 3–6

Parsons L, Macfarlane A, Golding J 1993 Pregnancy, birth and maternity care. In: Ahmad W (ed.) 'Race' and health in contemporary Britain. Open University Press, Buckingham

Patterson J, Barlow J, Mockford C et al 2002 Improving mental health through parenting programmes: block randomised controlled trial. Archives of Diseases in Childhood 87: 472–477

Pearce S, Erskine A 1989 Chronic pain. In: Pearce S, Wardle J 1989 The practice of behavioural medicine. BPS/Oxford University Press, Oxford

Pearce S, Wardle J 1989 The practice of behavioural medicine. Oxford Scientific Publications/BPS, Oxford

Pelosi AJ, Appelby L 1992 Psychological influences on cancer and ischaemic heart disease. British Medical Journal 304: 1295–1298

People First Scotland 1997 People First UK Conference 1997. Edinburgh, People First Scotland, The McDonalds Business Centre, Edinburgh

Petrie KJ, Weinmen J, Sharpe N, Buckley J 1996 Role of patients' view of their illness in predicting return to work and functioning after myocardial infarction: longitudinal study. British Medical Journal 312: 1191–1194

Petty RE, Cacioppo JT 1986 The elaboration likelihood model of persuasion. In: Berowitz L (ed.) Advances in experimental social psychology. Academic Press, New York, pp. 123–205

Philo G 1999 Media and mental illness. In: Philo G (ed.) Message received. Longman, London

Philo G, Henderson L 1999 Why go to casualty? Health fears and fictional television. In: Philo G (ed.) Message received. Longman, London

Pieterse ME, Seydel ER, De Vries H, Mudde AN, Kok GJ 2001 Effectiveness of a minimal contact smoking cessation program for Dutch general practitioners: a randomised controlled trial. Preventive Medicine 32: 182–190

Pilnick A 2002 Genetics and society: an introduction. Open University Press, Buckingham

Plant M, Peck D, Samuels E 1985 Alcohol, drugs and school leavers. Tavistock, London

Platt JJ, Husband SD, Taube D 1991 Major psychotherapeutic modalities for heroin addiction – a brief overview. International Journal of the Addictions 25: 1453–1477

Platt S 1985 Measuring burden of psychiatric illness on the family. An evaluation of some rating scales. Psychological Medicine 15: 383–393

Platt S, Martin, CJ, Hunt, SM. Lewis CW 1989 Damp housing, mould growth and symptomatic health state. British Medical Journal 298: 1673–1678

Platt S Pavis S Akram G 1999 Changing labour market conditions and health: a systematic literature review (1993–98). Dublin. European Foundation for the Improvement of Living and Working Conditions. Retrieved from www.eurofound.ie/publications/files/EF9915EN.pdf

Polivy J, Herman CP 2002 Causes of eating disorders. Annual Review of Psychology 53: 187–213

Porter AMD, Howie JGR, Forbes JF 1989 Stress in general medical practitioners of the UK. In: McGuigan FJ, Sime WE, Macdonald Wallace J 1989 Stress and tension control, 3rd edn. Plenum Press, London

Prior L 1995 Chance and modernity: accidents as a public health problem. In: Bunton R, Nettleton S, Burrows R (eds) The sociology of health promotion. Routledge, London

Prochaska JO, Diclemente CC 1983 Stages and processes of self-change of smoking: toward an integrative model of change. Journal of Consulting and Clinical Psychology 51: 390–395

Puri B, Laking PJ, Treasaden IH 1996 Textbook of psychiatry. Churchill Livingstone, Edinburgh

Radcliff C, Lester H 2003 Perceived stress during undergraduate medical training: a qualitative study. Medical Education 37: 32–38

Radley A 1994 Making sense of illness: the social psychology of health and disease. Sage, London

Raistrick D, Hodgson R, Ritson B 1999 Tackling alcohol together. The evidence base for a UK alcohol policy. Free Association Books, London

Raw M, White P. McNeill A 1990 Clearing the air. A guide for action on tobacco. WHO/BMA, London

Raw M, NcNeill A, West R 1999 Smoking cessation: evidence based recommendations for the healthcare system. BMJ 318: 182–185

Registrar General's Mortality Statistics 1994 HMSO, London

Richards HM, Reid ME, Watt GCM 2002 Socioeconomic variations in response to chest pain: qualitative study. British Medical Journal 324: 1308–1312

Richards M 1993 The new genetics: some issues for social scientists. Sociology of Health and Illness 15: 567–586

Richards T 1990 Chasms in communication. British Medical Journal 301: 1407–1408

Richardson JTE 2000 Hormones and behavior: cognition, menstruation and menopause. In: Ussher SM (ed.) Women's health. Contemporary international perspectives. BPS Books, Leicester, pp. 278–282

Rintala M, Mustajoki P 1992 Do mannequins menstruate? British Medical Journal 305: 1575–1576

Roberts H, Smith S, Bryce C 1993 'Prevention is better . . .' Sociology of Health & Illness 15: 447–463

Rogers A, Pilgrim D, Lacey R 1993 Experiencing psychiatry: users' views of services. Macmillan in Mind Publications

Rovelli M, Palmeri D, Vossler E, Bartus S, Hull D, Shweizer R 1989 Compliance in organ transplant recipients. Transplantation Proceedings 21: 833–844

Royal College of Physicians and Royal College of Psychiatrists 1995 The psychological care of medical patients. Royal College of Physicians and Royal College of Psychiatrists, London

Rudd P, Price MG, Graham LE, Beilstein BA, Tarbell SJ, Bacchetti P, Fortmann SP 1986 Consequences of worksite hypertension screening: differential changes in psychosocial function. American Journal of Medicine 80: 853–861

Ruiter RAC, Abraham C, Kok G 2001 Scary warnings and rational precautions: a review of the psychology of fear appeals. Psychology and Health 16: 613–630

Rushforth H 1999 Communication with hospitalised children: review and application of research pertaining to children's understanding of health and illness. Journal of Child Psychology and Psychiatry 40: 683–691

Ruston A, Clayton J, Calnan M 1998 Patients' actions during their cardiac event: qualitative study exploring differences and modifiable factors. British Medical Journal 316: 1060–1065

Ruta DA, Garratt AM, Russell IT 1999 Patient centred assessment of quality of life for patients with four common conditions. Quality on Health Care 8: 22–29

Sabat SR, Harre R 1992 The construction and deconstruction of self in Alzheimer's disease. Ageing and Society 12: 443–461

Sacks O 1986 The man who mistook his wife for a hat. Picador, London

Saile H, Burgemeir R, Schmidt LR 1988 A meta-analysis of studies on psychological preparation of children facing medical procedures. Psychology and Health 2: 107–132

Sapolsky RM 1993 Endocrinology alfresco: psychoendocrine studies of wild baboons. Recent Progress in Hormone Research 48: 437–468

Saunders C, Sykes N 1993 The management of terminal malignant disease, 3rd edn. Edward Arnold, London

Savage R, Armstrong D 1990 Effects of a general practitioner's consulting style on patients' satisfaction: a controlled study. British Medical Journal 301: 968–970

Scambler G 1997 Sociology as applied to medicine. Saunders, London

Scambler G, Hopkins A 1986 Being epileptic: coming to terms with stigma. Sociology of Health and Illness 8: 26–43

Scambler G 2002 Health and social change. Open University Press, Buckingham

Schachter S 1964 The interaction of cognitive and physiological determinants of emotional states. In: Berkowitz L (ed.) Advances in experimental social psychology, vol. 1. Academic Press, New York

Schachter S, Singer JE 1962 Cognitive, social, and physiological determinants of emotional state. Psychological Review 69: 379–399

Schaffer HR 1990 Making decisions about children: psychological questions and answers. Blackwell, Oxford

Schaie KW 1990 The optimization of cognitive functioning in old age: prediction based on cohort-sequential and longitudinal data. In: Baltes PB, Baltes MM (eds) Successful aging: perspectives from the behavioural sciences. Cambridge University Press, New York

Schaie KW 1996 Intellectual development in adulthood. In Birren J E and Schaie KW (eds) Handbook of the psychology of aging. Academic Press, London

Schwarzer R (ed.) 1992 Self-efficacy; thought control of action. Hemisphere Publishing Corporation

SCIEH 1997 Answer (AIDS News Supplement to the Weekly Report) Issue 7 (AM-37)

Scott J 2001 Cognitive therapy for depression. British Medical Bulletin 57: 101–113

Secretary of State for Health 1999 Smoking kills. The Stationery Office, London

Senior P, Bhopal RS 1994 Ethnicity as a variable in epidemiological research. British Medical Journal 309: 327–330

Seyle H 1956 The stress of life. McGraw-Hill, New York, NY

Shalev AY, 2001 Post-traumatic stress disorder. Disorder takes away human dignity and character. British Medical Journal 322: 1301, 1303–1304

Shalev AY, Schreiber S, Galai T, Melmed RN 1993 Post-traumatic stress disorder following medical events. British Journal of Clinical Psychology 32: 247–253

Shapira K, McClelland HA, Griffiths N R, Newell DJ 1970 Study of the effects of tablet colour in the treatment of anxiety states. British Medical Journal 2: 446–449

Shapiro DA, Shapiro D 1983 Meta-analysis of comparative therapy outcome studies: a replication and refinement. Psychological Bulletin 92: 581–604

Shapiro RS, Simpson DE, Lawrence SL, Talsky A M, Sobocinski KA, Schiedermayer DL 1989 A survey of sued and nonsued physicians and suing patients. Archives of Internal Medicine 149: 2190–2196

Sharma U 1990 Using alternative therapies: marginal medicine and central concerns. In Abbot P, Payne G (eds) New directions in the sociology of health. Falmer Press, Basingstoke

Sheeran P 2002 Intention–behavior relations: a conceptual and empirical review. European Review of Social Psychology 12: 1–36

Sidell M 1995 Health in old age: myth, mystery and management. Open University Press, Buckingham

Slack MK, Brooks AJ 1995 Medication management issues for adolescents with asthma. American Journal of Health-system Pharmacy 52: 1417–1421

Slade P 1984 Premenstrual changes in normal women: fact or fiction. Journal of Psychosomatic Research 28: 1–7

Smith R 1987 Unemployment and Health. Oxford University Press, Oxford

Snodden R 1992 The good, the bad and the unacceptable. Faber and Faber, London

Snoek F, Skinner TC (eds) 2000 Psychology in diabetes care. Wiley, Chichester

Social Trends 26 1996 HMSO, London

Social Trends 27 1997 HMSO, London

Social Trends 32 2002 HMSO, London

Spearman C 1923 The nature of intelligence and the principles of cognition. Macmillan, London

Spiegel D, Bloom JR, Kraemer HC, Gottheil E 1989 Effect of psychosocial treatment on survival of patients with metastatic breast cancer. Lancet 334: 888–891

Stationery Office 1998 Independent inquiry into inequalities in health (the Acheson Report). The Stationery Office, London

Stevenson BS, Coles PM 1993 A breast cancer support-group: activities and value to mastectomy patients. Journal of Cancer Education 8: 239–242

Stewart M 2001 Towards a global definition of patient centred care. British Medical Journal 322: 444–445

Stewart M, Brown J, Donner A, McWhinney I, McWilliam C, Freeman T 1995 Patient-centred medicine: transforming the clinical method. Sage, London

Stewart MA, McWhinney IR, Buck CW 1979 The doctor–patient relationship and its effect upon outcome. Journal of the Royal College of General Practitioners 29: 77–82

Stock J, Cervone D 1990 Proximal goal setting and self-regulatory processes. Cognitive Therapy and Research 14: 483–498

Stone J, Aronson E, Crain AL, Winslow MP, Fried CB 1994 Inducing hypocrisy as a means of encouraging young adults to use condoms. Personality and Social Psychology Bulletin 20: 116–128

Stroebe M, Schut H 1999 The dual process model of coping with bereavement; rationale and description. Death Studies 23: 197–224

Stroebe W, Stroebe M S 1987 Bereavement and health: the psychological and physical consequences of partner loss. Cambridge University Press, Cambridge

Stuart-Hamilton I 1994 The psychology of ageing. Jessica Kingsley, London

Stubbs P 1993 'Ethnically sensitive' or 'anti-racist'? Models for health research and service delivery. In: Ahmad W (ed.) 'Race' and health in contemporary Britain. Open University Press, Buckingham

Sudnow D 1967 Passing on: the social organization of dying. Prentice Hall, New York

Summerfield D 2001 The invention of post-traumatic stress disorder and the social usefulness of psychiatric category. British Medical Journal 322: 95–98

Swanston M, Abraham SCS, Macrae WA, Walker A, Rushmer R, Methven H 1993 Pain assessment with interactive computer animation. Pain 53: 347–351

Taylor KM 1988 Telling bad news: physicians and the disclosure of undesirable information. Sociology of Health and Illness 10 (2): 120–132

Taylor S 1986 Health psychology. Random House, New York

Tew M 1990 Safer childbirth? A critical history of maternity care. Chapman & Hall, London

Thomas L 1995 The youngest science. Penguin, New York

Thompson T 1996 The beast: a journey through depression. Plume/Penguin, New York

Thomson H, Petticre M, Morrison D 2001 Health effects of housing improvement: systematic review of intervention studies. British Medical Journal 323: 187–190

Thorpe G 1993 Enabling more dying people to remain at home. British Medical Journal 307: 915–918

Tizard B, Hughes M 1984 Young children learning. Fontana, London

Tones K, Tilford S 1994 Health education: effectiveness, efficienty and equity. Chapman & Hall, London

Townsend J, Frank AO, Fermont P et al 1990 Terminal cancer care and patients' preferences for place of death: a prospective study. British Medical Journal 301: 415–417

Townsend P, Davidson N, Whitehead M (eds) 1992 Inequalities in health: The Black Report and The Health Divide. Penguin, Harmondsworth

Trieman N, Leff J, Glover G 1999 Outcome of long stay psychiatric patients resettled in the community: prospective cohort study. British Medical Journal 319: 13–16

Tuckett D, Boulton M, Olsen C, Williams A 1985 Meetings between experts: an approach to sharing ideas in medical consultations. Tavistock, London

Tudor Hart J 1971 The inverse care law. The Lancet 27: 405–412

Tuomilehto J, Lindstrom J, Eriksson JG et al for the Finnish Diabetes Prevention Study Group 2001 Prevention of type 2 diabetes mellitus by changes in lifestyle among subjects with impaired glucose tolerance. New England Journal of Medicine 344: 1343–1350

Turner B 1995 Medical power and social knowledge, 2nd edn. Sage, London

Turner B 2000 The history of the changing concepts of health and illness: outline of general model of illness categories. In: Albrecht G, Fitzpatrick R, Scrimshaw C (eds) Handbook of social studies in health and medicine. Sage, London

Turner JA 1982 Comparison of group progressive-relaxation training and cognitive-behavioural group therapy for chronic low back pain. Journal of Consulting and Clinical Psychology 50: 757–765

Twigg J, Atkin K 1991 Evaluating support to informal carers. Social Policy Research Unit, York

Twycross R 1994 Pain relief in advanced cancer. Churchill Livingstone, Edinburgh

Twycross R 1999 Introducing palliative care, 3rd edn. Radcliffe Medical Press, Oxon

UK Prospective Diabetes Study (UKPDS) Group 1998 Intensive blood-glucose control with sulphonylureas or insulin compared with conventional treatment and risk of complications in patients with type 2 diabetes (UKPDS 33). The Lancet 352: 837–853

Usherwood TP 1991 Development and randomised controlled trial of a booklet of advice for parents. British Journal of General Practice 41: 58–62

Valliant GE 2003 A 60-year follow up of alcoholic men. Addiction 98: 1043–1051

Vallis J, Wyke S, Cunningham-Burley S 1997 'She's good that one down there'. Views and expectations of community pharmacists in a Scottish commuter town. Pharmaceutical Journal 258: 457–460

Vincent C, Furnham A 1997 Complementary medicine: a research perspective. Wiley, Chichester

Waddell G 1998 The back pain revolution. Churchill Livingstone, Edinburgh

Wadsworth MEJ, Montgomery SM, Bartley MJ 1999 'The persisting effect of unemployment on health and social well-being in men in early working life.' Social Science and Medicine 48: 1491–1499

Waldron D, O'Boyle CA, Kearney M, Moriarty M, Carney D 1999 Quality of life measurement in advanced cancer: assessing the individual. Journal of Clinical Oncology 17: 3603–3611

Walker A 1993 Poverty in old age. In Bond J, Coleman P, Peace S (eds) Ageing in society: an introduction to social gerontology. Sage, London

Warr PB 1978 Work, unemployment and mental health. Oxford University Press, Oxford

Watson JB and Raynor R 1920 Conditioned emotional responses. Journal of Experimental Psychology 3: 1–14

Weich S, Lewis G 1998 'Poverty, unemployment and common mental disorders: population based cohort study.' British Medical Journal 317: 115–119

Weinstein N 1982 Unrealistic optimism about susceptibility to health problems. Journal of Behavioral Medicine 5: 441–460

Weinstein N 1984 Why it won't happen to me: perceptions of risk factors and susceptibility. Health Psychology 3: 431–457

Weinstein N 1987 Unrealistic optimism about susceptibility to health problems: conclusions from a community wide sample. Journal of Behavioural Medicine 10: 481–500

Weinstein ND, Lyon JE 1999 Mindset, optimistic bias about personal risk and health-protective behaviour. British Journal of Health Psychology 4: 289–300

Wellings K 1988 Perceptions of risk – media treatment of AIDS. In: Aggleton P, Homans H (eds) Social aspects of AIDS. Falmer Press, London, pp. 83–85

Wellings K, Wadsworth J, Johnson AM et al 1995 Provision of sex education and early sexual experience: the relation examined. British Medical Journal 311: 417–420

Wells CG 1983 Talking with children: the complementary roles of parents and teachers. In: Donaldson M (ed.) Early childhood development and education. Blackwell, Oxford

Wessely S, Rose S, Bisson J 1999 A systematic review of brief psychological interventions ('debriefing') for the treatment of immediate trauma related symptoms and the prevention of post traumatic stress disorder. Cochrane Library

West P, Sweeting H 1992 Distribution of basic information from 1990. Follow-up of the Twenty-07 Study Youth Cohort. MRC Medical Sociology Unit, Working Paper No. 32. MRC, Glasgow

West P et al 1990 Social class and health in youth findings for the West of Scotland. Twenty-07 Study Social Science in Medicine 30 (6): 665–673

Westergaard J, Noble I, Walker A 1989 After redundancy: the experience of economic insecurity. Polity Press, Cambridge

Whalley LJ, Deary IJ 2001 Longitudinal cohort study of childhood IQ and survival up to age 76. British Medical Journal 322: 1–5

White A, Freeth S, O'Brien M 1992 Infant feeding 1990. OPCS, Social Survey Division. HMSO, London

White CA 2001 Cognitive behaviour therapy for chronic medical problems: a guide to assessment and treatment in practice. John Wiley, Chichester

White Paper, Secretaries of State 1989 Caring for people. Community care in the next decade and beyond. HSMO, London

WHO 1990 Cancer relief and palliative care: report of a WHO expert committee. World Health Organization Technical Report Series 804. World Health Organization, Geneva

WHO Division of Mental Health 1993 WHO-QOL study protocol: the development of the World Health Organization quality of life assessment instrument (MNG/PSF/93). Geneva

WHOQOL Group 1998 The World Health Organization quality of life assessment (WHOQOL): development and general psychometric properties. Social Science and Medicine 46: 1569–1585

Wight D, Henderson M, Raab G et al 2000 Extent of regretted sexual intercourse among young teenagers in Scotland: a cross-sectional survey. British Medical Journal 320: 1243–1244

Wilkinson RG 1992 Income distribution and life expectancy. British Medical Journal 304: 165–168

Wilkinson RG 1998 Unhealthy societies: the afflictions of inequality. Routledge, London

Williams C, Kitzinger J, Henderson L 2003 Envisaging the embryo in stem cell research: rhetorical strategies and media reporting of the ethical debates. Sociology of Health and Illness 25(7): 793–814

Williams G 1984 The genesis of chronic illness: narrative reconstruction. Sociology of Health and Illness 6: 175–200

Williams RL 1973 Black intelligence test of cultural homogeneity. Newsweek, December 19th, p. 109

Williamson VK, Winn CR, Pugh ALG 1992 Public views on an extended role for community pharmacy. International Journal of Pharmacy Practice 1: 223–229

Willis E 2002 Public health and the 'new' genetics: balancing individual and collective outcomes. Critical Public Health 12: 119–138

Winokur G, Pitts FN 1965 Affective disorder VI: a family history study of prevalences, sex differences and possible genetic factors. Journal of Psychiatric Research 3: 113–123

Winterton Report 1992 Maternity Services Second Report Vol 1 (Health Committee) HMSO, London

Woelk H 2000 Comparison of St John's wort and imipramine for treating depression: randomised controlled trial. British Medical Journal 321: 536–539

Wong D, Whaley L 1986 Clinical handbook of pediatric nursing, 2nd edn. Mosby, St Louis

Wood W, Kallgren CA, Priesler RM 1985 Access to attitude-relevant information in memory as a determinant of persuasion: the role of message attributes. Journal of Experimental Social Psychology 21: 73–85

Woodroffe C, Glickman M, Barker M, Power C 1993 Children, teenagers and health: the key data. Open University Press, Buckingham

Worden JW 1991 Grief counselling and grief therapy. A handbook for the mental health practitioner. Routledge, London

World Health Organisation 1946 Constitution. World Health Organisation, Geneva

World Health Organization 1980 International classification of impairments, disabilities and handicaps. WHO, Geneva

Wright J, Williams R, Wilkinson JR 1998 Development and importance of health needs assessment. British Medical Journal 316: 1310–1313

Yardley SJ, Davis CJ, Sheldon F 2001 Receiving a diagnosis of lung cancer: patients' interpretations, perceptions and perspectives. Palliative Medicine 15: 379–386

Yellowlees PM, Ruffin RE 1989 Psychological defences and coping styles in patients following a life-threatening attack of asthma. Chest 95: 1298–1303

Zigler E, Valentine J 1979 Project Head Start: a legacy of the war on poverty. Free Press, New York

Index